DIAGNOSIS
AND
EVALUATION
IN
SPEECH PATHOLOGY

second edition

DIAGNOSIS AND EVALUATION IN SPEECH PATHOLOGY

LON L. EMERICK
Northern Michigan University—Marquette

JOHN T. HATTEN
University of Minnesota—Duluth

Prentice-Hall, Inc., *Englewood Cliffs, New Jersey 07632*

Library of Congress Cataloging in Publication Data

EMERICK, LON L.
   Diagnosis and evaluation in speech pathology.

   Includes bibliographies and index.
   1. Speech, Disorders of—Diagnosis.
I. Hatten, John T., joint author.
II. Title. [DNLM: 1. Speech disorders—
Diagnosis. WM475 E52d]
RC423.E58 1978   616.8'55'075   78-13593
ISBN 0-13-208512-7

© 1979 by Prentice-Hall, Inc., Englewood Cliffs, N.J. 07632

Printed in the United States of America

10 9 8 7 6 5 4 3 2 1

Editorial/production supervision and interior design by Penny Linskey
Cover design by Jerry Pfeifer
Manufacturing buyer: Phil Galea

PRENTICE-HALL INTERNATIONAL, INC., *London*
PRENTICE-HALL OF AUSTRALIA PTY. LIMITED, *Sydney*
PRENTICE-HALL OF CANADA, LTD., *Toronto*
PRENTICE-HALL OF INDIA PRIVATE LIMITED, *New Delhi*
PRENTICE-HALL OF JAPAN, INC., *Tokyo*
PRENTICE-HALL OF SOUTHEAST ASIA PTE. LTD., *Singapore*
WHITEHALL BOOKS LIMITED, *Wellington, New Zealand*

Contents

3
THE CLINICAL EXAMINATION AND
TESTING PROCEDURES *52*

4
DIAGNOSIS OF LANGUAGE DISORDERS
IN CHILDREN *91*

5
LANGUAGE DISORDERS IN CHILDREN:
DETERMINING THE ETIOLOGY
DIRECTING THE CLINICAL EFFORT *128*

6
ARTICULATION DISORDERS *157*

Preface

With this second edition we invite a new group of students to look over the shoulder of a speech clinician as he goes about his appointed diagnostic rounds. We were pleased that so many readers of the first edition found in it the imprint of clinical relevance, that they too shared our primary concern with *people,* not speech defects or complex analytical models of communication. As working clinicians and teachers, we have gained much from the novel insights, open enthusiasm and challenging questions of our clients and students—and it is to them that this book is dedicated.

L.L.E.
J.T.H.

1

Introduction

The demands placed upon the speech clinician are many and varied and require a variety of skills, knowledge, and personal characteristics. Each active clinician finds himself working as case selector, case evaluator, diagnostician, interviewer, parent counselor, teacher, coordinator, record keeper, researcher, and student. The boundaries between these various professional duties are not clearly defined; and since clinicians must move continuously from one area to another, it is inevitable that no individual can expect to be equally competent in all areas. The ultimate goal is to maximize one's strengths in all areas to provide the best possible service to the communicatively handicapped.

Diagnosis is among the more comprehensive and difficult tasks of the clinician. The demands for clinical skill are as great as in any other undertaking. Since speech is a function of the entire organism, the canny diagnostician must take all relevant aspects of behavior into account. The student soon learns that he is not working with speech sounds or the sounds of speech, but rather with changing people in a changing environment. The mature diagnostician does not look at objective scores of articulatory skill, point scales of vocal-quality disorders, or language age as ends in themselves but rather as aspects of an individual's communication ability—we diagnose communicators, not communication! That revelation is a major factor in the transition from technician to professional.

Because our diagnostic tools are crude, being largely in the experimental stages, and because communication disorders are by nature complex and perplexing, many of our diagnostic undertakings are incomplete and ambiguous. The lack of absolute and definitive answers to the various questions of diagnosis is often frustrating and demoralizing to the clinician. The ambiguous findings that sometimes culminate a diagnostic evaluation must be dealt with in a fashion which perpetuates the evaluative undertaking rather than closing the door on further probing. Diagnosis is a continuous and open-ended venture that results in answers or partial answers which themselves are open to revision with added information.

DIAGNOSIS DEFINED

There are essentially three interrelated and overlapping aspects to diagnosis:

1. Determination of the reality of the problem;
2. Determination of the etiology of the problem; and
3. Providing clinical focus.

Diagnosis to Determine the Reality of the Problem

The first task of diagnosis is to determine whether the presenting speech pattern does indeed constitute a handicap.[1] Before this is possible, however, it is necessary to have a clear idea of what constitutes a speech disorder. Van Riper's definition of a speech disorder is widely quoted (1972:29): "Speech is defective when it deviates so far from the speech of other people that it calls attention to itself, interferes with communication, or causes its possessor to be maladjusted." We propose further that there are three essential aspects of the communicative act which are important in defining defective speech: the acoustic characteristics of the individual's speech signal; the influence of the acoustic signal on the intelligibility of the message; and, finally, the handicapping condition that results from the first two aspects. A communication *difference* involves signal alterations, a communication *disturbance* involves a breakdown of message transmission, and a communication *disorder* involves a handicapping condition. The first relates to speech signals, the second to information transmission, and the third to people.

The speech signal. The physical characteristics of the speech signal are subject to quantification through recording, measurement, and observation. Speech spectrographs, pitch meters, and other instruments are available to help the diagnostician obtain an objective measure of the acoustic nature of the individual's speech. Such data are of little value, however, if no interpretation is made of the impact of the speech behavior. We must look at the physical characteristics of the speech signal and judge its *quality*.

---

[1]Schultz (1972) has developed a model of clinical decisionmaking. Compare Schultz's "decision axis" concept with the present discussion.

The state of the art has not progressed to where we can simply take the quantified data, compare it with established numberical norms, and determine the correctness of the speech sample. Unfortunately, there is no registered standard /s/ phone; thus, each diagnostician must develop his own frame of reference. The physician is able to scrutinize data from a laboratory test and make an immediate diagnosis regarding the normalcy of an individual's blood count, but this kind of reference information is not yet available to the speech clinician. The question of whether the presenting speech difference is different enought to be of concern thus becomes a matter of human judgment. This judgment involves filtering incoming data through many synaptic junctions whose thresholds may have worn thin by bias and experience. An inordinately critical or uncritical acoustic system is a hazard with far-reaching implications.

Each clinician must find some way to realistically judge adequate speech production. Pronovost (1966:179) asks, "Do we consider ourselves self-appointed enforcers of society's standards of speech?" Even more perplexing is the question of whether we should appoint ourselves *determiners* of that standard. Should we protect some absolute standard of speech production? Is that the function of our profession or the function of society? If the speech difference we hear appears to have no impact upon the speaker or his environment, should the speech clinician consider it a problem and set out to correct it?

Many speech clinicians in the schools have recently begun to abandon the traditional screening process for case detection in favor of parent and teacher referral. This trend reflects an awareness that the determination of how much of a difference is important in speech production is primarily made by society rather than professionals. Some states have been even more restrictive in their definition of speech handicap by mandating that clinical speech services only be provided to those children whose communicative differences have a proven detrimental effect upon their educational growth. By this criteria many or all of the traditional articulation disorders and voice disorders would not qualify for clinical speech services.

Studies of the incidence of speech disorders provide a great deal of information about the researchers as well as the subjects. One has only to compare the often-quoted figure (7 to 10 percent) of the incidence of speech disorders as provided in speech pathology literature with the 0.65 percent figure which was obtained in a Public Health Service report cited by Newman (1961). Although the Public Health Service data no doubt is open to some criticism, it was obtained from a house-to-house interview study and may more accurately reflect the general population's concept of defective speech. Incidence figures are notoriously self-fulfilling prophesies; they are also reports about someone *by someone*. If you *expect* that 10 percent of all grade-school children will have speech disorders, the probability that you will find just that percentage is greatly enhanced.

Johnson (1946) has emphasized the concept of the "participants of a problem," implying that in the final analysis the diagnostician becomes a part of the defect by identifying and labeling it. The widely varying estimates of the percent-age of children in the schools with speech defects underscore the point that speech disorders are sometimes born in the ear of the listener as well as in the mouth of the speaker) In his admonishing and thought-provoking article, Van Riper (1966) emphasizes the importance of the client's self-image in rehabilitative efforts. If our diagnosis fixates a self-image and perpetuates the error rather than helping to eradicate it, then our selection criteria must be broadened to include more than simply the acoustic nature of the speech. We are charged with the responsibility to prevent or reduce abnormality, not to cause it.

What constitutes normal behavior? There are several definitions available (Johnson *et al.*, 1963), but we will discuss only two, representing the diverging philosophies with which each clinician must contend in establishing his own concept. The first theory we shall call the concept of *cultural norms:* the assump-tion is that there are behaviors that society considers aberrant in terms of *group* characteristics. According to this model, each bit of behavior can be judged against a real or theoretical standard, the nature of which is independent of the individual's personal idiosyncrasies. The second theory we shall call the concept of *individual norms*. Advocates of this model assume that each individual has made his unique adjustment to life based upon his own previous experiences, his physical limitations, and his environment's reactions to him. Any judgment as to the normalcy of a bit of behavior must be contingent upon individual characteris-tics such as age, intelligence, and experience.

Taken to the extreme, of course, the latter model would assert that each person is normal no matter what he does, since his behavior is the end product of all that plays upon his being; and to this extent the concept of individual norms loses meaning. But a case example may help to clarify and give perspective. The audiologist who examines the hearing of a seventy-five-year-old individual and obtains the "typical" presbycusic audiometric curve could make a case for the judgment that this person has "normal" hearing. According to personal norms, this is average or normal behavior for a person of seventy-five; but according to cultural norms, the individual's hearing level is below the average for the total population. Follow-up procedures would be based, then, partially upon the practi-cal matter of getting a more efficient communication system for the individual and also upon providing counseling so that the person will understand the nature of his hearing. Therefore, both cultural and personal norms play a part in diagnostic judgments and rehabilitative programs.

A severely retarded ten-year old with a frontal lisp may not be judged to have defective speech, whereas an eight-year old presenting a similar speech pattern, but a different intellectual potential, may be enrolled. Such judgments have implications for case selection, and the clinician must reconcile the variances between the physical differences in the sounds involved and individual variables in conjunction with what is normal for the population as a whole. Each clinician must continually use both concepts of normalcy in his diagnostic work. Every five-year-old "lisper" who leaves the kindergarten classroom for his semiweekly speech therapy session is most probably a victim of a one-dimensional definition of normal.

Far too many clinicians view diagnosis simply as a labeling process, but the actual labeling, or categorizing, is only a small part of the total assessment process. Classification systems within our profession are poor at best, and high-level abstractions (for example, lisping) tend to emphasize the similarities within a population rather than the individual differences. The keen diagnostician looks upon classifications as communication conveniences to be viewed with suspicion; he is continually alert for "hardening of the categories." Of course, the convenience factor is important, and each clinician making a determination of the reality of the problem must be willing to label it. This must of necessity, however, follow an orderly description of the characteristics of the disorder so that it can be clear what route the diagnostician took in arriving at the final classification. A diagnosis that only describes the characteristics of the problem, without judging its type or class, is a dead end. The opposite path is also dangerous; however, the diagnostician who is willing to begin his evaluation by labeling the problem has reversed the orderly sequence of acquiring knowledge and often effectively closes his mind to factors that may later point away from his premature "diagnosis."

Intelligibility of the message. The intelligibility of a speech signal relates to the degree of agreement between what the speaker intends and what the listener perceives. Many factors play a part in both the encoding and decoding process, and the diagnostician must be capable of representing the standard for his society when listening and making judgments. The essential judgment to be made is, how well did the intentions of the speaker match the perceptions of the listener, and what are the factors which effect this? Are there attributes of the signal which distract the listener, thus altering the message? Is the signal indistinct, thus allowing only partial transmission of information? Is the signal distinct but conveying a message other than that intended by the speaker? Is the signal distinct but conveying a message (albeit the one selected by the speaker) which is inappropriate for the context?

We have, in the main, been content with clinical insight and intuitive estimates when we have judged the impact of speech differences upon intelligibility. Only a few research investigations have been concerned with this important problem (Garwood, 1952, and others). No research has so far clearly quantified the effect of a lateral lisp, for example, and yet each working day practicing clinicians must decide on the importance of such acoustic characteristics. What is needed is a massive study of how each type of speech disorder influences the transmission of information to the listener. The speech clinician is able to count the phoneme errors, quantify the number of repetitions per sentence, and establish a type-token ratio, but as yet he is unable to assess the intelligibility of the transmitted message with any degree of reliability.

Handicapping condition. The most important variable in determination of the reality of a communication problem is the determination of whether anyone is handicapped by the signal or intelligibility differences. The diagnostician does not simply identify the error and assess its influence upon the intelligibility of the message; he must also prepare a description of the person and the ways in which the symptoms shape the individual's adjusting characteristics. In the final analysis this third aspect justifies the existence of our profession. If the speech difference has no discernible impact on the child's behavior, and ultimately on his adjusting abilities and learning potential, there is little justification for concern on the part of the speech clinician. Although it is not feasible to compile a listing of all of the possible conditions under which a communication difference would become handicapping, it is generally agreed that communicative differences are considered handicapping when—

Who's to
Say it won't
in future?

> the transmission and/or perception of messages is faulty;
>
> the person is placed at an economic disadvantage;
>
> the person is placed at a learning disadvantage;
>
> the person is placed at a social disadvantage;
>
> there is a negative impact upon the emotional growth of the person; or
>
> the problem causes physical damage or endangers the health of the person.

Among the three factors taken into account in determining the reality of a disorder, a variety of relationships are possible (See Figure 1.1). Condition *A* of Figure 1.1 represents a condition in which the speech signal is significantly aberrant, although intelligibility and impact upon the communication is minimal; this may be the case with certain voice disorders. In condition *B* there is little signal variation and similarly negligible impact upon the intelligibility, but the communicants are significantly affected by the difference.

> Mrs. N. brought her four-year-old son into our office ostensibly for evaluation of his speech. Initial testing revealed an inconsistent frontal lisp which was easily stimulable to correction. Our first inclination was to simply inform Mrs. N. that her child's speech was within normal limits and conclude the session, but better judgment prevailed. It was noted earlier in the interview that Mrs. N. was firmly convinced of the existence of the problem and considered it quite severe.

The last condition in Figure 1.1 reflects a situation which may be a bit more controversial. Some would argue that the severely retarded individual who lacks effective communication is not handicapped by this condition since the impairment is not central to his disability. The addition of communication skill, it is postulated, would not effectively alter his condition. Taking this line of thinking to its logical conclusion, it would then be possible to have an individual with significant signal differences which have a marked impact upon intelligibility but which do not handicap the speaker.

> Does this last situation reflect current thinking? Relate condition C in Figure 1.1 to the dictates of P.L. 94-142.

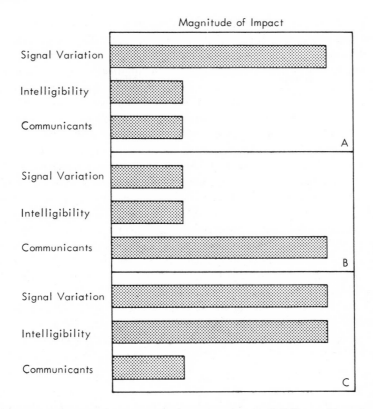

Figure 1.1 Possible relationships of signal distortion, intelligibility, and impact upon communicants.

Diagnosis to Determine the Etiology of the Problem

"Cause" has different meanings depending on its distance from the problem. As you look at a client in a diagnostic session, you search for reasons for his presenting behaviors. In fact many of these reasons may be buried in the past and can only be revealed by painstaking effort. Not only must we search through the client's past experience in order to uncover events that may help us alter current behaviors, but we must also guard against looking for causes in only one dimension of behavior. Johnny's brain damage, once identified, is probably not the only etiological factor, because speech is a complicated human function. Social factors, learning, motivation, and many other factors enter into the total process.

Classically, etiology has been defined in terms of *predisposing, precipitating*, and *perpetuating* factors. Agents that dispose or incline an individual toward communication impairment are designated as predisposing causes. Precipitating factors actually bring about the onset of the problem, while perpetuating variables are responsible for the persistance of the abnormality.

Predisposing factors are generally thought to be important because of their potential link with a third agent. A classic example of predisposing factors is the higher than normal incidence of left-handedness among stutterers. The left-handedness itself is of little consequence, but the implication of basic underlying neurological differences has perplexed researchers for decades. The wary diagnostician must watch for factors that occur with high regularity in association with certain communication disorders. Such data could ultimately be instrumental in uncovering some basic information regarding the nature of the disorder.

Precipitating factors are generally no longer operating and, as such, may or may not be identifiable. There is a philosophical question of whether we need to search for precipitating factors if they are not still operating, and the point is well taken. Each moment, however, there is created a new set of precipitating factors which, acting as characteristics of the past, perpetuate behaviors of the present. Speech disorders generally are not static entities developed at a given point and perpetuated without modification through time; rather they are ever-changing characteristics that are constantly influenced by intrinsic and extrinsic factors. Precipitating factors are best considered as the agents that brought the disorder to its present state.

The perpetuating factors are those variables which are currently at work on the individual. Almost without exception, habit strength is a prime perpetuating factor in developmental speech disorders. Other factors are also crucial, however, and it is the diagnostician's task to uncover the environmental and physical factors that are reinforcing and thus perpetuating the disorder.

> Mrs. M. was an alert, intense person with an extremely high energy level. The referring physician's report described her as "hyper," and the description was apt indeed. Although such people do not always develop vocal nodules, they certainly seem predisposed to them. Mrs. M.'s vocal nodules had been surgically removed but were beginning to show signs of recurrence when we first saw her. In the initial interview several facts became apparent. First, it was evident that Mrs. M. was overwhelmed by the pressures of motherhood (five children under seven years of age) and the routine and often unfulfilling chores of the daily household. She had, over the past five years, developed a method of control over the children which could best be described as the "holler and hit" technique. Unfortunately for Mrs. M.'s vocal folds, she resorted to too much hollering and too little hitting.
>
> Mrs. M.'s case illustrates the importance of all three types of etiological factors. The personality characteristics clearly predisposed her to the resulting disorder; the intrusion of children into her life precipitated the vocal disorder by raising her anxiety and greatly increasing her vocal output; and the perpetuating influence of habit strength and the continuation of the original "irritants" were currently evident.

Diagnosis to Provide Clinical Focus

Although it is important to know the causes of the disorder, it is substantially more important to know the causes of the correction of the condition. It is at this point that diagnosis and clinical management overlap. Finding the cause of the cure is an ongoing process which incorporates sound testing and evaluative procedures along with clinical management. Determining what will bring about change raises many questions which are both diagnostic and clinical in nature:

What do I know about this condition?
  What are the usual etiologies?
  What are the usual effective procedures for correction?
  What is the typical prognosis?
  etc.
What do I know about this person?
  What is the level of impact upon the person?
  What are the person's strengths and weaknesses?
  What do I know about other important personal variables—age, sex, environment, etc.?
  How is this person like others I have worked with?
  How is this person different from others I have worked with?
  etc.
What do I know about my own skills in management of this person and this disorder type?
  How do I effectively approach similar problems?
  How do I effectively approach similar people?
What do I know about the services of other professionals available for this person?
  What referrals need to be made?
What factors need to be removed, altered, or added to improve the possibility of correction?
  What inhibiting environmental factors exist?
  What organic factors need alteration?
  What new motivating procedures could be effective?
  etc.

If diagnosis is to be of utmost benefit it must be goal-oriented. Every classroom teacher has experienced the frustration of receiving a report from a school psychometrist stating that the child she referred because of behavioral problems does, indeed, have behavioral problems. Such a diagnosis fails to provide the crucial final link: recommendations for remedial procedures. Diagnosis is an empty exercise in test administration, data collection, and client evaluation, if it fails to provide logical suggestions for treatment.

There are several major diagnostic philosophies that the speech clinician must be aware of in order to formulate his own logical and professionally comfortable personal model.

The *medical*, or *disease*, *model* of diagnosis appears to be based upon a few solidly entrenched tenets. First, diagnosis must be completed *before* treatment. The assumption is that curative procedures are much more efficient if the etiological factors are known. Symptomatic medicine is considered tantamount to quackery. This model holds that diagnosis and treatment are two discernibly different tasks. Seldom is it possible for a physician to engage in a procedure that serves both diagnostic and therapeutic functions.

Another assumption of the medical model is that physical disturbances are generally related to organic causes. If the temperature is high, there is a structural explanation to be pursued within the soma. Identification of the site of the lesion is thus paramount in determining the cause-effect relationship. Classifications generally pertain to the site of the lesion, and it is generally assumed that the lesion is within the client. The application of this model to speech and language has been criticized because it restricts the scope of the investigation.

Medical diagnosis is generally concluded in an *absolute* manner. Hypotheses regarding etiology, nature of the problem, and prognosis are generally presented to other professionals and to the client as facts. This most useful technique serves to build confidence and may actually hasten the recovery process. Few of us would return to a physician who vacillated regarding the diagnosis of our ailment. The therapeutic value of an omniscient clinical demeanor is a lesson well learned by most physicians. Absolutism is indeed a luxury, but at times a very useful one.

There is no single *educational model* of diagnosis, but recent discussions by Ysseldyke and Salvia (1974), Bateman (1967), and others have described a variety of philosophies. Ysseldyke and Salvia describe the *ability training model* in which the teacher attempts to identify strengths and weaknesses in order to prescribe remedial approaches. Teaching is carried out using careful diagnosis and prescription with the assumption that knowledge of the cause and work on underlying skills will have a positive impact upon target behaviors. Since we have not determined what particular abilities are necessary for each educational skill, much of what is currently being done in this area is experimental in nature. Englemann (1967) criticizes such approaches because they end up teaching splinter tasks which may be irrelevant to the actual educational goal. Most speech clinicians would identify the ITPA, Frostig, or perceptual motor programs with this model.

The *task analysis* model of diagnosis could logically be included as a behavioral model, but it is often presented as a separate concept. The advocates of the task-analysis viewpoint stress the need to know where the child is along the ladder of skills necessary for achievement of a particular terminal behavior. The child's performance is not judged relative to norms but relative to the sequence of tasks assumed to be a part of the final product. Crucial counterparts of task-analysis training are clearly presented behavioral objectives and the development of *behavioral philosophies. Task-analysis teaching,* and *behavioral objectives* written in clearly defined terms have enjoyed a mutually supporting growth.

Another closely related model of educational diagnosis and teaching is *data-based instruction.* The basic tenets of this contribution are that intervention procedures should be based upon continuous and systematic measurement of child performance on relevant behaviors. Instructional goals are directly related to the level of performance, and the criteria for moving from one performance level to another are determined by reference to a task ladder and to child performance. Obviously, this model is directly related to the task analysis model.

The *operant,* or *behavioral paradigm,* offers several applicable concepts which speech clinicians are beginning to incorporate into their working philosophies (Sloane and MacAulay, 1968). Typically, the operant model disavows interest in the factors that intervene between stimulus and response, since such factors are at best only hypothetical. Probably the primary characteristic of the model is the belief that discriminative stimuli and resultant behaviors are observable, measurable, and quantifiable, and the establishment of "baseline," or presenting, behaviors is paramount to futher therapeutic measures. The second major undertaking is to determine what reinforcers exist for the person. In other words, the diagnostician must determine what systematic relationship exists between behaviors and the variables that control those behaviors. Detailed examination of the subject, his environment, and his current behavioral repertoire should lead the diagnostician to some conclusion regarding the terminal behaviors desired. This task is of vital importance in operant theory and, strangely, has been neglected in much of the speech therapy literature. Once goal behavior has been described, it will be necessary to delineate the exact progression of steps necessary to achieve the goal. Precision recording is necessary in order for the diagnostician to guide the clinician's work toward the proper level of difficulty and appropriateness.

Although there is no single *clinical speech model* of diagnosis, elements of many of the previously mentioned models are frequently found in the literature of speech pathology. Our profession has historically had a keen interest in etiology and has based much of its remedial programs upon the assumptions of the ability training model. As an example, many articulation approaches are based upon diagnostic findings of poor auditory discrimination skills, on the assumption that auditory discrimination is an underlying skill which has an impact upon articulation. In fact, elements of every diagnostic model are found in the working skills of most speech clinicians. Each concept makes a contribution to the diagnostic venture and each presents major pitfalls which must be avoided. For further information on models of communication as they apply to diagnosis refer to the works of Nation and Aram (1977) and Schultz (1972).

The philosophy of diagnosis dictates the uses of diagnostic information; however, there are several widely accepted ways in which diagnosis helps direct the clinical effort. The diagnosis should identify the problem, indicate the logical entry level for clinical work, identify the etiological factors which impact upon the problem, identify the avenues of input and output which will best serve the individual, determine the most appropriate methods to approach the problem, establish a most logical setting and timetable for clinical work, determine the appropriate stimuli and reinforcers, and determine the level of motivation and desire for change.

DIAGNOSIS—SCIENCE AND ART

Diagnosis demands a unique blending of science and art. The scientific method is applicable to our work as diagnosticians, both in guiding our procedures and in focusing our attitude of operation. The scientific method directs the diagnostician to observe "all" of the available factors, formulate testable hypotheses using clearly stated and answerable questions, test those hypotheses to determine their validity, and formulate conclusions based upon the tested hypotheses. The method demands rigorous adherence to standardized procedures and has as its favorable characteristics objectivity, quantifiability, and structure. The "scientific" diagnostician tends to rely upon tests, test data, and other procedures that lend themselves to quantification.

As an attitude of operation the scientific method implies that the diagnostician has not predetermined his test findings and that he is not biased in seeking the proof or disproof of his hypotheses. The diagnostician sees his hypotheses as something to be tested rather than something to be defended. Many things are implied in this attitude. We have all experienced the biased clinician who finds what he expects to find in each diagnosis. The self-fulfilling prophecy is a lethal but almost univeral human characteristic; it must be counterbalanced by a scientific approach to testing. The writers are familiar with one youngster who had traveled all over the country in search of a diagnostic explanation for his delay in language development that would be compatible with his parents' precepts. When we saw the child, his father brought with him a case file thick with reports from various noted authorities (the "fat folder" syndrome). Each report revealed more about the examiner than the child as it cited facts in support of a theory of etiology congruent with the diagnostician's particular specialty. Such youngsters—or diagnostic vagabonds, as we might call them—are victims of misguided, but persistent parents and nonscientific diagnosticians.

The beginning student must also guard against the "recent article" syndrome to which we all fall prey upon occasion. Typically, the behavioral pattern goes something like this: you read an article that depicts a particular syndrome and explains the distinctive characteristics of a disorder; for a few weeks thereafter every child you see appears to fall into the pattern described in the publication.

Speech pathology witnessed a significant increase in the incidence of "apraxia" in children following the publication of a series of articles on the topic. The way to overcome the "recent article" syndrome, of course, is to be aware that it exists and, incidentally, to have a thorough understanding of the nature of human perception.

> In nearly all matters the human mind has a strong tendency to judge in the light of its own experience, knowledge, and prejudices rather than on the evidence presented. Thus new ideas are judged in the light of prevailing beliefs (Beveridge, 1951: 103).

The strict adherence to fact that is demanded by the pure scientific method is often a bit confining. That, in part, may explain why we all practice the ''art'' of diagnosis at times. The artistic approach has several specific characteristics. The ''artist'' is less dependent upon specific observations for the formation of hypotheses than upon his casual and nonstructured scrutiny. This type of clinician is perfectly willing to disregard formal test results or standard testing procedures in favor of what appears obvious to him on the basis of his clinical expertise. The hunch, or clinical intuition, plays a significant part in such evaluations. The diagnostician will contend that facts can be approached from several directions and that he is capable of assessing the same kinds of behaviors that are measured by formal tests. Such contentions are disconcerting to the test-bound person who has come to expect that the only valid way to gain information is through standardized procedures.

It is obvious that, in the extreme, there are weaknesses in both approaches. The scientist may tend to become so dependent upon his objective methods of measurement that he fails to see the client through the maze of percentile scores and age norms. The whole is greater than the sum of its parts, and every diagnostician must guard against simply measuring the isolated characteristics without getting a full picture of the individual. The client is often made to fit the test results even when circumstances clearly contraindicate such a conclusion. We recently received a report from a clinician who claimed great frustration with a particular child because ''his ITPA results are not consonant with his classroom performance. He is not as low in psycholinguistic abilities as his test performance would indicate.'' This person believed that the child had poorer abilities than his classroom performance indicated and that there must have been something invalid about his daily behavior. Could it not be that the test results do not tell us as much as the child's everyday performance? Test data become an artifact of the child's total behavior and should be so judged, while the daily behavior may hold much more meaning for the future remedial program. Don't build altars to any testing device; every objective instrument was once only a hunch in someone's mind.

The other end of the science-art continuum is just as precarious, if not more so. The possibility of a diagnostician projecting more than a modest amount of himself into his evaluation is greater when he is less scientific in his approach. Clinical intuitions are often simply clinical biases, and it is very easy to make new evidence fit old categories. The diagnostician must find the proper admixture of each philosophy in establishing his own diagnostic procedures.

The Diagnostician as a Factor

Ultimately, however, the most important diagnostic tool is the diagnostician himself. The children we assess have seldom read the test manual, and the rigid structures of the testing situation may not be compatible with the child's fluid and nonstructured style of behavior. (Tests are abstractions of behavior, and as such they represent only a fraction of the child's total repertoire of responses to his environment.) What better measure of an individual's behavior than that behavior itself? Thus, the diagnostician becomes an important aspect of the evaluating situation as he selects, interacts, responds, and assembles information.

What skills are necessary to develop in order to become an effective, nontest-bound diagnostician? How do you develop them? There are no easy answers to these questions. Experience in the diagnostic process is an absolute necessity, but experience in terms of number of children seen is not enough; there is little value in one diagnostic experience reduplicated 1,000 times. The diagnostician must be able to gain from new experiences, and this demands *flexibility*. The stereotyped and stagnant diagnostician learns little from increased exposure to people and new situations, but those who use their experience as a pattern to be compared against, rather than as a mold into which all new experiences must fit, will continue to grow and learn.

The diagnostician must be flexible enough within the testing situation to shift from predetermined plans to new modes of evaluation as the client presents unpredicted behaviors. The examiner who steadfastly plods through a series of tests even though a child has not interacted in any significant degree may well have lost the opportunity to gain information by other means. It is not atypical for beginning speech clinicians to panic in the face of an unexpected performance and become intransigent in their application of a series of formal tests. In this regard, continued experience in diagnosis may provide the flexibility needed to move freely to other avenues of information.

> A graduate student was recently observed attempting to administer a comprehensive language inventory to Mr. D., a sixty-three-year-old aphasic. Despite the student's determined attempts to complete the formal testing, Mr. D. continued commenting on the test room, the diagnostician, and other subjects irrelevant to the test. His most persistent topic was his altered life circumstances and his frustrations. The diagnostic session ended with two unfulfilled participants. The student could not understand why Mr. D. would not cooperate and came away with none of the data he desired regarding the client's language ability. Indeed, upon later discussion it became evident that the student even failed to gain much insight into the patient's current concerns because he worried only about completing predetermined procedures. Mr. D., on the other hand, left the session feeling that the diagnostician lacked any understanding of his problem, thereby adding to his feelings of futility.

Practicing clinicians often eagerly accept new and novel techniques as they become available. We have noted a generation gap within the field of speech pathology in the past few years. As the profession moves into new and uncharted areas of concern, many new materials, tests, and techniques have become available. The old guard tends to scoff at something new, and the young clinicians bristle with frustration at the inflexibility of the veteran therapists. New techniques must not be accepted or rejected carte blanche but rather must be scrutinized for their merit. Techniques grossly foreign to experience tend to threaten and bewilder the inflexible diagnostician because he perceives them as attacks upon his trusted and time-proven methods. Is it possible that training programs which emphasize testing and therapy techniques and materials are more likely to produce an inflexible therapist than those programs which emphasize theory, problem-solving ability, and creativity?

A clinician must possess many important personal attributes. Rogers (1942) speaks of empathy, congruency, and unconditional positive regard as necessary characteristics of the clinician, and they most certainly apply to the diagnostic process as well. Generally these qualities must be nurtured through consistent effort and proper guidance. Video- and audio-tape equipment now allows the developing clinician to observe his own behaviors in the testing situation in order to more fully understand his own performance. Equally important in developing these important characteristics is skillful guidance from a master diagnostician.

If the term *sensitivity* may be defined as a keenness of sense or a heightened awareness of incoming sensory data, then this much-maligned term has meaning for the diagnostician. He must be able to detect subtle physical, psychological, or interactional changes in a client's behavior; as these small changes have the most significant meaning in the diagnostic process. For further reading in advancing awareness skills see the works of Gunther (1971) and Schultz (1967).

Insight into the meaning of behaviors must be developed from a thorough grounding in the basic processes requisite for the speech act. Each diagnostician must become so familiar with the normal process of language acquisition and normal speech functioning that he has a built-in set of standards upon which to base judgment. The insightful clinician is the knowledgeable professional who is capable of quickly comparing the client's behavior with the norm.

The development of an *evaluative attitude* is often a rather difficult task for the beginning clinician. We are, to a large extent, slaves to our experience; each clinician tends to bring the "social attitude" into the testing setting. Rather than looking upon the client's performance as having meaning for the evaluative process, we consult our own responses and formulate our own points of view in the give-and-take of the conversation. The critical, questioning attitude must be developed so that the clinician looks upon the behaviors in terms of their meaning rather than in terms of the response expected of him. Social interaction lends itself to superficiality, whereas the flow of the diagnostic interaction must, by design, lend itself to uncovering the meaning of the incorporated behavior. Effective diagnosticians tend to question the surface validity of behaviors and search for motivations, explanations, and interpretations that are not readily apparent.

Closely allied with the concept of the evaluative attitude is the idea of *persistent curiosity.* The diagnostician must develop an inquisitiveness that will make him persistent in his search for explanations. Answers are seldom apparent at first, and continuous effort is imperative. The directors of training institutions foster weakness in this area when they assign clients to students and expect therapy to get underway in a "reasonable" period of time. They are so bound to the rigid university timetables that therapy is often discontinuous. In an attempt to give each student a variety of clinical experiences, they often tend to sever clinical undertakings with a client at each semester's end, knowing full well that the diagnostic or therapeutic process is not best served in this way. The student may not always understand that these have been decisions based upon program convenience rather than client need, and may develop the notion that diagnosis is a temporary therapy-initiating exercise to be completed in an hour or two. The curious and persistent clinician, however, continues to place the client in situations that will permit additional scrutiny.

Objectivity comes from practicing the art of controlled involvement. The diagnostician must cultivate objectivity because he is subject to human errors. He must be warm, understanding, and accepting on the one hand and objective, evaluative, and detached on the other. Without some degree of balance between the two extremes the diagnostician may so severely distort the interaction between himself and the client that he obtains little of value. Objectivity demands more than simply guarding against undue emotional involvement. The examiner must be objective about *himself,* his skills, knowledge, and personal characteristics. He must, in other words, know himself to a sufficient degree that he can judge his own successes and failures and continue to grow in professional skill.

Rapport may be defined as the establishment of a working relationship, based upon mutual respect, trust, and confidence, which encourages optimum performance on the part of both client and clinician. Rapport is developed over a period of time and is not easily established in a single session or during a few minutes at the initiation of one therapeutic encounter. Rapport must not only be developed, it must be maintained and this calls for continued effort. The list of characteristics that enhance rapport is endless, but the factor which we have found to be universally important is the *ability to maintain a nonthreatened posture throughout the testing session.* The student or clinician who is easily threatened in interpersonal interaction tends to have greater difficulty establishing rapport than one who can work with people and experience little threat from unpredictable or hostile reactions. The link between this characteristic and egostrength is probably quite strong and should be seriously contemplated by the beginning diagnostician.

Although much standardization is possible through strict adherence to test routines, the lowest common denominator in diagnostic evaluations is the examiner himself. Test results are the product of the subject, examiner, test, and test circumstance, each of which has certain influence. A baseball player's batting average is judged against many factors, including how many "at bats" he had (was this a continuing performance?) and the league he played in (who administered the tests?) to name but a few. Examinations are clearly selected as a result of the experiences and biases of the examiner. Just as the answers we receive to questions are in part a function of the questions we ask and how we ask them, the diagnostic findings we obtain are in part a function of the tests we administer and the way they are administered. A "defective speech pattern" may be partially due to a defective testing pattern or a defective tester.

Diagnostic Observation

How can the clinician receive the kinds of data that he needs except by formally administering tests? That question should be foremost in the mind of every examiner because it forces him to look to the test itself and ask what behaviors this test is measuring and the pertinence of those behaviors to speech and language functioning. Among the most crucial methods of obtaining information is *observation*. Observational skills are the product of many hours of hard work. There is no shortcut to developing these skills, and each student must practice by testing his skills against established measures of subject performance. There are five aspects to observation which are necessary for the orderly acquisition of useful information: focus, depth, description, interpretation, and implication.

Focus. Probably the most difficult aspect of observation for the beginning student is focusing on the pertinent aspects of behavior. It is important for the student to remind himself that *no behavior has meaning unto itself,* and thus not only must he look at the presenting conduct of the client, but he must also determine what aspects of the environment serve as stimuli or antecedent events to that behavior and what aspects serve as perpetuators. Quantification of behaviors forces the observer to become objective and he should carefully analyze the effect of the action on the environment. If the behavior is of high incidence, the events which succeed it must be suspect as maintainers and as such are of prime importance. The casual and untrained observer usually cannot focus on the descriptive level. He tends to categorize behavior as good or bad, normal or abnormal, cooperative or uncooperative, shy or outgoing, and so forth. The first step in observation, then, is to focus on a very descriptive level so that the examiner can present the actual behaviors the client exhibited rather than generalizations regarding the meaning of those actions. In order to underscore the importance of focusing attention in the observational task, we often ask students to observe some single aspect of behavior in a therapy session and report on that one characteristic. Recently five students were assigned to observe one of the following aspects of a given therapy session: (1) how much of the session was consumed by the clinician talking; (2) the amount of eye contact between child and clinician; (3) the percentage of the total therapy session in which goal directed behaviors were exhibited by both the clinician and child; (4) the mother's facial expressions and remarks as the session progressed; and (5) the entire therapy process. The interesting result of this experiment was that each of the first four students later came up with suggestions which were pertinent to the therapy process, while the last student could only add general suggestions. These microscopic observations must eventually enable the student to make general conclusions from the total situation; our experience has led us to believe that it is best to start with such a finite focal point.

Depth. The depth of the observation is determined to a large degree by circumstance, but the diagnostician must find ways to observe the client interacting with many different people and stimuli. The diagnostician cannot expect to gain a great deal of information from fleeting observations; he must be willing to spend the time and energy necessary to observe a significant amount of behavior.

In student-training programs it is often possible to afford certain luxuries which the clinician in other settings would not have available. In some of our diagnostic evaluations, teams of students work together to test and gather information. One such team established an observational design that paid huge benefits. One student sat in the waiting room and "casually" observed the interaction between parent and child as they waited for the forthcoming diagnostic session. Following the formal session the parent was brought into the testing room, and the child was allowed to play with the puzzles in the waiting room. A student inconspicuously observed the child interacting first with toys and eventually with other children. The language sample gained during observation outside of the testing room more than tripled the total language sample obtained through formal testing procedures. Not only do such experiences convince the student of the value of in-depth observation, they also underscore the importance of using caution in interpreting small segments of child behavior.

Observation of the child in many and varied settings must have a reference point and that point must be normal behavior. Never let an exception to a general state go unnoticed! The unexpected may take any one of several forms. It may be bizarre and out of place with no observable precipitant, it may be the lack of response where one is naturally expected, or it may be expected in terms of the stimuli presented but bizarre in some other aspect such as intensity, frequency, or length of response.

Description. Simply selecting the proper focus and observing ample and varied behavior is not going to lead to a productive session; the diagnostician must attempt to put those observations into words. The translation from observation to description is often a much more difficult step than the novice suspects. In the early stages the diagnostician must train himself to describe behavior in writing as objectively, explicitly, and completely as possible. During these first attempts to communicate the findings of the observation, the clinician must withstand the temptation to jump to conclusions. He must stick to what he observes and what he can describe. The authors recently assigned several students to the same diagnostic session and asked them to record their observations; here are two samples of their reports:

> *Student A*. Timmy entered the testing room and was very shy and unhappy. He was afraid of the examiner and wanted his mother. He continued to act in this spoiled manner until his mother was brought into the room. Once Mrs. H. was in the room, Timmy began to behave himself, and the testing could be undertaken.
>
> *Student B*. Timmy stood in the doorway, held his head down, and refused to move into the room for three or four minutes until the clinician physically picked him up and closed the door. Timmy stood by the door and cried, while the clinician attempted to engage him in such play activities as card games, lotto, and ball. Timmy continued to cry for approximately fifteen minutes throughout all of these attempts until the clinician went out and brought Mrs. H. into the room. Timmy immediately crawled up on his mother's lap, and the clinician gave the articulation testing cards to the mother to show Timmy. After five minutes of encouragement by the mother, Timmy began to name the pictures.

Careful examination of these two accounts shows that one student was willing to make judgments, classify behavior, and generally draw conclusions without clearly specifying just what behavior was observed; the other student made a valiant effort to report the observables. Either approach can be taken to an extreme and thus interfere with the orderly transmission of information, but we strongly recommend that the beginning clinician make every attempt to keep the early accounts of his observations descriptive.

Interpretation. Once all pertinent behaviors have been described, it is incumbent upon the observer to make *interpretations*. Without moving to this level, the observations are of little value (unless the worker is willing to allow someone else to make an interpretation based upon his descriptive data). At this point the observer makes inferences regarding the meaning of behaviors; he attempts to generalize and classify behaviors and draw conclusions as to the meaning of what he observed. All of this can only be done, however, after sufficient purely descriptive information has been compiled. Interpretations drawn from objective quantified data are much more easily checked against reality than are interpretations made from desultory observations.

While making interpretative statements it is generally best to provide the reader with specific examples of the types of observational information which lead to such conclusions. For example, the examiner concludes that Mrs. K. is having some difficulty with behavior management which may have an influence upon Jason's language disorder:

> During the interview session Jason emptied his mother's purse on the floor, pulled the testing materials off the table, took his shoes and socks off and pinched his mother's leg until large red marks appeared. Following each of these episodes Mrs. K. twice asked Jason to stop, with no result.

Implications. Finally, the observer is expected to explain the *implications* of the observed behavior. Implications may be found by evaluating the consistency of the disorder in various settings, the degree of intelligibility in contextual speech, and so on. Information on the etiology of the problem may also be available through observation, and such interpretations as are warranted must be ventured. Similarly, the observed behavior can be assigned a meaning in order to direct the therapeutic effort.

It should be evident to the reader that we have attempted to apply the "abstraction process" to the task of observation (Weinberg, 1959). The diagnostician moves from the nonverbal level of sensing and observing to the verbal levels of describing, labeling, and interpreting; and finally he draws conclusions and states some implications. Leaving out the middle verbal steps of description would be undisciplined because it allows too much distorting subjectivity and projection on the part of the observer. Strict adherence to the logical order of observation leads to accurate and more defensible conclusions.

Our rather extended discussion of the various skills and abilities necessary for efficient diagnosis is designed to impress upon the reader the necessity of mediating between the scientific and artistic elements of diagnosis. We are neither computers coldly collecting and collating data, nor are we just friends sitting down for a social chat. The diagnostician must possess warmth and compassion as well as observational skill and a scientific attitude.

PUTTING THE DIAGNOSIS TO WORK

As mentioned previously, the most important variable in the success of a diagnosis is the diagnostician. The available body of knowledge and set of skills set the stage for success or failure. The diagnostician brings knowledge of individual behavior, normal human behavior, normal speech and language development, concepts of testing and evaluation, test selection, communicative disorders, and a variety of other information, all of which culminates in skillful application of test administration, interviewing, and observation. The most knowledgeable and skillful diagnostician, however, may fail to achieve adequate results if he lacks the inquisitiveness necessary to encourage continuous effort and if he does not have the professional integrity to serve each individual to the maximum of his potential. Each of us is subject to individual variations in daily behavior which can have a direct effect upon performance; however, it is incumbent upon every professional to control those variations so as to provide each individual with the best professional service available.

Perhaps the most demanding of all diagnostic ventures is the ultimate synthesis of findings into a coherent statement of the nature of the problem. The skilled clinician draws the findings together using the data available, past experience, knowledge, and intuition to formulate a total picture of the condition. At this point textbooks, research findings, and academic lectures fail to provide all of what is needed to succeed. Maturation of skills will only develop in an extensive practicum under the close supervision of a knowledgeable diagnostician.

The essence of the synthesis process is comparison of what is observed with what we expect to observe from our knowledge of the normal process. The incongruities between the observed and the normal provide the building blocks for completion of the picture. Figure 1.2 identifies diagnosis as a synthesis of findings, and shows a number of outcomes to which this synthesis might lead.

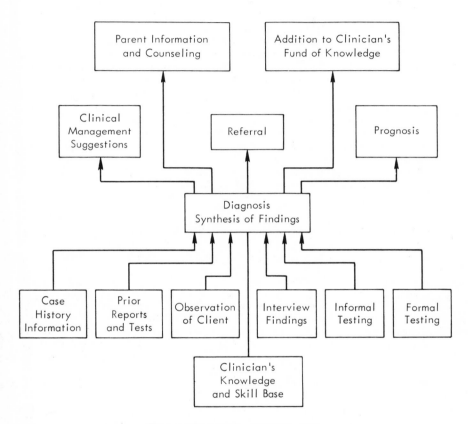

Figure 1.2 Paradigm of Diagnosis.

SUMMARY

Diagnosis is the most demanding and possibly the most exhilarating of clinical experiences. The rewards from careful and accurate diagnosis have far-reaching effects upon the client and his family by providing answers to basic questions and providing appropriate direction to the clinical effort. The research base and data orientation which hallmark all great professions is best exemplified in speech pathology through our diagnostic efforts.

PROJECTS AND QUESTIONS

1. The current emphasis on accountability is exacting a heavy tool on many professions. (Siegel, 1975a) Having been thrust upon speech pathology from several directions, accountability has become a time- and energy-consuming component of each clinician's working day. Although the net result should be improved services to the handicapped, there may be instances where the need to be accountable to some administrative guideline or dictate decreases actual quality and quantity of service. Two elements of accountability—efficiency and measurement—are of major interest to speech clinicians. The major method for achieving efficiency is the determination of the best technique for improving behavior with the least expenditure. Diagnosis plays a major part in the measurement of change by providing exact pre-test and post-test data necessary for evaluation of change. The recent surge of interest in accountability has forced diagnosticians to incorporate objective quantifying types of measures which allow comparison from one point in time to another. Unfortunately, not all of the parameters of communication lend themselves to quantification, thus some of the procedures are a bit contrived. It is an unfortunate reality of today's accountability trend that efficiency is measured through objective data on variables which may be neither objectified nor counted.

   Read the following articles and then formulate your concepts of accountability in relation to the following: cost accounting, Public Standards Review Organization, preparing clinical objectives, professional honesty, and variables of the speech signal.

CACCAMO, J. (1973). "Accountability—A Matter of Ethics?" *ASHA*, 15: 411–412.
MOWRER, D. (1972). "Accountability and Speech Therapy." *ASHA*, 14: 111–115.
RICHARDSON, S. (1974). "Accountability to the Child With a Disorder of Communication." *ASHA*, 16: 3–6.
SIEGEL, G. (1975). "The High Cost of Accountability." *ASHA*, 17: 796–797.

2. There are several types of speech disorders which lend themselves to objective and quantitative measurement. List some, describe how they might be quantified, and relate that quantification to a determination of the normality or abnormality of the problem.
3. Compare the traditional etiological and symptomatic systems of classifications of speech disorders with the system devised by Milisen (1971). Of what value are classification systems? Could you devise one with some novel characteristics that are of value to your understanding of speech disorders?
4. What implications for diagnosis do you find in the theory that speech is essentially an overlaid function?
5. Have society's changing definitions of aberrant behavior influenced speech therapy's definitions of speech disorders? How? Is there a relationship between our definition of what constitutes defective speech and the clinical approach to public-school clinical speech work?
6. We have all observed other professionals undertaking diagnostic evaluations. Make a descriptive analysis of three individuals who you feel were most proficient. What characteristics typify these persons? How would you rate them on a ten-point scale of objectivity (scientific) versus subjectivity (artistic)?
7. Most speech-pathology texts quote speech-impairment incidence figures of 5 to 10 percent of the public-school population; yet Newman (1961) quotes a Public Health Service report revealing only 0.65 percent of the population as being speech impaired. What implications does this have for our definition of what constitutes defective speech?

8. The volume of information regarding human behavior has made it impossible for any individual or profession to stand alone. The need for interdisciplinary cooperation in the evaluation and treatment of handicapped individuals has been tacitly acknowledged but not particularly enthusiastically embraced by many professions. Interdisciplinary ventures very often end up being multidisciplinary in nature, with each profession seeking to protect its own professional turf. Speech pathology, because of its rather favored position within special education over the years, has been aloof to other professions and may, as a result, find that interprofessional cooperation must be fostered through conscious effort. Professions and professionals should place the needs of the individual at the forefront in establishing improved channels of communication for interdisciplinary work. What professions should be included in an interdisciplinary approach to diagnosis of the child with a communication disorder?
9. What is the difference between criterion-referenced and norm-referenced tests? What purpose do each play in the diagnostic process?
10. The term diagnosis comes from a German word meaning, "to decide." What are the decisions to be made in a diagnosis?
11. A common danger in diagnosis is seeing only what you expect to see. Familiarity with tests and typical test responses may help or hinder objective examination. Without looking, draw the palm of your right hand . . . how accurate were you? No matter how familiar you think you are with something, it always pays to observe carefully prior to making judgments.
12. Compare the models of diagnosis offered by:

SCHULTZ, M., and M. CARPENTER (1975). "The Bases of Speech Pathology and Audiology: Selecting a Therapy Model." *Journal of Speech and Hearing Disorders*, 38: 395–404.
BROWN, J. (1972). "A Communication Model for Evaluation and Remediation." *Exceptional Children*, 38: 385–394.
MYSAK, E. (1976). *Pathologies of Speech Systems*, Baltimore: Williams and Wilkins, Chapter 2.

13. In order to formulate your concept of the difference between a speech difference and a communication defect, trace the impact of communication skills upon the lives of Dwight Eisenhower, Truman Capote, Charles Darwin, Billy Budd, Barbara Walters, and Leigh Hunt. Did a speech difference exist? What was the influence of the speech pattern upon the life of the individual?

BIBLIOGRAPHY

BATEMAN, B. (1964). "Learning Disabilities—Yesterday, Today, and Tomorrow." *Exceptional Children*, 31: 167–177.
——— (1967). "Three Approaches to Diagnosis and Educational Planning for Children with Learning Disabilities." *Academic Therapy Quarterly*, 3: 11–16.
BEVERIDGE, W. (1951). *The Art of Scientific Investigation*. New York: W. W. Norton & Co., Inc.
DARLEY, F. (1964). *Diagnosis and Appraisal of Communication Disorders*. Englewood Cliffs, N.J.: Prentice-Hall, Inc.
DIETZ, H. (1952). "A Study of the Understandability of Defective Speech in Relation to Errors of Articulation." Master's thesis, University of Pittsburgh.
DUFF, R. and A. HOLLINGSHEAD (1968). *Sickness and Society*. New York: Harper & Row.

GARWOOD, V. (1952). "An Experimental Study of Certain Relationships Between Intelligibility Scores and Clinical Data of Persons with Defective Articulation." Doctoral dissertation, University of Michigan.

GREY, S. (1963). *The Psychologist in the Schools*. New York: Holt, Rinehart & Winston, Inc.

GUNTHER, B. (1971). *What to do Till the Messiah Comes*. New York: Macmillan.

HADLEY, J. (1958). *Clinical and Counseling Psychology*. New York: Alfred A. Knopf, Inc.

JOHNSON, W. (1961). "Are Speech Disorders 'Superficial' or 'Basic'?" *ASHA*, 3: 233.

——— (1964). *People in Quandaries*. New York: Harper & Row.

———; F. DARLEY; and D. SPRIESTERSBACH (1963). *Diagnostic Methods in Speech Pathology*. New York: Harper & Row.

LOVITT, T. (1967). "Assessment of Children with Learning Disabilities." *Exceptional Children*, 34: 233–239.

MILISEN, R. (1971). "Methods of Evaluation and Diagnosis of Speech Disorders," in *Handbook of Speech Pathology and Audiology*, ed. L. Travis. New York: Appleton-Century-Crofts, Inc.

NATION, J., and D. ARAM (1977). *Diagnosis of Speech and Language Disorders*. Saint Louis: The C. V. Mosby Company.

NEWMAN, P. (1961). "Speech Impaired?" *ASHA*, 3: 9–10.

PRONOVOST, W. (1966). "Case Selection in the Schools: Articulatory Disorders." *ASHA*, 8: 179–181.

REESE, E. (1966). *The Analysis of Human Operant Behavior*. Dubuque, Iowa: Wm. C. Brown.

ROGERS, C. (1942). *Counseling and Psychotherapy*. Boston: Houghton Mifflin Company.

SCHULTZ, M. (1972). *An Analysis of Clinical Behavior in Speech and Hearing*. Englewood Cliffs, N.J.: Prentice-Hall, Inc.

SCHUTZ, W. (1967). *Joy: Expanding Human Awareness*. New York: Grove Press, Inc.

SIEGEL, G. (1975a). "The High Cost of Accountability." *ASHA*, 17: 796–797.

——— (1975b). "The Use of Language Tests." *Language Speech and Hearing Services In Schools*, 7:211–217.

——— (1966). "Evaluative Reactions and the Pathologies of Speech." *Quarterly Journal of Speech*, 52: 70–73.

SLOAN, H., and B. MACAULAY, eds. (1968). *Operant Procedures in Remedial Speech and Language Training*. Boston: Houghton Mifflin Company.

VAN RIPER, C. (1972). *Speech Correction: Principles and Methods*. Englewood Cliffs, N.J.: Prentice-Hall, Inc.

——— (1966). "Guilty?" *WMU Journal of Speech Therapy*, 2: 2–3.

WEINBERG, H. (1959). *Levels of Knowing and Existence*. New York: Harper & Row.

YSSELDYKE, J., and J. SALVIA (1974). "Diagnostic-prescriptive Teaching: Two Models." *Exceptional Children*, 41: 181–185.

2

Interviewing

While clinical evaluation obviously involves more than proficiency at conducting interviews, to be an effective diagnostician a worker must be skilled in communicating with parents and clients. In order to assess and treat persons with disorders of oral language, it is essential that we know how to talk with them in a manner which reflects our expertise and inspires confidence and trust.[1]

THE IMPORTANCE OF INTERVIEWING

The ability to conduct professional interviews is central to the role of the diagnostician. The client is initiated into the clinical transaction by means of verbal exchange through which data are gathered, information is transmitted, and a working relationship is established. The interview is also the means by which treatment is carried out and, as such, serves as both a tool and a relationship (See Figure 2.1). For the clinical speech pathologist, interviewing is an extremely important activity.

Although widely used, interviewing is one of the least understood aspects of the worker's role. Prospective speech clinicians are expected to acquire an impres-

---

[1]This chapter is based upon Lon L. Emerick, *The Parent Interview* (Danville, Illinois: Interstate Printers and Publishers, Inc., 1969).

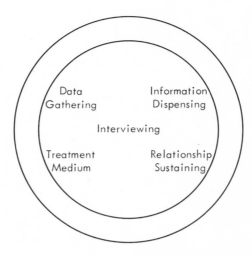

Figure 2.1   Interviewing is central in speech pathology.

sive array of knowledge, but often it is merely presumed that they know how to communicate effectively with clients. The mastery of interviewing is either taken for granted or expected to accrue somehow as an incidental artifact of required course work and practicum experiences. Some clinicians consider interviewing to be secondary; they use paper to replace personal interaction. An elaborate case-history form containing a plethora of questions is mailed to the parents, and they are requested to fill it out and return it before the diagnostic appointment. The rationale for this procedure is that it saves the clinician time and alerts him to problem areas he can then explore in the personal interview. Although the clinician certainly should get some idea of the problem before the diagnostic examination, he seldom needs a twelve-page questionnaire. There are several reasons for disenchantment with the paper approach: (a) the questions are generic—i.e., they cover *all* possible respondents—and thus are ambiguous or not applicable to many *particular* clients; a parent may not understand the relationship between the questions posed and his child's speech problem and demand, "Why does the clinician need to know *all of this* to cure Mary's speech?" (Irwin, 1965: 76); face-to-face interviews permit greater flexibility in formulating precise and germane inquiries; (b) the queries may be threatening or engender guilt, and the clinician is not present to observe these reactions or to support and assist the respondent as he searches for an answer. Does the mailed questionnaire allow time for the respondent to plan a defense? Is it more likely that we end up with a view of what the respondent wants us to see? More complete information can be obtained in an interview, where primary questions may be followed up with pertinent secondary inquiries; (c) the questions, if answered by the respondent in one particular way, may prevent him from developing any other possible answers. Spoken language does tend to create a reality for the individual, but writing lends an air of permanence. During an interview, however, the clinician can determine not only *what* a client says but also *how* he says it—for example, how does he assign priority to items, how does he associate items with one another, how does he reveal attitudes by vocal quality or body language? (d) mailed case-history forms also tend to bias the diagnostician to a set of expectancies that are difficult to change. The main objection, however, is the impersonal, routine nature of the procedure. It denies the uniqueness of each client and implies that the agency simply wants to compile a fund of information for its files.

THE NATURE OF INTERVIEWING

An interview is essentially a process, not an entity—a process of verbal and nonverbal intercourse between a trained professional worker and a client seeking his services. More specifically, an interview, in a clinical diagnostic sense, is a *purposeful* exchange of meanings between two persons, a directed conversation that proceeds in an orderly fashion to obtain data, to convey certain information, and to provide release and support. The professional worker, by reason of his position and clinical expertise, is expected to (and usually does) provide the direction for the verbal exchange. (Thus, an interview is not just an ordinary conversation in terms of a desultory exchange of opinions and ideas, but rather a specialized pattern of verbal interaction directed toward a specific purpose and focused upon specific content) The roles of interviewer and respondent are more highly specified in a professional interview than in a conversation. An interview differs from a social conversation in a number of other important respects (Kadushin, 1972): (a) the time and location of an interview is specified formally; (b) the inquiries are generally unilateral—the clinician may ask about the parents' relationship with their child, for example, but it is not expected that the client will reciprocate with questions about the worker's children; and (c) the clinician does not necessarily avoid unpleasant topics in the interest of social propriety.

In a good diagnostic interview, the clinician and client must become co-workers, multiplying their efforts by creating a mutual feeling of cooperation. It is futile to expect straightforward answers to simple questions. A good diagnostic interview always involves more than making queries and recording answers.

Interviewing is a unique kind of conversation. Perhaps for the first time the respondent can talk freely without fear of criticism or admonishment. Now, the *clinician* knows that an interview is a unique and distinct mode of verbal exchange, but does the client need to know? Probably not. Indeed, we typically advise students to refer to an interview as a "chat" or "a chance to share information" when they contact clients or parents to request an appointment time. An "interview" sounds rather ominous and frightening—perhaps even like a summons to account for one's failings.

In summary, a diagnostic interview is a directed conversation, carried out for specific purposes such as fact finding, informing, or altering attitudes and opinions. The clinician's efforts are directed toward the creation of mutual respect and team effort in the understanding and solution of the communication problem.

COMMON INTERVIEWING PROBLEMS

Several factors can prevent the establishment of effective communicative bonds between a speech clinician and those he interviews. Although the list could obviously be expanded, we have picked several aspects which in our experience are the most common interviewing barriers.

Fears of the Clinician

There are two points in a student clinician's career when his anxiety rises to very high levels: the confrontation with his first therapy case and his first diagnostic interview. It is—and should be—an awesome responsibility to undertake the professional treatment of a fellow human being. There is always an element of risk in offering help. As a matter of fact, if a student does not get somewhat tense in this situation, we suspect his suitability for the profession, since either he is so dumb he knows no fear or he doesn't care enough to be afraid. We certainly are not applauding anxiety, but we should accept and recognize our fears, specify their nature, and develop effective ways to channel the nervous energy into improving our performance. The client's needs, not the clinician's feelings of adequacy are salient.

Perhaps the most common fear expressed by beginning interviewers is that clients will not accept them in a professional role because of their youth. They doubt they can bridge the age gap, especially when they deal with parents: "Who am I to be asking questions and giving suggestions to them when they are older and more experienced?" They sigh, "Won't parents consider me a pipsqueak? Won't they look down on me if I don't have children?" Most of this is pure projection on the student's part. If the interviewer indicates his deep concern for the welfare of the child, then nearly every parent will respond in a positive manner, without scrutinizing the clinician for wrinkles, grey hairs, or diaper-pail hands. The clinician, of course, should not communicate the uncertainty he may feel in the interview situation, or he will never establish his competence or inspire confidence. The worker must abandon all thoughts of himself, his doubts and fears, how well he is doing, and channel all his energy into making the client feel that he is a co-worker.

Another common fear among incipient interviewers—and one that is also largely projected—is that the interviewee will become defensive or resentful during questioning. We have seen students omit a whole series of important questions when a client, especially a parent, responded curtly or showed mild annoyance. While it is not uncommon for parents to feel ashamed because they think of their child's speech disorder as an outward and visible sign of their own failure, few in our experience are resentful or defensive about the clinician's sincere efforts to determine the nature of the child's problem. The important point is, again, to make the interviewees feel that they have done the best they could do, and now, with some assistance from the clinician, they can do better. The best advice we can offer is this: *always assume a non-threatened posture in the clinical transaction.*

> During a recent diagnostic interview, a student clinician asked a routine question about a change of family residence and its relationship to the onset of the child's fluency problem. The mother's face flushed and she stiffened noticeably. "Why is that important—do you think the move had something to do with Marcie's stuttering?" she demanded. The clinician paused for a few moments, leaned forward in her chair toward the parent, and restated her feelings in a calm, even voice. Later, when Mrs. Martin had relaxed, she did relate how traumatic the family move had been for her then three-year-old daughter.

Many beginning interviewers are leery of questions directed at them. "What do you do when the client starts asking *you* questions?" the student interviewer frequently despairs. "Will I be able to explain to them adequately what they need to know? How will I know if I have gotten it across if they just sit there and nod?"

Finally, some beginning interviewers are frightened to deal with feelings and attitudes. Since Freud drew his vivid pictures of the mental monsters that lurk beneath everyone's psyche, many workers have maintained that the beginner should not tamper with the lids of these Pandora's boxes. Fearful of unleashing such dreadful forces, it is small wonder that many students conduct sterile, superficial interviews with their clients.

Memory failure. A common deterrent to communication in an interview is loss of memory. Clients will simply not remember things that the clinician needs to know in order to best plan a program of therapy.

Emotional barriers. Sometimes an interviewee cannot or will not give information because there are emotional blocks that prevent free communication. Self-disclosure is often difficult and the respondent may not be able to identify a payoff for revealing personal information.

Loath to find out. Physicians have reported that some patients coming for medical assistance tend to minimize or conceal their symptoms because they don't want to find out that they have something wrong. The same device can operate in diagnostic interviews.

The class barrier. Students in training are pretty much cloistered in a middle-class milieu. Rarely are they called upon to interact with persons from lower socioeconomic levels; often they are sufficiently shocked that they lose their effectiveness when dealing with these people and their unfamiliar life styles.

The language gap. The clinician must remember that laymen often have a markedly different way of talking about a speech or hearing problem. If there is a language gap and the clinician does not take steps to close it, the interview will be unsuccessful: the greatest barrier to communication is the assumption of it (Stewart and Cash, 1974).

The lack of specific purpose. Many beginning interviewers either have purposes that are too broad and general or interviewing goals that are too nebulous. It is important to carefully and rather explicitly write out the purposes for the interview before meeting with the client. We must know *why* we want the answers to the questions we ask. Specifying the purposes of an interview is also an effective way to reduce the interviewer's uncertainty and anxiety. Kadushin (1972: 2) summarizes the importance of planning in this way:

> To know is to be prepared; to be prepared is to experience reduced anxiety; to reduce anxiety is to increase the interviewer's freedom to be fully responsive to the interviewee.

The clinician should keep in mind, however, that thorough planning does not mean the application of an inflexible routine.

AN APPROACH TO INTERVIEWING

We now present an interviewing approach, an eclectic product of our experience in social work, speech pathology, and clinical audiology, together with an intensive study of relevant bibliographic materials. No doubt the reader will want to modify it to suit his individual setting. It is desirable that he do so, for only through critical self-evaluation and modification can any clinician acquire an interviewing procedure that is uniquely his own.

There are three basic goals in diagnostic interviews: to obtain information, to give information, and to provide release and support. For the purpose of discussion each goal will be considered separately, a procedure rarely possible to do in an actual interview.

Goal One: Obtain Information

Although it may seem rather obvious, it is worth restating that as clinicians we must listen before we speak. There are essentially three reasons for this: (1) it gives clients an opportunity to talk out problems, to ventilate fears and feelings, thus enabling them to better profit from the direction and advice which the speech clinician will offer; (2) it gives the clinician an idea of the nature and scope of the information the client will need; and (3) it allows the clinician to formulate hypotheses concerning the individual's communication disorder.

Setting the tone. The first important task of the clinician is to set the right tone for the interview, to get a structured conversation initiated and channeled in the proper direction. How does one go about that? Research by McQuire and Lorch (1968) has underscored the importance of proper structuring. Their findings indicate that the initial style of interaction may well determine the style of interaction for the entire interview (see all the work of Matarazzo and Wiens, 1972). We find that defining the roles is an effective procedure for setting the tone:

> Mrs. Seelos, I'm Miss Sullivan, Terry's speech clinician. I really appreciate the opportunity to chat with you about Terry and the things we are doing in speech. First, though, you can be of great help to me since you know Terry so much better than I do. There are several things about his early development and how his speech seems to be at home that I need to understand before planning a long-range therapy program. Before you came in today, I made some notes for myself so that we could best use this half hour before my next session.

It is helpful to think of the interview as a kind of role-playing situation. The clinician defines the roles for the client and indicates the rules and responsibilities that accrue to these roles. He tells who he is, what he intends to do, and what he expects of the client. In other words, the interviewer structures the situation by explaining the purposes of the interview—why the information is wanted and what will be done with it. Initially, of course, the client accepts the respondent role because of the nature of the situation and the official sanction of the interviewer's position. Then it is up to the worker to demonstrate his empathy and clinical expertise in order to solicit further cooperation. Two problems sometimes arise here. First, some clients may be inhibited by such explicit role definitions; respondents from lower middle or lower social classes have had little experience in holding directed conversations. In this case, a clinician can prolong the small-talk phase, emphasize the nature of the interview as a chat, and gently ease into the more structured situation as the relationship develops.[2]

The second, more difficult problem concerns the site of the interview. Although it is generally best to conduct interviews in a clinical setting, sometimes this is not possible and one has to seek out the client or his parents at home. This is rarely satisfactory not only because of the distractions inherent in the situation (children, pets, and neighbors) but also because the interview frequently becomes a social visit.

It is vital that the interviewer convey his sincere interest in the situation as the client sees it. He must demonstrate to the client that he is genuinely trying to comprehend what the problem is and what it means to the client personally. The clinician can show his interest by carefully attending to the respondent: assume a relaxed, natural posture; maintain eye contact; and offer minimal verbal encouragements which reveal that he is listening.

---

[2]When two or more people meet together, even for serious purposes, a certain amount of social and idle talk seems to foster positive attitudes toward continued interaction. Czikszentmihalyi (1975) describes this feature of group interaction as "flow".

Rapport, of course, is not a separate substance that one pours into a session; it is mutual respect and trust, a feeling of confidence in the clinician, and a large measure of understanding. Empathy, warmth, and acceptance are crucial aspects; the worker must strive for the ability to sensitively and accurately understand the interviewee's situation. He should also try to be genuine, not contrived, with a professional character armor that signals "clinician on duty." As a matter of fact, it is helpful to avoid interposing a desk—a symbol of authority—between the respondent and the interviewer (Sommers, 1969). The interview is more effective without such a barrier. In addition to the words spoken, a number of forces shape the interview. Some things are conveyed by the setting and by the dress, manners, and expressions of the participants. If our office is located in a boiler room or a storage area, we have already conveyed something of our attitude toward the client and his problem by the very physical space that we use. In professional interviewing, the goal is to provide an atmosphere that fosters communication between client and clinician (Staples and Sloane, 1976).

Asking the questions. Preferably, the clinician should use an interview guide rather than one of the more elaborate questionnaires—that is, instead of a formal set of questions written out to be read and answered, he should use a form that indicates areas to explore. The interview is much more spontaneous and meaningful if the speech clinician words his questions in keeping with his understanding of the individual's situation, rather than reading prepared ones. In most cases, formal questionnaires operate as another type of barrier or crutch for the insecure interviewer.

The specific content of the queries addressed to a respondent are dependent upon, among other things, the nature of the problem, the age of the client, and the purposes of the interview. There are, however, some generic areas of interest. What is the respondent's perception of the problem? When and under what conditions did the difficulty originate? In what ways has the communication disorder changed since its onset? What are the consequences (the handicapping conditions) of the problem? How have the client and his family attempted to cope with the difficulty? In order to obtain a description of a child's ongoing behavior, and how he fits into a family regimen, ask him to describe a "typical" day from the time he gets up until he goes to bed.

Students frequently ask what type of interviewers they should strive to be: directive, nondirective, behavioristic, psychoanalytic, neo-Freudian, and so forth. The best answer that we have been able to give—although it sounds facetious—is that he must use whatever techniques seem to be best for the job that he needs to do. Often we feel that a beginning clinician concentrates too hard on being behavioristic or Rogerian rather than focusing on what he must do to meet the needs of a particular client. Some writers feel that the direct interview is unpleasant, although there is no evidence to support this assumption. As a matter of fact, one research team (Richardson, Dohrenwend, and Klein, 1965) discovered that the lack of structure inherent in the pure nondirective interview produced anxiety in some respondents, especially the less educated ones. Actually, the whole matter is an academic question, because the good diagnostic interview is characterized by a shifting of styles: objective questions that ask for specifics, subjective queries that deal with feelings and attitudes, and finally the indeterminate questions like "tell me more" that keep the respondent going.

A far better question for the clinician to direct to himself is, "Why am I asking these questions?" He should have his purposes clearly in mind. Classically, the interviewer should start with the least anxiety-provoking queries, mostly objective questions that have high specificity (Woolf, 1971), and then proceed to more subjective questions as the relationship develops.

Quite often, however, we find it useful to employ a "funnel" sequence of inquiry during the course of a diagnostic interview—starting with broad, open-ended questions and then progressing to more specific or closed questions (Stewart and Cash, 1974). Here is an example of a funnel sequence from a recent parent interview:

- How does Jimmy function in the family setting?
- How does he get along with his siblings?
- How does his older sister "help" him to communicate?
- Can you describe an instance in which she talked for him?

The "inverted funnel" approach, proceeding from specific to general, is also useful. It is best to avoid the checklist or long series of "tunnel" questions which call for information on one level of specificity and all of which are asked in a similar style (for example, "Did your child have earaches; fevers; head injury, etc.").

Dexter (1956) found that the interviewer can elicit greater cooperation by vividly demonstrating that he is on the respondent's side—that is, by using the client's phraseology, his style and manner, the interviewer demonstrates he is "one of the crowd." This is sometimes effective with a very anxious or reluctant client.

The presenting story. Most persons who anticipate visiting a clinic or discussing a speech problem with a public-school speech clinician will have mentally rehearsed what they intend to say.[3] They may even, in some cases, have a pseudoconversation with the worker. We must allow this story to be unraveled, or the respondent will be left with a sense of frustration and lack of closure. A question such as, "What seems to be the problem?" will permit the flow of conversation to begin. The clinician should remember that this is how the *client*

[3]Often the interviewer will have to contend with events that occurred prior to the session—the family car failing to start, a burned breakfast, absence of a convenient parking place. A few words to reveal the worker's understanding of the distracting antecedents will generally assist the respondent in shifting then to the topic of the interview.

perceives the problem—it is his unique way of looking at the situation. It may be grossly inaccurate, but the interviewer should hear him out; nothing turns a respondent off more quickly than for the interviewer to suggest by word or action that his views are silly or misguided. Sometimes the presenting story will become a motif that recurs again and again during the course of the interview.

This is generally a crucial point in an interview. The interviewee may cautiously extend a portion of himself verbally, carefully scan the interviewer's response, and then decide whether or not to tell the whole story. Sometimes a respondent may even set up a straw man to see how the interviewer deals with it:

> Mrs. Dimitri, mother of Ivan, a fifth-grader who possessed a serious lateral lisp, appeared to see herself as a modern, informed parent. At our initial interview, she launched into a lengthy diatribe about the school reading program, explaining in great detail why Ivan couldn't read. We listened intently for a time and when she paused to recycle her complaints, we praised her for her concern and suggested that she bring this up at the next P.T.A. meeting and with Ivan's teacher. Apparently Mrs. Dimitri expected a debate, and she was much mollified that we had heard her out. We then proceeded to an excellent review of her insights into the child's speech problem.

This is not the proper time for the clinician to debate an issue with the client. His story can be accepted initially on the level of feeling, and later in the interview—when rapport is stronger—the point can be discussed more fully. We feel very strongly that these initial stories, these primitive theories, should be respected as the best possible answer clients have been able to come up with. This does not mean agreeing with their conclusions; it just means we accept their judgment with understanding so that we can form a basis for further communication.

Actually, the presenting information can be a very rich source of clinical hypotheses to be explored during the course of the interview. How do the client and parent present themselves (Goffman, 1959)—as long suffering, anxious, diffident? How do they associate ideas or items of information sequentially? What priorities do they assign to issues they raise? Do they seem to be realistic in their expectations regarding the diagnostic session and treatment?

Nonverbal messages. Respondents do not communicate by words alone, and the discerning clinician attends to body as well as oral language during an interview. As a matter of fact, some observers (Bosmajian, 1971; Hinde, 1972; Mehrabian, 1972; Harrison, 1974) suggest that a large portion of the total message—particularly messages involving strong feelings—is carried by nonverbal cues. However, the diagnostician should resist the urge to interpret a client's every twitch; each instance of nonverbal behavior should be related to the *content* of the oral message and the *context* in which it occurs (Birdwhistle, 1970; Knapp, 1972; Feldman, 1973):

> If a parent leaves her coat on during an interview it may mean she feels vulnerable and the garment provides a bit of protective armor. It may also mean that she has a spot on her dress, or that all the hangers in the waiting room were taken again by

forgetful students, or that the room is chilly. However, if she shifts her chair away from the clinician, sits with her arms and legs tightly crossed, avoids eye contact and responds to questions with one word answers, then it may be concluded that she is defensive and guarded in the clinical setting.

The issue here is to avoid making one item of nonverbal behavior the sole basis for interpretation; the interviewer should be on the lookout for patterns (Weitz, 1974).

Although research into the nonverbal facets of dyadic interviewing is still in its early stages, there are several useful questions which can assist the examiner's scrutiny of body language (Egolf and Chester, 1973):

1. What clues are evident during the initial contact with the client? Does he enter the room hesitantly and wait to be seated? What can be discerned from his clothing or personal grooming? Does he avoid eye contact and shake hands limply?

2. Is the respondent's facial expression congruent with the content of his oral message? Does his face flush or show other emotions when discussing different aspects of his speech problem? Does he reveal tension by constant bunching of his jaw muscles?

3. How does the respondent use eye gaze during the course of the interview? As a general rule, persons maintain less eye contact when talking than listening, particularly when responding to questions that provoke reflection and recall. The amount of mutual gaze between two individuals is increased markedly when they like each other and are involved in a joint concern. Keep in mind, however, that unwavering eye contact by the clinician, particularly when asking questions, may be interpreted as a threat signal or an attempt to dominate (Argyle and Cook, 1976).

4. Attend to the client's body movements and postural shifts: what is the rate and extent of movement, and the degree of tension shown? Does the respondent's postural shifting congruently mirror that of the interviewer?

5. How does the client speak with his hands? Does he use mainly pronated or supinated gestures? Are his hands tightly clasped? Does he wring them, or play continually with his ring? Does he use a number of "adaptors" (Knapp, 1972), such as adjusting his clothing, scratching, or inspecting his finger nails?

6. How does the respondent communicate by use of the available space? In which chair does a client choose to sit with respect to proximity with the interviewer?

7. What can be discerned by attending to nuances of the client's use of pitch, loudness, or vocal quality? Does his rate reflect apprehension, excitement, or depression? Is the respondent's recital of the presenting story punctuated by heavy sighs?

8. In what respect do the stigmata associated with various communication disorders (for example, stuttering, cerebral palsy) interfere with or confound nonverbal messages (Goffman, 1963; Eisenberg and Smith, 1971)? How does body language vary with respect to the factors of sex, age, and culture (Morsbach, 1973)?

The most important thing to look for may be lack of congruence between the respondent's verbal and nonverbal messages; in cases where the two conflict, body language is a more accurate indicator of how a person feels about an issue:

During a recent diagnostic session we opened the parent interview by asking the parent to describe the nature of his child's speech problem (the child was multiply handicapped). Before the parent responded verbally, he made a short, chopping gesture with his right hand, stamped his right foot, and wrinkled his face in a fleeting expression of disgust. However, he then proceeded to tell us calmly what a wonderful relationship he had with his son. The nonverbal message occurred so swiftly that later we were uncertain if we had really seen it; when we played back the videotape, however, the graphic body language was evident even to the father. This vivid self-confrontation seemed to release some long-repressed feelings, and the father then talked at length about how disappointed he was in his son, how much attention his wife devoted to the child—often, he felt, at his expense, and what a financial drain the various treatment programs had been. The consequence of the interview was a referral to a family service agency where both parents received the type of counseling they needed.

Although persons vary in terms of their skill at ''reading'' nonverbal cues, it is possible to improve with training (Rosenthal *et al.*, 1974). Since body language is continuous—there is no way to turn it off, not even the clinician's—the interviewer will want to investigate the topic of nonverbal communication more fully (Scheflen, 1972; Spiegel and Machotka, 1974; see also Project 1 at the end of this chapter).

Things to avoid in the interview. Beginning interviewers commit several common errors. The list that follows is not meant to be exhaustive, but does cover the most glaring mistakes.

1. It is usually best to avoid questions that may be answered by a simple yes or no. Although open-ended questions do produce longer responses in general, it is interesting to note that respondents from lower socioeconomic groups, who have less education, become more anxious as the questions become less structured. We have interviewed several clients who are confirmed yes-men. No matter what the clinician asks, no matter what comments he makes, these respondents simply nod in passive agreement. Perhaps they are fearful of exposing their ignorance and feel that it is better to remain silent and be thought a fool than to say something and make it obvious.

We find that requesting the client to rate himself on some simple scale is more effective than either-or questions. We frequently ask the client to tell us not whether something is difficult or easy but to what degree. A simple rating procedure, with low values (1 or 2) indicating relative ease and higher values (4 or 5) indicating relative difficulty may be used.

2. Avoid phrasing questions in such a way that they inhibit freedom of response. Do not say: ''You don't have any difficulty with ringing in your ears, do you?'' or ''You don't tell Billy to stop and start over again, do you?'' Such leading questions are not effective interviewing. The beginning interviewer tends to be anxious about asking open-ended questions. He is afraid that silence will result and that this will damage his relationship with the client. So, he will ask an open-ended question and then close it. For example, ''How do you feel about David's stuttering; does it bother you?'' Leave it open! Although open-end questions consume more time and may produce some rambling and irrelevant responses, there are many advantages to recommend their use:

> They let the respondent do the talking while the interviewer plays his role as listener and observer. The freedom to determine the nature and amount of information the

respondent will give may communicate to him that you are interested in him, as well as his answers, and that you respect his ability to give accurate and relevant data (Stewart and Cash, 1974: 28).

Try also to avoid abrupt shifts in your line of questioning. For example, if you are exploring the client's feelings or attitudes on a particular issue (subjective questions), don't suddenly ask an objective question. Inexperienced interviewers, fearful that they are too deep in an area, tend to jump around; often they persist with objective queries and, once a pattern of response is established, the client finds it difficult to shift to more elaborate answers.

3. Avoid talking too much. This is perhaps the most common mistake of the beginning interviewer. He feels he must fill up every pause with his own verbiage. It is much better to rephrase what the respondent has said or make some comment like, "I see," "Tell me more," or "Anything else?" Sometimes a smile and an understanding nod are effective when it is felt that the client has more to say but needs some silent time to conjure it up. If there is a positive attitude—a good rapport—and the person feels comfortable in the situation, then these encouragements increase the length of the response; if the topic or situation is neutral, these comments tend to expand the message. However, if the topic is negative or the individual feels uncomfortable, the "hmmmmhmmmm" may be taken as a criticism—that is, if he *cannot* respond at length, he will feel that he is being pressured to do so.[4] Parents with little education are perhaps the most vulnerable to this kind of pressure.

Be careful not to fall into stereotyped verbal habits. One of our students used "very good" as reinforcement so frequently with a severely aphasic patient that one day, after making a particularly effective response to a problem, the patient—who had said very little since his stroke—finished the clinician's "very" with a resounding "good," surprising them both.

4. Avoid concentrating on the physical symptoms and the etiological factors to the exclusion of the client's feelings and attitudes. There is a little bit of Dr. Kildare in all of us; we yearn to play the role of omniscient healer. This is further compounded by instructors who dwell interminably on causation in their courses dealing with speech disorders. But it is possible to track each suspicious symptom with such zeal that we fail to obtain a basis for understanding the emotional and environmental complications of a speech or hearing disability. The interviewer should remind himself to distinguish between items of information that are simply interesting and background information that he really needs to know.

5. Avoid providing information too soon. There will be plenty of time to clear up misconceptions later in the interview. The surest way to cut off the flow of information is to stop a parent, for instance, after he says, "I just tell Michael to stop, take a deep breath, and start all over again," and counsel him on the proper responses to nonfluency.

---

[4]The "activity" level of the clinician appears to be a critical factor in his perceived effectiveness: interviewers who talked more (and interrupted respondents more often) were rated at higher levels of accurate empathy (Matarazzo and Weins, 1972).

6. Avoid qualifying and hemming and hawing when asking questions. Ask them in a straightforward fashion and maintain eye contact. Rather than asking, "Did you find that, well, you know, when you were, ah, shall we say . . . with child—did you experience any untoward conditions?" say, "Did anything unusual happen during your pregnancy?" Instead of inquiring, "Did you discover, hmmmm, I mean, well, after your father, ah, passed away, did your stuttering problem increase?" say, "What impact did your father's death have upon your speech?"

7. Avoid negativistic or moralistic responses, verbal or nonverbal, to the client's statements (avoid even the response "good," as it implies a value judgment). The flow of information will stop rapidly and the relationship will be impaired severely if the individual senses that we find him or his behavior distasteful. We do not have to subscribe to a person's values or code of behavior for us to show compassion and understanding for his situation. Use inquiries that begin with "why" very sparingly since the word is often perceived as a challenge or a threat; it is too reminiscent of disciplinary sessions (Why were you late for class? Why can't you behave properly?). In a clinical setting we must not let our values obscure our perception of the client's frame of reference (Benjamin, 1974).

8. When the client causes the interview to wander, avoid abrupt transitions to bring it back to the point. Most of those whom you will interview have had little experience in directed, orderly conversation. They tend to follow chance associations and wander far afield. The experienced interviewer has the ability to make smooth transitions. How does one go about getting the interview back on the track? The best way is by building a bridge to the respondent's previous statements. For example: "That's interesting, Mrs. Davis, maybe we can come back to that in a little while; now earlier you were mentioning that your child's loss of hearing occurred suddenly. . . ." The key here is to use respondent antecedents—things that the person has said earlier in the interview. If we use only the interviewer's antecedents—questions that the interviewer has asked before—the client will not feel understood and will sense that what he has said was of little consequence. The inexperienced interviewer asks lots of questions either with no antecedents or with his own antecedents. He is afraid of losing control of the interview and thus becomes preoccupied with formulating the next question.

9. Avoid allowing the interview to produce only superficial answers. We need ways to get deeper, more significant responses from our clients. There are several interviewing devices, termed *probes,* that the clinician will find helpful:

Crosshatch, or *interlocking,* questions are useful when we need to elicit more detail about a topic that has been glossed over. Often there are discrepancies that must be resolved. Essentially, the way to go about this is to ask the same thing in different ways and at different points during the interview. For instance, the father of a young stutterer responded in a superficial manner to our query about his relationship with the child. He assured us that he had a "loving relationship" with his son and then complained at length about his working conditions. Later in the interview when we asked him to describe the sorts of things he did with the child, he was unable to mention a single one. We don't mean to imply that the clinician should attempt to catch the client lying and then demand an explanation. The clinician must check out discrepancies, however, in order to enhance his understanding of the problem, since they could have a significant effect on the mode of treatment.

Next, *pauses* can be very helpful. When there is a lull in the interview, it may mean simply that the client has exhausted his store of information, that a memory barrier has prevented further recall, or that he senses he is not being understood. It can also mean, however, that a sensitive area has been touched upon. Do not feel that pauses harm the interview. Much significant information can be forthcoming if we keep quiet and indicate with a smile or a nod that we expect more.

Another aid is to encourage *time regression* and *association*. Memories are weak. In order to pinpoint some significant data, we may have to take the person back in time to find a memory peg such as a wedding, a natural calamity, or the like, that may call forth more information. One father, a long-time air force sergeant, catalogued everything in terms of the make and model of car he was driving. Another client, an inveterate bird watcher, remembered incidents by the times he had seen the Marbled Godwit or the Prothonatary Warbler.

The *summary probe* is one of the best ways to keep the interview moving smoothly. The clinician summarizes periodically what the client has said, ending perhaps with a request for clarification or further information. Incidentally, this procedure also demonstrates to the person that the interviewer is indeed trying to understand his problem. We generally use "mini-summary probes"—echo questions—all the way through an interview:

Respondent: After my husband's stroke, my whole world collapsed.
Interviewer: You were overwhelmed by the sudden change in your life.
Respondent: Yes, one day he was happily planning our trip to Sanibel Island . . . and then, in just a moment, he was paralyzed and couldn't talk. Now, all our plans are up in the air . . . the new car, the checking account, he took care of all that.

The *stumbling probe* is a variation of the summary probe; we have found it helpful, especially with the reticent respondent. The interviewer rephrases a portion of the respondent's communication and then, attempting to interpret or comment upon it, he pretends to halt or stumble. For example, when interviewing the mother of a child allegedly beginning to stutter, the clinician might say: "Now, you were saying that Bruce first started to repeat and hesitate after he caught his finger in the car door. Under these conditions, it would be natural for you to . . . ah. . . ." This really works. The respondent's need for closure will precipitate significant information and, perhaps more important, significant insights.

Finally, the *assuming probe*. (This stems from the old incriminating question, "Have you stopped beating your wife yet?") Such a technique should, of course, be used sparingly and only after some interviewing experience; at times, however, it is the only way to get information out in the open. If the client has avoided an important area, if he has left much unsaid regarding his speech or hearing problem and what it means to him, then it is up to the interviewer to bring this out. One adolescent boy who had been vehemently denying that his stuttering bothered him, unburdened himself when we said, "It bothers you so much that you don't want anybody to know, do you?"

10. Avoid letting the client reveal too much in one interview. You may have had similar experiences: a good friend encounters severe trouble and you come to his aid, helping him through the crisis. A curious thing often happens when your friend recovers his equilibrium. He feels obligated to you; he felt exposed to you as a raw human being during the crisis, and now he is embarrassed, somewhat resentful, and perhaps even hostile. It is as if you are now an outward and visible sign of his former debacle. Sometimes a beginning interviewer makes the mistake of trying to get everything in one sitting. The client, sensing perhaps his first really understanding listener, may want to pour out his whole sad tale of woe. Later, however, the individual will feel embarrassed and foolish, perhaps even exposed and guilty at revealing so much of himself to this comparative stranger.

Bringing an interview to a graceful close can sometimes be more difficult than getting it started. In our experience, an interview is most effectively terminated by summarizing what has been discussed and reviewing the specific actions to be taken. It is probably best not to consider new material at this time when neither the interviewer nor the client can devote sufficient attention to it. It is always important, however, to leave the door open for future contacts (see Stewart and Cash, 1974: 197–201; and Kadushin, 1972: 207–214 for more information on leave-taking).

11. Avoid trusting to memory. Record the information as the interview progresses. Tell the client that you will take some notes during the interview so that you can plan his treatment program more effectively and make recommendations for other services. Such note-taking, or even recording devices, are rarely questioned. Indeed, we have found that clients expect you to write down some of the information they are giving you; they doubt that you would be able to remember all of their answers. You obviously would lose your relationship, however, if you scribbled furiously while the client was revealing some sensitive information. It is axiomatic that the respondent's confidence will be respected, but we have mixed feelings about mentioning this explicitly to the client. The clinician's manner should suggest that all information received is to be held strictly confidential. At times, the clinician can suggest the possibility that he might listen and tell others, and this had never entered the respondent's mind.

Put the clinical situation, procedures, observations, and recommendations in writing as soon as possible. Commit it to paper while the facial characteristics and voice inflections can still be remembered. Make the report "alive" so that others can experience most of the clinical situation just by reading about it. Watch during the interview for things that may have significance: how the client used time (was he late or early?), postures, sighs, association of ideas, word choice, retraction of statements, insights, and so forth.

Goal Two: Provide Information

The most common complaint of patients in modern hospitals and clinics is that they have not been kept informed of their condition and progress. Interviewing 214 patients, Pratt, Seligman, and Reader report (1958: 229): "Patients who were given more thorough explanations were found to participate somewhat more effectively with the physician and were more likely to accept completely the doctor's formulation than were the patients who received very little information." We have formulated a fundamental principle in this regard: *there is never too little information, there is instead misinformation*. Not one of us can stand uncertainty. All too frequently the information, if not supplied by the professional worker, will come distorted from other sources. When not correctly informed, parents become misinformed and this leads to confusion, misunderstanding, and further compounding of the problem. It is our responsibility, therefore, to provide accurate, unemotional, objective information on the status of the individual's speech and hearing problem. This is generally accomplished during the post-diagnostic conference (Martin, 1977).

Summarize the findings of the clinical examination in simple, nontechnical language; use common terms compatible with the person's background. We prefer to commence, if possible, with results which show a client's areas of normal functioning, to review findings which indicate what is good before describing deficiencies. It is good technique to proceed by a review of the support systems for oral language—auditory, sensory, motor, psychosocial—and then describe the findings of language, voice, articulation, and fluency assessments. Relate comments to normative values whenever possible. Clarify and help the respondent ask questions by using examples and simple analogies. If the interviewer is in doubt concerning the client's understanding of the diagnostic material (clients will rarely ask if they don't understand), he should talk more slowly, employ longer descriptions, and use more redundant language (Longhurst and Siegel, 1973). Recapitulation of a conference, by audio or videotape playback fosters even greater understanding (Marshall and Goldstein, 1969).

Avoid superficial statements of reassurance. Most people can see through this sort of sham. The individual's anxiety and uncertainty will be better relieved once he begins to understand his particular speech problem; the best antidote to fear and uncertainty is knowledge. Be sure, however, to avoid iatrogenic errors. Do not use terms or suggest consequences that will precipitate more stress for the client. One parent was told his child's hearing problem was caused by atrophy of the hearing nerve. It is difficult enough to have a hard-of-hearing child without worry about mysterious nerves atrophying, something about which the parent can do very little. Do not communicate your negative expectations regarding the outcome of therapy to the client. We are convinced that what the clinician thinks a client can do, that he shall do. In other words, after Parkinson, the client's behavior expands to fit the clinician's concept of his potential. Do we precondition our own therapeutic behavior when we make a prognosis? Is this communicated to the client and his relatives in some manner and on some level? We think it often is.

Below are six basic principles for imparting information to clients, which we have found useful:

1. Emotional confusion may, and often does, inhibit the person's ability to understand cognitively what you are trying to say. Just because you have once reviewed the steps of ear training is no reason to expect that its importance will be grasped.

2. Refrain from being didactic; do not lecture your clients. Focus on sharing options rather than on giving advice.

3. Use simple language with many examples and illustrations. If you must err, err in the direction of being too simple rather than complex. And repeat, repeat, repeat the important points—rephrasing each time.

4. Try to provide something that the client—especially a parent—can *do*. Action reduces the feelings of futility and anxiety. The activity should be direct, simple, and require some kind of reporting to the clinician.

5. Say what needs to be said pleasantly—but frankly. Do not avoid saying something that must be said on the assumption that the client cannot take it or that you will be rejected. People often display an amazing reserve of courage in difficult situations (Buscaglia, 1975).

6. Remember, however, that the one who finally communicates what the client may have been dreading to hear is often hated and maligned. If you are the first to say the feared words, you may become the focus for all the hostile, negative feelings thus aroused. As a professional worker, you will have to be strong enough to be the lightning rod for these emotions.

Clients and their parents expect to receive help from the clinician, but often will resist change. No matter how maladaptive a client's behavior may seem from an objective point of view, it represents his best solution; in fact, he will often resist attempts to alter his equilibrium, precarious as it may appear to others. Change is stressful; diagnosis and treatment imply change; therefore, assessment and therapy are stressful.

Goal Three: Release and Support

The clinician does not, of course, wait until the end of the interview to provide release for the frustrations and fears of the client. Most of the parts of the interview already discussed will serve this purpose. By helping the individual talk out his problems, the worker is providing an excellent escape for pent-up feelings. We maintain that our purpose is not just to remove discomfort but also to promote a state of comfort and well-being.

More than advice is needed during interviews for the purpose of helping clients take some specific action or move in a particular direction. They need help in sorting out the confusing choices before them. To support a respondent's real strengths, we need to make it clear that we understand what the situation means to him and that we uncritically sympathize with his feelings and attitudes. We can restore the client's self-esteem and his ability to function more appropriately if we convey our interest in him as a person and our solid acceptance of his importance. If the client feels appreciated and understood, he can sometimes drop his self-protective behavior and see how the experience will eventually benefit him.

There is an unfortunate tradition of "sweetness and light" in client counseling. A person has a problem. He is sad and depressed, and we try to cheer him up. Sometimes this degenerates into a debate, with the interviewer attempting to persuade the person that he should not feel miserable. When a person feels depressed, anxious, and fearful, he does not want to count his blessings. He wants you to feel miserable, too. He wants you to share and identify with him on his own level. Thus, the interviewer is given a basis for communication with the person. We start where he is, accept it as the proper place to start, and tell him that it is a sad state of affairs that would make anyone sad and depressed. Then, using this bond of identification, which becomes a basis for communication, we can assist him in solving the problem. The main ingredient is *empathy*, the capacity to identify oneself with another's feelings and actions. The best way to demonstrate our attempt to understand a client's point of view is by listening creatively.

According to Carkhuff and Berenson (1967) and others (Ginott, 1965; Gordon, 1970), the key feature of *creative listening* is the ability to scan a client's comments and respond in a way that fosters understanding and releases the potential for growth. Creative listening represents empathy in action: before anyone can or will listen, he must first be listened to.

The particular kind of understanding we are referring to involves two facets, a *cognitive* aspect (the content) and an *affective* aspect (the feelings). In order for genuine understanding to take place, both must be included in the interviewer's response to the client's statement. If the clinician is successful in crystallizing both aspects of his response, he has provided an *interchangeable base* which allows the interview to move forward to levels of helping that involve direct action. Here are some examples taken from diagnostic interviews:

Client: (in response to a query regarding his marital status): "No, I'm single . . . who would want to marry a clod who stutters like me?"

Clinician: "You feel rejected because of your speech problem, is that right?"

Parent: "We tried to be good parents, we really did . . . but somehow we messed up in helping Peter learn to talk."

Clinician: "You feel a sense of failure, perhaps even guilt, that your child has a speech problem."

> *Client:* "I stutter so badly that life is worthless . . . I can't get a job . . . the business of living just doesn't seem to meet expenses."
>
> *Clinician:* "You feel thwarted and frustrated by your speech problem; sometimes you wonder if you can go on . . ."

Note the clinician's responses carefully. He does not simply repeat the client's comment; he attempts to restate it in clarified form. Observe that the interviewer used the second-person-singular "you" in referring to the client's affect. Feelings are commonly stated first, since they are more important than content. We sometimes add a tag question ("Is that right?") to check on the client's intake of our responses.

How does one handle emotional scenes? They are bound to arise at some point in your interviewing experience. Some clinicians excuse themselves from the room and allow the respondent to recover his dignity alone. Others try to change the subject to something less emotional. Both of these approaches may, with certain clients, give the impression that the clinician is rejecting their feelings. It is more effective to indicate one's understanding of the feelings that are being expressed and accept them as natural human reactions. For example: "That's okay to let it come out, Mrs. Moody; you have been holding it back too long. Sometimes it helps to get it out in the open."

Not all clients seen by the speech clinician will need or even want extensive supportive interviewing. In some cases, the procedures discussed here would be grossly inappropriate. Visualize an interview as ranging along a continuum from affective concern such as feelings and attitudes to objective matters such as goals and advice. Some respondents simply need objective information so that they can do the job; others require considerable support and succor before they can take over and modify their behavior. The clinician's role in some interviews may consist of simply listening to and supporting a client.[5]

IMPROVING INTERVIEWING SKILLS

Hopefully, the material in this chapter will be useful to students majoring in clinical speech pathology and to our colleagues working in various settings. However, no one ever became proficient in interviewing solely by reading about it. It took us many years of constant searching and experimenting to evolve the interviewing approach presented here. And, by the indulgence of our clients and many long-suffering parents, we continue to explore for better ways.

We have included below a series of activities and projects for your own practice. Let them serve as the beginning steps in a continual learning effort toward

---

[5]We quite agree that love alone is not enough in a helping transaction; a good relationship is a *necessary* but not a *sufficient* condition for good interviewing.

improved interviewing. You will find that the time devoted to such training exercises is well spent. Now, consider these steps on how to improve your interviewing skills:

1. Read widely from a variety of sources. We have included a list of selected references to get you started. Find out what people are like by reading in sociology, psychology, anthropology, and philosophy. This is, of course, a lifetime project which we feel is delightful since there is always a new frontier, an open horizon on which we can set our sails. Our profession has arisen so abruptly, grown so rapidly, and been so concerned with the urgent scientific and clinical issues, that it has ignored the important issue—the development of a philosophical basis for our work. A speech-and-hearing clinician without a rationale is like a ship without a rudder. The fundamental and mandatory basis for sound, purposeful therapy is an overall point of view, a workable theory that does not necessarily include the specific activities that will be used to carry it out. Nothing is so pathetic as the clinician who, in a willy-nilly manner, empties a bag of therapeutic homilies on the client's lap, hoping somehow that one of them will work. Only a sequential system of logically interrelated theorems will enable us to evaluate our clinical effectiveness.

2. Listen to all sorts of people, to their dreams, their rationalizations, their insights—or lack of them—and their gripes. Get acquainted with the way common people think and talk, by following the example of Caldwell (1976) and others (Steinbeck, 1967; Walters, 1970; Coleman, 1974; Morris, 1972).

3. Form small heterogeneous groups of majors in speech pathology and audiology. Following the T-group format (a self-directed group with no set rules, which meets in a highly permissive atmosphere for prolonged intervals), conduct some sensitivity training, particularly as it relates to your self-concept, assets and liabilities, your responses to people, and your relationship with your own parents and other older adults (Kaplan and Dryer, 1974). The senior author finds, as a stutterer, that each time he works with parents of children beginning to stutter, he has a distinct tendency to summon up the "ghosts of his stuttering past." He must monitor his behavior by listening to recordings and scrutinizing interviewing protocols. In order to provide assistance to others, we must know our own foibles and potential blind spots and have them under reasonable control. Remember too that the way our academic preparation teaches us to explain a situation will tend to determine the way we perceive it: no one has immaculate perception.

4. Role playing is one of the best methods to prepare for interviewing (Cross, 1974). Set up several typical interview situations in front of a class and play, for example, the roles of the reluctant parent, the spouse of an aphasic patient, or the hostile father. Discuss the interaction, and replay the situations with others assuming the roles. Write out interview purposes prior to the role playing and determine, or have the class determine, how effectively the interviewer accomplished his avowed purposes. Whenever the viewers feel that the interview went wrong or the responses were ineffective, see how many different ways it could have been handled. This builds up the beginning interviewer's repertoire of

adaptive responses. You can do a surprising amount of intrapersonal role playing in your spare time. While we are waiting for a class to begin, for a light to change, or for our mother-in-law to cease talking, we frequently imagine ourselves in various interviewing situations and then explore alternate statements, probes, and so forth. Successful interviewing is largely a matter of attitude (Nideffer, 1976):

> Borrowing from a method of solitary practice devised by successful athletes, we use a simple technique to help students build clear cognitive maps of the clinical encounter. The prospective interviewer first assumes a comfortable posture, and breathes deeply for a few moments to induce a feeling of relaxation. Then, step-by-step, the individual mentally rehearses the interview: he pictures himself successfully orienting the client, encouraging communication by attending and responding in an empathic manner; he tries to visualize the scene as vividly as possible—even to the point of feeling the satisfaction of accomplishing the interview in an easy, efficient manner.

5. Make recordings of your first few interviews, then analyze them carefully with your clinical supervisor or a colleague (Adler and Enelow, 1966; Cannell, Lawson, and Hausser, 1975; Irwin, 1975). We believe that multiple interviewers simply do not work (although seeing multiple interviewees—such as a mother and father at the same time—can be useful and productive); hence, we would suggest that your supervisor not observe your performance in the same room, especially for your first ventures.[6] We have found that when the supervisor stays in the room, the student has a tendency to seduce him into taking over the role of interviewer; and if he refuses to assume the mantle, he can only sit there looking at the clients as if they were bugs in an insect collection. We have no role sanction in our social structure for the silent scrutinizer, and his presence can seriously impair the effectiveness of the interview.

Play back your interview again and again, revising statements, underscoring errors, and scanning for the good parts. Have typed protocols prepared from some of these tapes—the errors really leap out at you from the printed page—and discuss them with your instructors, fellow students, or colleagues. Use the set of questions devised by Stewart and Cash (1974: 201–202) as a guideline for evaluating your performance (See also Project 2 for this Chapter).

Persistent errors, such as stereotyped verbal habits, can be eradicated by using negative practice. One student was required to use his substandard "this here" and "that there" in every third utterance for a month; this procedure (and an extra thick chocolate malted as a reward) succeeded in breaking him of the habit. More substantive problems can be dealt with by using role playing.

We would like to end this chapter with a challenge to the reader. We challenge you to utilize the interviewing approach delineated above, find the

---

[6]In a dyadic interview there are only two possible directions for communication ($1 \times 2 = 2$). When a third party is added it increases the potential interaction to six ($1 \times 2 \times 3 = 6$). Add yet another person and the possibilities for communicative exchange reach unwieldy proportions ($1 \times 2 \times 3 \times 4 = 24$).

errors, the things that just don't work for you, and then develop your own methods. We have given you the foundation blocks; can you use them to create stepping stones?

PROJECTS AND QUESTIONS

1. Expand your awareness of nonverbal communication through the following activities:
   a. In what way does body language reveal deception (Ekman and Friesen, 1972; Baskett and Freedle, 1974)? Prepare a list of twenty questions including informational items ("What is your favorite television show?") and items which evoke stress ("Have you ever cheated on an examination?"). Videotape several persons responding to the questions, using the following procedure: the individuals answer the first ten items truthfully, then they lie in responding to the last ten questions. View the film in class and discuss nonverbal cues associated with deception.
   b. Invade the personal space of several persons in public places (libraries, cafeterias) and record their nonverbal behavior.
   c. Prepare a list of questions alternating between those which call for a cognitive response ("How far is it from Los Angeles to New York?") and those which call for an emotional response ("What sort of things make you feel angry or resentful?"). Interview several persons with the list of questions, noting carefully the direction in which their eyes shift when formulating an answer (Harrison, 1974: 125).
2. Devise a checklist of specific behaviors which are basic ingredients of a diagnostic interview. Table 2-1 is a form prepared by members of a graduate class (based on the work of Ivey, 1971). See if you can improve upon it. Note: do not expect beginning interviewers to remember, let alone exhibit, all the skills delineated on the checklist; have them practice on only a few at a time, and provide constructive feedback on their performance.

Table 2-1   Checklist of Interviewing Competencies

  I. *Orienting the respondent*
     A. Attends to comfort
     B. Engages in appropriate flow talk
     C. Explains purposes, procedures
     D. Structures roles
 II. *Engendering Communication*
     A. Attending behavior
        1. relaxed, natural posture
        2. appropriate eye contact
        3. responses which follow the client's comments
     B. Open invitation to share (open-end questions)
     C. Non-distracting encouragement to continue talking
        1. verbal ("Yes," "I see," etc.)
        2. nonverbal (nodding, shifting posture toward client)
III. *Use of questions and recording*
     A. Orderly, sequential questions
     B. Non-distracting note taking

IV. *Active listening*
    A. Reflects feelings
        1. matches affect
        2. matches content
    B. Periodic summarizing of affective and content messages
V. *Monitoring nonverbal clues*
    A. The diagnosticians
    B. The respondents
VI. *Skills in presenting information*
    A. Transmission of information
        1. content
        2. style and language
    B. Appropriate use of humor, flow talk
VII. *Closing the interview*
    A. Summary, review of findings
    B. Recommendations
    C. Supportive comments
VIII. *Analysis of the Information*
    A. Major themes in the client's presentation; association of ideas; inconsistencies and omissions.

3. Explore the use of humor as an interviewing tool (Rosenheim, 1974).
4. Make an analysis of systems for cataloging responses given to statements made by interviewees (Harris, 1967; Johnson, 1972; Bales, 1953).

BIBLIOGRAPHY

ADLER, L., and A. ENELOW (1966). "An Instrument to Measure Skill in Diagnostic Interviewing: a Teaching and Evaluation Tool." *Journal of Medical Education*, 41: 281–288.

ARGYLE, M., and M. COOK (1976). *Gaze and Mutual Gaze*. London: Cambridge University Press.

BALES, R. (1953). "The Equilibrium Problem in Small Groups." In *Working Papers in Theory and Action*, eds. T. Parsons, R. Bales, and E. Shils. New York: Free Press.

BANAKA, W. (1971). *Training in Depth Interviewing*. New York: Harper & Row.

BASKETT, G., and R. FREEDLE (1974). "Aspects of Language Pragmatics and the Social Perception of Lying." *Journal of Psycholinguistic Research*, 3: 117–131.

BASSETT, G. (1965). *Practical Interviewing*. New York: American Management Association.

BENJAMIN, A. (1974). *The Helping Interview*. 2nd ed. Boston: Houghton Mifflin Company.

BENNY, M.; D. REISMAN; and S. STAR (1956). "Age and Sex in the Interview." *American Journal of Sociology*, 62: 143–152.

BERMOSK, L., and M. MORDAN (1964). *Interviewing in Nursing*. New York: Macmillan.

BIRDWHISTLE, R. (1970). *Kinesics and Context*. Philadelphia: University of Pennsylvania Press.

BINGHAM, W., and B. MOORE (1959). *How to Interview*, 4th ed. New York: Harper & Row.

BOSMAJIAN, H., ed. (1971). *The Rhetoric of Nonverbal Communication*. Glenview, Illinois: Scott-Foresman Company.

BUGENTAL, J. (1954). "Explicit Analysis: A Design for the Study and Improvement of Psychological Interviewing." *Educational and Psychological Measurement*, 14: 552–565.

BUSCAGLIA, L. (1975). *The Disabled and Their Parents: A Counseling Challenge*. Thorofare, N.J.: Charles B. Slack.

CALDWELL, E. (1976). *Afternoons in Mid-America*. New York: Dodd, Mead & Co.

CANNELL, C.; S. LAWSON; and D. HAUSSER (1975). *A Technique for Evaluating Interviewer Performance*. Ann Arbor, Michigan: Institute for Social Research.

CAPLOW, T. (1956). "The Dynamics of Information Interviewing." *American Journal of Sociology*, 62: 165–171.

CARKHUFF, R., and B. BERENSON (1967). *Beyound Counseling and Therapy*. New York: Holt, Rinehart & Winston.

COLEMAN, R. (1974). *Blue-Collar Journal: A College President's Sabbatical*. New York: Lippincott.

COUCH, A., and K. KENISTEM (1960). "Yeasayers and Naysayers." *Journal of Abnormal and Social Psychology*, 60: 151–174.

CROSS, C., ed. (1974). *Interviewing and Communication in Social Work*. London: Routledge & Paul.

CZIKSZENTMYHALYI, M. (1975). *Beyond Boredom and Anxiety*. San Francisco: Jossey-Bass.

DAVIS, J. (1971). *The Interview as Arena*. Stanford, Calif.: Stanford University Press.

DEUTCH, F., and W. MURPHY (1955). *The Clinical Interview*. New York: International Universities Press.

DEXTER, L. (1956). "Role Relationships and Conceptions of Neutrality in Interviewing." *American Journal of Sociology*, 62: 153–157.

——— (1970). *Elite and Specialized Interviewing*. Evanston, Illinois: Northwestern University Press.

EDINBURG, G. (1975). *Clinical Interviewing and Counseling: Principles and Techniques*. New York: Appleton-Century-Crofts.

EGOLF, D., and S. CHESTER (1973). "Nonverbal Communication and the Disorders of Speech and Language." *Journal of American Speech and Hearing Association*, 15: 511–518.

EISENBERG, A., and R. SMITH (1971). *Nonverbal Communication*. New York: Bobbs-Merrill.

EKMAN, P., and W. FRIESEN (1972). "Hand Movements." *Journal of Communication*, 22: 353–374.

ENELOW, A., and S. SWISHER (1972). *Interviewing and Patient Care*. New York: Oxford University Press.

FEAR, R. (1973). *The Evaluation Interview*. New York: McGraw-Hill.

FELDMAN, S. (1973). *Mannerisms of Speech and Gestures in Everyday Life*. New York: International University Press.

FENLASON, A. (1952). *Essentials in Interviewing*. New York: Harper & Row.

GARRETT, A. (1942). *Interviewing: Its Principles and Methods*. New York: Family Service Association.

GINOTT, H. (1965). *Between Parent and Child*. New York: Macmillan.

GOFFMAN, E. (1959). *The Presentation of Self in Everyday Life*. Garden City, N.Y.: Doubleday & Co.

——— (1963). *Stigma: Notes on the Management of Spoiled Identity*. Englewood Cliffs, N.J.: Prentice-Hall, Inc.

GORDON, R. (1956). "Dimensions of the Depth Interview." *American Journal of Sociology*, 62: 158–164.

——— (1969). *Interviewing: Strategy, Techniques and Tactics*. Homewood, Illinois: Dorsey Press.

GORDON, T. (1970). *Parent Effectiveness Training*. New York: Peter H. Wyden, Inc.

HARRIS, T. (1967). *I'm OK—You're OK*. New York: Harper & Row.

HARRISON, R. (1974). *Beyond Words: An Introduction to Nonverbal Communication*. Englewood Cliffs, N.J.: Prentice-Hall, Inc.

HINDE, R. (1972). *Nonverbal Communication*. New York: Cambridge University Press.

IRWIN, R.B. (1965). *Speech and Hearing Therapy*. Pittsburgh: Stanwix.

———— (1975). "Micro-counseling Interviewing Skills of Supervisors of Speech Clinicians." *Human Communication*, 4: 5–9.

IVEY, A. (1971). *Microcounseling: Innovations in Interviewing Training*. Springfield, Illinois: C.C. Thomas.

JOHNSON, D. (1972). *Reaching Out*. Englewood Cliffs, N.J.: Prentice-Hall, Inc.

KADUSHIN, A. (1972). *The Social Work Interview*. New York: Columbia University Press.

KAHN, R., and C. CANNELL (1959). *The Dynamics of Interviewing*. New York: John Wiley & Sons, Inc.

KAPLAN, N., and D. DREYER (1974). "The Effect of Self-awareness Training on Student Speech Pathologist-Client Relationships." *Journal of Communication Disorders*, 7: 329–342.

KNAPP, M. (1972). *Nonverbal Communication in Human Interaction*. New York: Holt, Rinehart & Winston.

LANGDON, G., and I. STOUT (1954). *Teacher-Parent Interviews*. Englewood Cliffs, N.J.: Prentice-Hall, Inc.

LONGHURST, T., and G. SIEGEL (1973). "Effects of Communication Failure on Speaker and Listener Behavior." *Journal of Speech and Hearing Research*, 16: 128–140.

MARSHALL, N., and S. GOLDSTEIN (1969). "Imparting Diagnostic Information to Mothers: A Comparison of Methodologies." *Journal of Speech and Hearing Research*, 12: 65–72.

MARTIN, A. (1977). "Post-diagnostic Parent Counseling by a Speech Pathologist and a Social Worker." *Journal of American Speech and Hearing Association*, 19: 67–68.

MATARAZZO, J. (1965). "The Interview" in *Handbook of Clinical Psychology*, ed. B. Wolman. New York: McGraw-Hill.

————, and A. WIENS (1972). *The Interview: Research on its Anatomy and Structure*. Chicago: Aldine-Atherton.

McDONALD, E. (1962). *Understand Those Feelings*. Pittsburgh: Stanwix.

McQUIRE, M., and S. LORCH (1968). "A Model for the Study of Dyadic Communication." *Journal of Nervous and Mental Disease*, 146: 221–229.

MEHRABIAN, A. (1972). *Nonverbal Communication*. Chicago: Aldine-Atherton.

MORGAN, H., and J. COGGER (1973). *The Interviewers Manual*. New York: The Psychological Corporation.

MORRIS, T. (1972). *The Walk of the Conscious Ants*. New York: Alfred A. Knopf.

MORSBACH, H. (1973). "Aspects of Nonverbal Communication in Japan." *Journal of Nervous and Mental Disorders*, 157: 262–277.

NIDEFFER, R. (1976). *The Inner Athlete*. New York: Crowell Company.

PAYNE, S. (1951). *The Art of Asking Questions*. Princeton, N.J.: Princeton University Press.

PRATT, L.; A. SELIGMAN; and G. READER (1958). "Physicians' Views on the Medical Information Among Patients," in *Patients, Physicians and Illness*, ed. E. Jaco. New York: The Free Press.

RICH, J. (1968). *Interviewing Children and Adolescents*. New York: Macmillan.

RICHARDSON, S.; B. DOHRENWEND; and D. KLEIN (1965). *Interviewing: Its Forms and Functions*. New York: Basic Books, Inc.

ROSENHEIM, E. (1974). "Humor in Psychotherapy: an Interactive Experience." *American Journal of Psychotherapy*, 28, 584–591.

ROSENTHAL, R., et al. (1974). "Body Talk and the Tone of Voice: The Language Without Words." *Psychology Today,* 8: 64–68.

SCHEFLEN, A. (1972). *Body Language and Social Order.* Englewood Cliffs, N.J.: Prentice-Hall, Inc.

SIEGMAN, A., and B. POPE eds. (1972). *Studies in Dyadic Communication.* New York: Pergamon Press.

SHOUKSMITH, G. (1968). *Assessment Through Interviewing: A Handbook for Individual Interviewing and Group Selection Techniques.* New York: Pergamon Press.

SPIEGEL, J., and P. MACHOTKA (1974). *Messages of the Body.* New York: The Free Press.

STAPLES, F., and R. SLOANE (1976). "Truax Factors, Speech Characteristics and Therapy Outcome." *Journal of Nervous and Mental Disorders,* 163: 135–140.

STEINBECK, J. (1961). *Travels with Charley.* New York: Viking Press.

STEWART, C., and W. CASH (1974). *Interviewing: Principles and Practices.* Dubuque, Iowa: William C. Brown.

SOMMERS, R. (1969). *Personal Space.* Englewood Cliffs, N.J.: Prentice-Hall, Inc.

WALTERS, B. (1970). *How to Talk with Practically Anybody About Practically Anything.* Garden City, N.Y.: Doubleday & Co.

WEITZ, S., ed. (1974). *Nonverbal Communication: Readings with Commentary.* New York: Oxford University Press.

WILSON, D.; H. GINOTT; and S. BERGER (1959). "Group Interview: Initial Parent Contact." *Journal of Speech and Hearing Disorders,* 24: 282–284.

WOOLF, G. (1971). "Informational Specificity: A Correlate of Verbal Output in Diagnostic Interview." *Journal of Speech and Hearing Disorders,* 36: 518–526.

3

The
Clinical Examination

Some types of information can be obtained only through direct scrutiny of the client—by testing, measuring and examining. The interview provides us with a view of the presenting problem as the client or his parents perceive it; it also allows the clinician to observe the client's behavior and formulate hypotheses which can then be evaluated in a more structured form of interaction. In this chapter we present an overview of the clinical examination, a procedure for inspecting and testing the impressions generated during the intake interview.

The overall purpose of the clinical examination is to assemble sufficient information to provide a working image of the client. More specifically, the clinical examination is guided by the following interrelated purposes:

1. To describe the problem—what are the dimensions of the communicative disturbance with respect to voice, fluency, language and articulation?
2. To estimate its severity—how large a problem is it?
3. To identify factors that are related to the problem—what are the antecedents and consequences of it?
4. To estimate prospects for improvement—what estimate can we make of the extent of possible recovery and the time frame of treatment?
5. To derive a plan of treatment—what are the specific targets for therapy and how can the client best be approached?

Thus, we are concerned with the systematic collection, organization, and interpretation of information regarding an individual and his particular communication disorder. All of this activity is carried out to provide a basis for predicting the outcome of treatment and to guide the nature and scope of the therapeutic regimen.[1]

ASPECTS OF THE CLINICAL EXAMINATION

There are several important aspects of the clinical examination with which the beginning clinician should be acquainted. We have selected the most salient factors for discussion; all are potential pitfalls for the unwary.

The Interpersonal Context

We see three major constituents in any clinical transaction: interpersonal dynamics, the sequence of goals, and the activities (see Figure 3.1). The most crucial factor in conducting a successful diagnostic session is the client-clinician relationship. When a person works with another, there is always human impact; even when clients are treated by computers, they come to accord human attributes to the machines. No matter how well prepared and rehearsed an examiner may be, if his approach to people is poor, he is bound to experience failure. All tests, all examinations, all so-called objective diagnostic procedures are mediated by person-to-person contact (Emerick and Hood, 1974).

We can be seduced into grave errors by test norms, percentile scores, and standard examination procedures: man is a total functioning unit and the various tests are multiple and fragmented. The instruments we use are relatively precise, and we are often deluded into thinking that the patient is functioning with the same degree of precision in the testing situation. But human elements may disturb the validity of the tests no matter how refined the scoring procedures or how calibrated the machines.

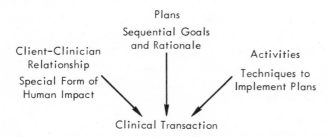

Figure 3.1 Basic constituents of the clinical transaction.

[1]Repeated testing during therapy will also enable the clinician to judge the efficacy of the plan of treatment. Moreover, testing may be helpful for appropriate placement in group therapy. Finally, some speech pathologists urge more extensive testing of each client in order to provide additional scientific information on the various communication impairments.

Impersonal, test-oriented clinical examination sessions can also make treatment more difficult since there is no absolute division between diagnosis and therapy. The first contact with a client initiates treatment. During a diagnostic session he is forming opinions and conceptions about the clinician and the total clinical situation. Barker and his colleagues (1953: 310) have warned that "while to the medical practitioner, diagnosis and therapy are often routine technical jobs, to the patient the situation never has such limited personal meaning. To him diagnosis and therapy are a route to highly important life conditions."

Not all clients will require the full impact of this interpersonal dimension. Indeed, some individuals simply want to find out what is wrong and then rectify the situation. The point is, however, that the clinician should be able to discern what the client needs and then adjust his style appropriately.

Age factors. Although all age levels present unique diagnostic problems, three groups in particular—young children, adolescents, and to a lesser extent, older or aged clients—require special effort and expertise.

YOUNG CHILDREN. Preschool (and kindergarten) children are often difficult to test and examine. Unlike most older children and adults, they just don't see the payoff for all the questioning and prodding. The main problem is dealing with the child's fear of the clinical situation. This apprehension may stem from one or more of the following related factors: (1) Inadequate preparation for the examination, which produces, (2) uncertainty as to what will be done to or with him by the clinician, (3) vivid memories of trauma during visits to dentists and physicians, (4) the contagious anxieties and uncertainties experienced by the parents, and (5) stress and conflicts engendered by past listener reactions to the speech impairment. Children confront the speech examination in a variety of ways, but the two most trying responses are shyness and withdrawal and, at the other extreme, aggressiveness and hyperactivity.

The shy ones are the most difficult to deal with clinically because there is no output—no speech or language to evaluate. The lack of response per se is behavior, too, however, and has meaning we must judge; the child is always telling us something even when he isn't talking. If he cannot or will not respond to our attempts to discern his capabilities, we have to employ special procedures to get him involved with the tasks. It is fascinating to witness how our students and colleagues attempt to deal with the reticent child:

> The impulse is to swarm the child's defenses with instant rapport, superficial bonhomie, or glib reassurance that everything is going to be all right. But youngsters don't want to be overwhelmed any more than adults do. One clinician, who claims to be able to obtain all manner of information from shy children, swoops down upon a youngster, holds him on her lap, fondles him, and chatters incessantly, repeating questions over and over at close range. Emerging from these somewhat explosive sessions, she is able to detail behavioral responses that equally competent clinicians cannot confirm. We finally discovered how she does it when we videotaped her

during a diagnostic session. She is simply receiving her own stimuli as reflected by the bewildered child and is mistaking these images for the youngster's responses. She is literally answering her own questions; small wonder she confirms her own predictions.

Most clinicians advocate a low key, easy-does-it approach with shy children, who must see that the diagnostician is not a threat and can be trusted. But that does not mean adopting a coy, childlike demeanor:

> One speech pathologist of our acquaintance adopts a vocal pitch at least a half octave above his normal pitch level and correspondingly childish inflections and immature motor behavior when he works with preschoolers. It was sometimes difficult to tell who was the client, and even the children seemed annoyed, bemused, or embarrassed by this cloying cuteness.

How *do* you get a small child to talk? Questioning is a common procedure but we must agree with Van Riper:

> Questions are demands. They immediately place the child in a subservient role, with the questioner in the position of power. Even when the child responds appropriately, the resulting relationship is one which immediately puts the questioner into the same category with other authority figures who have been controllers, a relationship which often regenerates the conflicts the child has previously experienced in threatening communication. If you ask what something is called and the child cooperates, he must either think that you must be stupid not to know its name or that you suspect he doesn't know it (which implies stupidity), or that you must want him to do a little verbal dance for your pleasure. . . . Moreover, the eliciting of speech by questions often yields very impoverished samples. At best, you'll get just a vocabulary item, not a good speech sample. Or, if you ask him a yes-no question, you'll get a yes or no answer, often the latter. Like a marriage, we do not feel that a therapeutic relationship should start with an invitation to say no. If the question is more elaborate ("What did you have for breakfast this morning?" "What did you do in school today?") the child has probably forgotten or finds it difficult to formulate, or feels that it is none of your business, anyway. Especially with children for whom the acquisition of speech has been no easy accomplishment, any question tends to pose some threat. They have been bedevilled by too many questions from too many questioners and, when they have answered, their listeners have not always understood them or have rejected them. For these children, the interrogative inflection is almost as potent a signal as the tone that makes the rat jump in expectation of shock.[2]

Eschewing questions, then, we recommend a simply play activity—a box of common farm animals or a doll house with miniature furniture is excellent—and the use of *self-* and *parallel-talk*.

> How then should one begin? We suggest that you should simply greet the child, then do some simple self-talk, commenting on what you are doing, or perceiving, and with plenty of moments of comfortable silence interspersed, until you have him playing with his box of toys. And then, in the role of the adult playmate, you can play with those in your own box—silently at first. No questions. No demands. *Solo play!*

---

[2]Charles Van Riper, *Speech Correction: Principles and Methods,* 5th ed. © 1972, pp. 108–110. Reprinted by permission of Prentice-Hall, Inc., Englewood Cliffs, N.J.

Once the child is comfortable in this activity, you should begin to put some self-talk into your own solo play; first noises (those of trucks, animals, etc.), then single words, then short phrases and simple sentences. All of these refer to what you are experiencing at the moment. Usually the child will begin to follow suit. His noises and his self-talk begin to flow. Next you should shift to contact play very gradually. Let your toy truck occasionally touch his fire engine, or help him find a block, or put another one on his toppling pile, or straighten it up a bit so he can make it higher. When you feel the time is ripe in this *tangential contact play,* begin to accompany it with some noises or commentary, using *parallel talk,* telling him what he is doing, perceiving, or feeling, again making sure you have more silence than speech. From tangential play, you can often proceed rapidly to *intersecting play* in which your activity becomes a part of his. (Let your truck go over the bridge he has built or feed your doll or toy dog a piece of the play fruit he has put on the play-house table). Verbalize what you are doing. Next seek to achieve *cooperative play,* assisting him in what he is doing. (Have your truck bring him the blocks he needs to build his tower.) Usually by this time, the child is speaking very easily and often copiously, your own verbalizations primarily confined to reflecting what he has said. From this point onward, the communication can proceed fairly normally and naturally. We hope we have not given the impression that this process is too time-consuming. Often we can accomplish all the progressive interaction in a single session and build a very warm communicative relationship in less than an hour. There are, of course, many children for whom such a careful approach may not be vitally necessary, children who have learned that big people always seem to have to ask stupid questions, children who are willing to dance when the interrogative strings are pulled, children who relate easily. Yet even with these children this approach seems to work very well. The relationship established is less superficial, more satisfying. We do not meet with as many moments of resistance or negativism later on in therapy (Van Riper, 1972: 108–110).

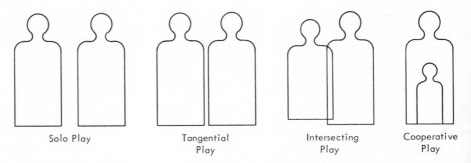

| Solo Play | Tangential Play | Intersecting Play | Cooperative Play |

Figure 3.2 Diagram of Interaction Between Clinician and Child (Van Riper, 1972: 109). Reprinted with permission.

But what do you do with the aggressive, active ones, the children who cannot or will not sit still, who demand to structure the situation in the way they desire? First, and most important, the clinician must retain control of the situation. He does this, basically, by defining the limits for the child and by a firm, but accepting manner. The child must see clearly that he cannot test the examiner, that the examiner is not threatened and has no intention of acquiescing. We do not mean a rigid intransigence, for it is often desirable to alter the testing situation to fit the child. To be sure, much of the behavior manifested by these children is for testing the limits of the situation; they want to know the rules of the game before they will cooperate. On some occasions, with a highly distractible child, we have had to reduce the stimuli in the room; we may have the child sit facing a plain wall, draw the window shade, and keep all test materials out of sight until used. We have even turned off lights in a room to force the child to focus on us. In a few instances we have found it necessary to take the child out of the testing situation and go for a walk before returning to the clinical tasks:

> Tim migrated restlessly from the window to the door of the examining room, whining belligerently. When an item was presented to him, he either threw it away or ignored it. We then took the child for a walk about the clinic; we looked into each room while carrying on a running commentary about what was going on. Then Tim was able to return to the examining room and was content to move through the various tasks we had planned.

With a few genuinely hyperkinetic children we have resorted to mild physical restraint, generally holding them close to us (Baxley and LeBlanc, 1976). They seemed to need and actually like external controls on their flighty behavior that they could not control from within. Although we don't recommend the procedure, we know one highly successful clinical audiologist who, when confronted with a recalcitrant child, firmly squeezes the youngster's trapezius muscle as he guides him toward the examining booth.

Second, don't plead or cajole the obstreperous child. If he ducks beneath the table and announces he will not cooperate, we go ahead with the various tasks, using self-talk. Don't reinforce crying or whining by soothing or placating. It is, however, a good practice to distract the child with some interesting task and then praise his attentiveness (Hubbell, 1977).

There are obviously many other considerations that could be discussed; additional suggestions will be offered in the several chapters concerning various disorders. But for the present, here are several basic precepts on the management of children in a clinical examination:

1. Help the parents prepare the child for the diagnostic session. It is a good idea to call prior to the date of the examination and provide the parents with information about the experience. Suggest that they tell the child he will be going to a special school where he will look at pictures and play games of various sorts. If the parents report that their child is particularly shy, ask them to bring along his favorite toy or stuffed animal.

2. Play, rather than talk, is the natural medium of expression for children. Try to arrange the diagnostic tasks with this in mind.

3. As a general rule, ask less and observe more (Rowen, 1973). Children usually lack the insight and cooperation necessary to analyze their problem rationally and objectively.

4. The prospective diagnostician should learn everything possible about normal children in order to provide a baseline for observations of youngsters presenting problems (Blumenfeld, Thompson and Vogel, 1971; Dreikurs, 1972; Perske, 1973;

Knobloch and Pasamanick, 1974). This can be done by taking courses, studying relevant norms, but most of all by extensive scrutiny of children in nursery schools and other settings. The prospective diagnostician should have a good idea of the typical or modal behavior for children at various age levels. One student claimed that a four-year-old client was in grave need of psychiatric appraisal and treatment. We remembered the child and were somewhat puzzled by this recommendation. We demanded a rationale. It seems that the child had an imaginary companion, a wrinkled green elephant that served as a scapegoat and alter ego. We chuckled and then sent the student scurrying to the Gesell profiles to see how common such fantasies are in four-year-olds.

5. Limit the choices you offer a child. Don't ask if he would like to go with you, do this or that, unless the alternatives do not conflict with the examiner's goals. He will invariably say "no" and you will be left with egg on your face.

6. Be flexible in your use of tests and examinations. If you cannot employ the rigid standardized format for administration, use the test to obtain all the data you can. If the child refuses to name the pictures and objects, you might be able to get a language sample from the items he has in his pockets.

7. Absolute honesty and candor is important in working with children. Don't make promises unless you can keep them. Children function better knowing the truth than they do with mystery, dread, or uncertainty.

8. Children relate very well to animals, and the clinician might consider having a hamster, rabbit, or an affectionate dog in the examining room. Puppets—or better, muppets from Sesame Street—are also very useful in establishing a relationship with a young child (Dodson, 1970).

9. The whole assessment does not have to be done in one session; marathon diagnostics tend to be counterproductive. Remember that all we can hope to obtain in one time frame is a sample of a child's behaviors. It is better to terminate (if possible, on a light, pleasant note) than to continue an unproductive session.

10. You should keep in mind that parents are people, too, not just vehicles to assist diagnosis or carry out therapy (Buscaglia, 1975).

ADOLESCENTS. Experienced clinicians frequently report that adolescents— the classical teenagers, especially in grades 7 through 11—are often difficult to examine and resistant to therapy. The main problem seems to be getting through to the person. There is no magic formula for this, but we would like to make some suggestions that we have found helpful in guiding our work with adolescent clients:

1. Acquire an understanding of the myriad of pressures and changes the teen is experiencing: rapid physical growth, sexual maturity, conflicts between dependence and independence, the development of self-confidence and interpersonal skills necessary to make decisions, definition of a new ego-ideal, a search for identity and life work, intense group loyalty and identification, and many more. It is a turbulent, trying period of behavioral extravagance and excess (Ginott, 1969; Ohlsen, 1974). Small wonder that teenagers are often overloaded with personal concerns and do not always welcome an overture of clinical assistance. Empathy that flows from understanding is a powerful force in establishing a working relationship.

2. There is an intense desire to be like others, not to stand out from the group in any way that would suggest frailty. Hence the adolescent will find it extremely difficult to

reveal a speech impairment, even if he does want help. Often he is simply *sent* to treatment. In some instances, the teenager with a chronic problem may have been in therapy for a long time and is weary of continued treatment. He will tend to cover up his true feelings with a sullen bravado or a dense "it-doesn't-bother-me" shell. Denial is his particular forte. "Coolness" and image are very important. You can neither beat this down nor simply dismiss the individual with a shrug. Nor is silence a particularly effective tool in dealing with adolescent resistance. We advocate a straightforward approach: acknowledge the forces that are bearing on the individual; point up objectively the paths that others have taken; provide information about the economic and social penalties that accrue to the speech-defective person (have him talk to older clients). The young client may need more time to become accustomed to the idea of therapy. Basically, try to demonstrate by your demeanor and what you say that you care about him: a growing ego needs lots of nourishment; personal involvement and commitment are key factors.

3. Don't try to "swing" with teenage clients; empathy is not identification. Don't abandon your professional role for that of a teenager. Be yourself. As Will Rogers pointed out, if they don't like you the way you are, they are sure not going to like you the way you are trying to be:

> One public-school clinician had a painful experience in learning to maintain her role and status as adult therapist. While waiting one day for a fourth member of a therapy group to arrive, she attempted to enter a rap session with three teenage males. She wanted to know the meanings of several "in" words, but the boys demurred and looked rather curiously at her. She responded by saying, "Look, teenagers want to know all about the adult world, right? So, turnabout is fair play, why shouldn't I learn about yours?" One of the bolder adolescents suggested that they were becoming adults and thus they needed to know—but was the clinician going to be a teen?

4. Approach adolescents with tolerance and good humor. Don't be shocked or annoyed by their overstatements and superlatives; don't over-react to expressions of hostility or tempests of other emotions. Sometimes they will, in order to uphold their protective armor, resort to all sorts of strategies to confuse, defeat, or anger the clinician. The ability to laugh at yourself and to use humor in a gentle, needling manner is an asset. Remember, though, to always treat the adolescent with dignity—don't make fun of his intense and idealistic views. Young people typically are hopeful that they can change the world for the better: how could you use this trait in treatment?

5. Talk person-to-person, not station-to-station (Ginott, 1969). Respond to the *individual*, not to the *group* of which he is a member. Try to describe rather than judge. Avoid commenting about long hair, (sometimes outrageous) costumes, slouching posture, and so forth.

6. Demonstrate your competence and confidence to deal with the person and his problem. We like to do this by explaining what we are about, the reasons for the various tests and examinations, how we will use the information, and the process of checking out our hypotheses. However, don't be a know-it-all or talk about the obvious in the voice of adult mystery. We encourage the adolescent to challenge and question what we are doing. Finally, we usually give him an idea of the route we would follow when therapy commences; we enumerate the steps and even do some trial therapy.

7. Avoid the teacher image as much as you can. Unfortunately, many of our schools are more concerned with keeping order than with learning or with human relationships. Teacher is always right in some schools. We eschew this image by our style of

interaction, by keeping the person's confidences, by listening to him when he complains about a teacher or a course. We don't enter into the criticism or side with the client against the school, nor do we try to defend the institution or retreat to moralisms.

8. When praise is offered, make it specific rather than general. Tell him that you like how he persisted on a particular diagnostic task rather than simply saying he is a good worker.

9. Discuss the results of the evaluation with the client before talking with the parents or school personnel. Be sure to let him know exactly what you intend to tell his parents and teachers (we sometimes make audio tapes of parents conferences so the teenage client can check on our veracity).

These recommendations have been distilled from our clinical experience and are not presented as magical touchstones for all diagnosticians or all clients; nor do they represent the full range of possibilities for successful interaction with teenage clients. We present them here to provoke other workers to develop clinical generalizations on the basis of their experience.

OLDER OR AGED CLIENTS. Older clients present some rather special problems for the diagnostician. Although the concept of "aged" is relative, we refer here to persons in their sixties or older. The clinician should be alert to fatigue, disorientation, failing eyesight, and hearing loss. With advanced age, the person may find it more difficult to focus his attention on a task, and he generally has trouble remembering directions because of short-term memory decline. We need, therefore, to explain each step of our clinical procedures at greater length and repeat instructions several times to insure understanding. Our pace should be geared down, if necessary, to the client's slower level. Organize the testing sequence carefully to reduce distractions, noise or interference. Older people are more cautious and have a greater need to be certain before they respond, so adapt the tasks with this in mind; following standard procedure may not be as important as providing an environment in which the person is able to perform at his optimum level. Since many older clients tend to feel useless and discarded in our youth-oriented culture, and resentful that their bodies are betraying them, we may find it important to spend some time listening to their memories of past achievements.

As with children and adolescents, the diagnostician should know as much as possible about aging (see Project 4). Further, the clinician should recognize and have under control his own ambivalence toward growing old. Let us state it more forcefully: the number of people over sixty-five comprises a significant proportion of the population and we can not afford to perpetuate the stereotype that old people are expendable, that they should be relegated to a demeaning idleness (Comfort, 1976). Finally, it is absolutely imperative that a multiprofessional approach be employed in rendering services to older clients (Leutenegger, 1975).

The factor of sex. In what manner does the sex of the diagnostician influence the clinical examination and testing situation? Do young children relate better to female clinicians? Do adolescent boys feel more comfortable, and hence more able to reveal information about themselves, with male diagnosticians? We know of no scientific basis on which we can answer these questions, and no doubt it is often a highly individual matter. However, in our own practice, in the supervision of student clinicians and extensive consultation with colleagues working in various settings, we have observed several principles at work:

1. Female clients of all ages, with the possible exception of adolescents, seem to experience little difficulty with a male diagnostician. This might be the product of countless experiences with male dentists and physicians.

2. Adolescent females, girls in the process of becoming women physically and psychologically, seem to be more comfortable and open with a female clinician; likewise male adolescents seem to work better with male clinicians.

3. Female clinicians of college age sometimes find it difficult to maintain a clinical context when performing diagnostic examinations on men of the same age level. College-level male clinicians may experience some of the same difficulties in diagnosis with female students.

Obviously, the factors of age and sex are interrelated in a complex manner in the clinical relationship. We do know that the interpersonal context does influence the *kinds* of responses clients will give to various tasks; it also may influence the *amount* and *style* of response. Men talking together assume a rather distinct verbal style (the "locker room" set) as do women (the "bridge club" set). Since the clinician can do little about his or her sex at this point, he should inspect his value systems to see that this particular facet does not become obtrusive in the clinical setting.

The work setting. Ideally the speech clinician performs his professional role as he has been trained to do, regardless of where he works. However, diagnosticians working in schools often report several difficulties: (1) The speech clinician is identified in the child's mind with the teachers, some of whom may be penalizing or disturbing listeners. In addition, the clinician may find himself identified with authority figures, and this hampers the development of a clinical relationship. (2) The type of diagnostic regimen best suited for the client may be difficult to implement within the school. (3) The child usually has no choice about entering the examining situation; he is brought for diagnosis by his parents, referred by a teacher, or is "screened out" by the speech clinician. (4) It seems more difficult to secure active parental participation when children are seen in school. Some parents are suspicious of the authority which a school represents; they may harbor resentment for alleged bad treatment when they attended school. Inherent in this is the natural resistance manifested by many persons toward official institutions of government. The clinician may find that he has been tarred by the same brush, and may be unable to obtain the cooperation of some parents.

Some clinicians, however, give up too easily; with a resigned shrug, they suggest that it is impossible to do careful, thorough diagnostics in the schools with the heavy caseload requirements. But *the nature of the child's problem, not the characteristics of the work setting*, dictates the nature of the clinician's responsibility. The needs of the client, not the arbitrary and often antiquated state codes or educational policies of the school, should and must determine the scope of the speech clinician's professional activities. To be accorded professional treatment, one must behave as a professional. The hallmark of professionalism is doing what needs to be done for the good of the client. A clinician's responsibilities do not end when the last school bell rings.

The ideal (seldom achieved) setting for conducting an evaluation is, most importantly, physically and psychologically comfortable. Many examining facilities we have seen unfortunately reflect an austere, clinical aura—banks of fluorescent lights, large mirrors, microphones, videotape cameras, sterile decor. In our experience, rooms which are furnished with soft chairs, end tables, table lamps, and are tastefully decorated create a zone of comfort and safety; thus, they are conducive to self-revelation and exploration. The rooms should be free of distractions—noise, clutter, intrusions, and the diagnostic facility should provide an efficient working space for the clinician.

We have attempted to show how three factors—age, sex, and work setting—influence the clinical examination. There no doubt are many other conditions which also impinge: the timing of the diagnostic examination should coincide with the individual's readiness for help; the manner of referral; and idiosyncratic aspects such as the motives and fantasies of some clients. Additional comments will be presented in the discussion below dealing with test selection.

THE SELECTION OF TESTS

There are many diagnostic instruments to assess all aspects of a client and his communication abilities. Thus, it becomes a matter of critical selection among the diverse tests available. What factors are employed in making a selection? In addition to such obvious criteria as the purposes of the evaluation, the amount of time available, the nature of the client's presenting problem, the client's age and level of intelligence, the constraints of the setting, and the diagnostician's training, the following factors should be considered:

1. Does the test provide information that cannot be obtained by interviewing or by less structured observation? All diagnostic instruments cause a certain amount of stress to the client; if it is feasible within reasonable time limits to obtain data by indirect means, then the clinician should be wary of using the test. We find that observation of ongoing behavior affords us a better idea of a child's typical behavior (what he usually does) than do many formal tests that assess abilities (what he can do in maximum performance). It must be stressed, however, that both observation and test information are hypothetical constructs which provide only samples of the client's total repertoire.

2. Is it possible to convey the instructions without lengthy and complicated explana-

tions? The more intricate the introduction to a task, the greater the possibility that a client's errors in performance are an artifact of the instructions.

3. Is the test relatively easy to administer and score? Some diagnostic instruments are so complicated that unless used daily, the clinician may forget how to administer them. Complexity in a diagnostic tool does not necessarily correlate with precision or validity. Further, it is important to keep in mind the purpose of testing: beyond a certain point, precision is meaningless and clinically irrelevant.

4. Is the test economical in terms of the client's time and energy? Is it efficient? How much time does it consume relative to the quality and quantity of data obtained?

5. Are the theoretical constructs upon which the test is constructed congruent with the examiner's beliefs? It is difficult to use an instrument clinically unless the examiner is convinced of its explanatory adequacy.

6. Does the test permit objective scoring? Although the important decisions, clinically as well as scientifically, are judgmental, the basis for making the judgments is sounder to the degree that human bias is at least identified and, hopefully, limited (Weiner and Hoock, 1973). Is the test standardized—are the procedures and materials fixed so that, regardless of where or by whom a client is evaluated, the same methodology can be employed?

7. Will the test actually make a difference in solving the person's problem? Is it practical in the sense that the results lead logically to a program of treatment?

8. Does the test suggest to the client that he might have additional problems? A diagnostic procedure should not be iatrogenic. The inadequacy of some attitude scales and personality inventory scales is that the respondent can recognize the acceptable and the nonacceptable answers.

9. Does the test violate the client's integrity? We would not use a picture-naming test of articulation with adult clients; some violations are less obvious:

Perhaps there should be a bill of rights for adult aphasics; more ill-considered activities have been used with them than with almost any other group of persons with communication handicaps. Many of the tasks on widely used language inventories are patently infantilizing—they rather blatantly impugn the client's mental status.

10. Does the diagnostic instrument permit the development of clearly defined and reportable concepts regarding the client and his communication disability? Does the test yield clinically relevant descriptive information about the person's problem?

11. Is the instrument reliable? Does it give consistent measures when administered repeatedly to the same client? Do separate examiners arrive at the same conclusions from this instrument when making independent judgments?

12. Is the test valid? Does it test what it says it does? Obviously, an instrument must be reliable—you must evoke the same "something" each time—before it can be valid; for example, if every time we said "corn" a client responded "tree," he would be reliable but consistently wrong. There are several types of validity: content validity (how well does the test *sample*—all tests obtain only a sample, not a parameter or whole—the particular aspect in which we are interested?); predictive validity (how well does the test predict performance?); concurrent validity (how well does the test data we have check with other evidence available?); and construct validity (how well does the test show or reflect some trait, quality, or construct presumed to underlie performance on the test?).

13. In what manner was the test standardized? What types of norms are set forth and on what population are they based? Is it "fair" to give a measure of verbal intelligence, based on suburban, middle-class vocabulary, to an Ojibway Indian child?

Space limitations do not permit a review and analysis of the many diagnostic instruments available. The reader will want to consult the work of Cronbach (1960) and that of others (Anastasi, 1968; Burros, 1972; Davis, 1975) for a comprehensive discussion of psychometric testing and a compendium of measurement devices in print. We now turn to a review of possible dangers involved in testing persons with communication disorders.

DANGERS IN TESTING

At some point in the future, the speech-and-hearing clinician might have a massive diagnostic computer system for rapidly assessing speech and language disorders. Into the maw of this marvelous machine, the diagnostician will feed certain key signs, and error-free diagnosis, with suggestions for remediation, will emerge following a short wait. But, alas, this is a mythical beast, at least for the present.[3] We must rely on the fragile magic of human perception.

It is axiomatic that no testing device or examination procedure is any better than the person who administers it. *The efficacy of an evaluation rests on the calibration of the diagnostician.* A test is merely a systematic way for obtaining, describing, and comparing a sample of behavior under rather structured conditions; every test was once a system for observing clients that one person had in mind. Tests are tools, after all, and can be used wisely or foolishly. In this section, we focus on some of the dangers involved in using tests: overtesting, undertesting, and other assorted dangers.

Overtesting

Many clinicians employ a shotgun approach to diagnosis. They administer several tests and collect a plethora of data on the assumption that quantity is the key issue—the more information they have, the more likely they are to have something relevant. This type of procedure is especially evident in some training programs where the unfortunate client is poked and prodded in the interest of clinical experience. We do not favor the battery concept of assessment: each diagnostic procedure should have a rationale, a clearly stated goal or hypothesis.

The worst aspect of overtesting is the tendency to fragment the patient into a series of clinical artifacts and, in the process of sorting out the scores and profiles, to lose his unique wholeness. It is possible to become engrossed in test scores and forget our mission. A test score is simply an estimate of a client's performance under a particular set of conditions—it is not a fixed trait. *We may overlook the person for the percentiles.*

[3]The medical profession is moving rapidly to computerized diagnosis. Normman Anderson of the Argonne National Laboratory is developing a machine capable of diagnosing 900 different disorders ranging from cancer to genetic disease on the basis of blood or urine samples.

Overdependence on the process of testing and test scores may prevent us from seeing important clues about the person and his life situation. By placing too much emphasis on the formal diagnostic instruments we can ignore how the client and his family see the problem.

Another danger, also a form of overtesting, is delaying treatment. The structure afforded by the administration of various diagnostic instruments does provide a sense of security to the clinician.

Finally, since diagnosis and treatment are part of the same continuous process, we should carefully consider how tests may structure relationships in an undesirable way. Extensive test batteries may lead the client to suspect that his problem will be handled in a detached and authoritative manner.

Undertesting

Grave errors may also be committed by not having sufficient information on a given client. Many clinicians who work in schools operate as if they have made a diagnosis when they state that a child has a frontal lisp; this is a description—and a superficial one at that—not a diagnosis. It is certainly not the basis for a therapeutic program.

Consider the child who was enrolled in speech therapy year after year for a "simple" functional disorder of articulation. More extensive assessments revealed sensory problems, mild motor impairments, psychological conflicts, and other learning disabilities—all hiding behind the "simple lisp" label. The ubiquitous diagnosis of "functional articulation problem" may result from insufficient scrutiny of the client. Obviously, then, a very real danger in undertesting is the fact that you may well overlook something serious if you do not investigate beneath the obvious. Also, you will not have enough information to convey in reports to experts in the field when you want to refer a client; perhaps you may not even know when there is a need for referral.

Finally, certain tests, when judiciously used, can prevent us from creating speech defects where none exists:

> Many first-grade children have "maturational speech differences" which, in most cases, will clear up by the end of the school year. Some, of course, will not. There is no need to include all first graders with lisps in speech therapy, to catch the few who will not mature into better speech. By using a screening test to identify those in need of help, we not only conserve our efforts but also prevent the development of a self-concept that includes "I have trouble with /s/."

Assorted Dangers

In addition to the polar dangers of over- and undertesting, there are several other possible risks involved in the use of tests. They are all interrelated:

The client's participation. No diagnostic procedure is a one-way street; if the client cannot or does not participate in the testing to the level required—because of attitudes, moods, his personal background—the results may be spurious. We are, in a very real sense, at the mercy of the respondent's cooperation. The relationship with the client is critical. What is the client's frame of reference for the testing situation? Does he consider it a threat, a challenge, a silly adult game? Does he feel anxious or manipulated? Some highly structured tests are so formal that a clinical relationship is strained; the style in which the tasks are administered tend to make the client feel uncomfortable, inhibited, even ridiculous. We must remember to always consider the test results in light of the person's total behavior.

The competence of the examiner. The prospective diagnostician should be thoroughly familiar with a diagnostic instrument before he attempts to administer it. The test manual should be carefully studied and several trial attempts with normal-speaking individuals completed before assessing a client.

The magic of tests. Some clients feel that a test will do something for them; once the test has been administered, someone will be able to figure out the exact cause of their problem and pinpoint a solution. Tests, thus, often raise false hopes.

The mean scores. Most diagnostic instruments have tables for interpreting given scores obtained; these norms are generally based upon the average performance of a large number of subjects. Hence, their application to a given individual is problematical.

The presumption of the test. Some tests are contraindicated because they presume normal speech and hearing. Their application to clients with communication problems is suspect:

> Our favorite aphasic client, perhaps our all-time favorite client, was Charles S. Hanford. Following a thrombotic stroke, with resultant auditory aphasia, his employer demanded a psychological appraisal, fearful of the possibility of brain damage. Mr. Hanford was taken by his wife to a local clinical psychologist, who gave him a comprehensive intelligence measure. The psychologist, although noting the aphasia, did not modify the test instrument. He made recommendations on the basis of the test results, including an IQ score of 54, which was remarkable in terms of Mr. Hanford's degree of auditory aphasia at the time. The client's wife was told that "he had suffered extensive brain damage, would be unable to work or drive again [he had no paralysis] and would not be able to make judgments with regard to family finances, etc." When Mr. Hanford eventually learned of this, he was furious. In retribution for the psychologist's actions, he paid the twenty-five-dollar fee in quarters and other small change over an interval of eighteen months, always demanding a receipt and always indicating that if the psychologist left town he would immediately pay his bill in full.

Looking where the light is. The joke about the drunken man looking for his lost watch under the bright illumination of a street light rather than in the darkened alley where it was lost applies to the way some clinicians use tests. They have a pet instrument which they apply willy-nilly to each client without regard to his particular needs.

Following the fads. It is very difficult to identify the beginning and end of a particular fad or intellectual *Zeitgeist* when you are in the middle of it. There are some workers who make a total commitment to one way of assessing and talking about a particular communication impairment and cannot change to meet the needs of a client who does not fit the mold of the test in vogue. In fact, some clinicians focus narrowly on a particular test, not on the client; instead of using the instrument as a tool, they defer to it as their master (Keenan and Brassel, 1975). We urge you not to abrogate your responsibility for exercising clinical judgment with respect to test results. A test *describes* certain aspects of behavior, but it does not *explain* the level of performance.

Hardening of the categories. Following the fads can easily lead to that dread clinical disorder, "hardening of the categories." This involves being able to see behavior only through well-worn perceptual grooves with regard to identification and classification of clients and their responses.

With all these possible pitfalls it is easy to see why some impressionistic diagnosticians, the artisans described in Chapter 1, eschew formal tests. Many of these individuals feel that tests tend to traumatize clients. There is little hard evidence that this has to be true. Indeed, Schuell, Jenkins, and Jimenez-Pabon (1964: 159–176) observe that when the tasks are presented in the spirit of mutual exploration, they can be factors in correcting misapprehensions and misinformation. This is to say that a diagnostic session can be therapeutic; the client explores himself and the dimensions of his problem with the objective support of the clinician. The unknown begins to take on limits and definition; the client is no longer faced with a global failure. Testing can and should reveal the client's strengths as well as weaknesses.

PROGNOSIS

Prognosis may be defined as a prediction of the outcome of a proposed course of treatment for a given client: how effective therapy will be, how far we can expect the client to progress, and perhaps, how long it will take. Since diagnosis is a continuing progress, prognosis should, like therapy planning, have both long-range and immediate facets. Immediate prognosis covers what the person can do now, what steps in therapy are possible, what is the best route to take. Prognosis for specific communication disorders will be discussed in subsequent chapters; in this section we will present some generic purposes and a possible danger involved in predicting a client's response to therapy.

The basic purpose in making a prognosis is to economize our therapeutic efforts. There is only so much time and energy, and we must focus it upon those clients who show the greatest promise of improvement. This seems to be difficult for speech clinicians to do. Perhaps because we are such a young profession, we feel we must help all clients; we try too hard and hate to give up even when the client is plainly signaling that he has had enough:

> Mrs. Bachman was sixty-nine and had global aphasia. In addition to a severe cerebral vascular episode, she was hypertensive and diabetic. The speech clinician had been seeing the client for several weeks before she asked for our consultation. We examined the individual thoroughly and, in our judgment, decided that it would be better to work out patterns of communication with her environment (the end result of therapy is not always speech). We advised that Mrs. Bachman's husband should be shown how to provide language stimulation and that the medical social worker should be consulted with regard to family readjustment. The clinician demurred and continued to work with the client, maintaining that she saw a certain something in Mrs. Bachman's eyes that would not allow her to "give up." One later session which we observed entailed the repetition of the phrase, "I wear a size 34C bra" at least twenty-three times by actual count. Not only is that a phrase that would be rather difficult to fit into a conversation, its use suggested to the physician and other members of the treatment team that the clinician was not employing good professional judgment in her insistence on not terminating therapy.

Prognosis also provides direction for treatment; we must know where we are going so that we will know when we have arrived. Some predictive factors are specific to a particular speech or language disability and will be discussed in the appropriate chapters. There are, however, a number of general factors that the clinician must consider when making predictions: the client's age, habit-strength, the existence of other problems, the type and intensity of reactions from significant persons in the client's environment, the client's motivation, and secondary gains the client may derive from the problem.

Accurate prognoses can help establish our credibility with other professions. The ability to predict with reasonable precision is perhaps the highest form of scientific achievement. Needless to say, however, these predicitions should be based on something more than clinical intuition. Impressionistic conclusions, especially when made by experienced workers, can often be startlingly accurate, but they should always be labeled as impressionistic: a prognosis should be supported by a substantial amount of information.

In what sense might a prognosis be dangerous? We have become suspicious of what these predictions can do to our therapeutic interaction with the client; we are becoming increasingly convinced that the clinician's expectations regarding the case's potential influences the treatment program. It is certainly possible that our negative prognoses can be communicated to a client and affect the course of therapy.

SOME TESTS AND EXAMINATION PROCEDURES COMMON TO MANY DIAGNOSTIC UNDERTAKINGS

A number of tests and examination procedures are clinically useful regardless of the client's particular communication impairment. In order to avoid repetition in the chapters that follow, these commonly utilized assessment techniques are discussed here; in the chapters dealing with the various disorders, we shall present diagnostic procedures that are pertinent to the specific speech problem.

The Oral Peripheral Examination

It is a common practice to inspect a client's oral structures to determine their structural and functional adequacy for speech.

To provide an example of typical data gathered during an oral peripheral examination, we have included notes hastily scribbled during an evaluation of a nine-year-old boy with a hoarse voice and several articulation errors:

> Lips look okay. No asymmetry of face. Slight open bite; poor dental hygiene (lots of cavities and tarter buildup). Tongue has good mobility, no paralysis or sluggishness; can protrude, wiggle from side to side swiftly, and touch the alveolar ridge; can even curl and groove. Hard palate seems OK, no scars. Soft palate has good tissue supply; elevates fine, no asymmetry. Palatine tonsils are *really* enlarged, filling the whole isthmus between the fauces. Pharynx looks inflamed (possible postnasal drip?). Good gag reflex. Wonder why he has mandible thrust to left side on /sh/ and /ch/?

Note the systematic nature of the inspection. Although the period of observation was relatively brief—an oral examination is generally completed in less than two minutes—the clinician has a sound basis for making a referral to a laryngologist. Now we shall present a rather detailed procedure for conducting an oral examination.

Tools you will need. You will need a light source; a small flashlight is good (we avoid the head mirror because it makes us look like a physician). Next, obtain a supply of plain applicator sticks. We dislike tongue depressors because of their association with doctors; in addition they are so blunt they do not permit evaluation of point-to-point sensitivity in the oral area. If you do use tongue depressors, the individually wrapped ones are best for sanitary purposes (it is curious that no one has yet invented a flavored tongue blade). Finally, your kit might include several pads of cotton gauze (for holding onto tongues), a few candy suckers, and a mirror.

How to get into a small child's mouth. Most older children and adults will open their mouths on request. Small children, however, are sometimes rather reluctant to let the clinician examine their tongue and teeth:

> Jimmy cooperated, cautiously but willingly, in all the diagnostic tasks until the clinician brought out a tongue depressor. He clamped his little jaw shut in bulldog

fashion and tears began to form in the corners of his huge brown eyes. The clinician unwrapped the wooden blade and produced a small pen light, chatting amiably all the time. "Let me see, here is my mirror. I wonder if that little black dot is still on the back of my tongue. Hmmmm. Only three boys have ever seen it. . . ." (The clinician opened his mouth and looked intently with light and mirror.) Then, turning to Jimmy, the clinician requested, "Say, can you help me find that black dot? It's way on the back of my tongue. That's right, here's the flashlight." Jimmy, curious now, looked cautiously into the clinician's mouth. The clinician giggled and suggested he look further back. "I taw it, I taw it," Jimmy said triumphantly. "Hmmmm. You did? Say, I wonder if . . . no, I bet you don't . . . but maybe you do, maybe you have a black dot, too?" suggested the clinician. The child handed the light to the clinician and opened his mouth, erasing a small grin.

There is another method we have used which, although slightly indelicate, is more universally effective:

Children are engrossed with magic and guessing games. We make a wager—some small token will do—that he cannot guess what we had for breakfast (or lunch). Then, after he scrutinizes our oral cavity and makes a guess, we agree, with shocked surprise at his wizardry. Now we ponder aloud what he might have had for the most recent meal. Generally, their mouths pop open like baby starlings. Our first guess is usually something outlandish (like sardines and Bermuda onions) which provokes much mirth and a chance to look and guess again.

With some especially shy children or those for whom the oral examination conjures vivid memories of past trauma, we have used another technique. It may take more time, but children almost always like to play follow-the-leader games. Using a large mirror so that we can see each other, we go through a series of comical movements of our arms, legs, and torso. Gradually we shift the focus of movement to our head, using our eyes and lips. Finally, we open our mouths and make weird movements with our tongue. The children usually follow in this "play," and we end up peering into each other's mouth before the glass.

What to look for. It is important to be *systematic* and *swift* when conducting an oral examination. This demands considerable practice. Use every opportunity to scrutinize normal-speaking persons, not only to perfect your technique and observational skills, but also to establish a frame of reference on the range of structural and functional variation. The following outline is presented as a guide for conducting oral peripheral examinations.[4]

1. Lips and lip movement: inspect the lips first for relative size, symmetry, and scars. Can the client smile, pucker his lips, and retract them? Can he close his lips tightly for the sounds /p/, /b/, and /m/? Can he utter the nonsense syllable "puh" at least once per second (Fletcher, 1972)?

2. Jaws: scrutinize the client's jaws in a state of rest; observe for symmetry. Can he open and close his mandible at least once per second? Does his mandible deviate to the right or left on opening?

[4]Laryngoscopic examination is the professional responsibility of the physician. While the speech pathologist usually describes breathing patterns, and examines the external musculature of the larynx for tension, an assessment of the vocal folds must be undertaken by a laryngologist.

3. Teeth: inspect the client's bite during a state of rest. A normal dental bite is characterized by the upper incisors overlapping the lower incisors by not more than one half of their vertical dimension. Is there an open, under-, or overbite? Does the client have cavities, jumbled teeth, gaps between teeth, or more than the normal complement of teeth? Does he wear a dental prosthesis?

4. The tongue: note the size of the tongue relative to the oral cavity. Observe for symmetry in structure and during movement. Is there scarring, atrophy, or fasiculations? Can the client protrude and retract his tongue, wiggle it from side to side, and touch the alveolar ridge without random movement or extraordinary effort? Inspect the tip of tongue and the frenulum for any evidence of tongue tie. Some children, especially those presenting neuromuscular problems, may find it difficult to elevate the tip of their tongue to the alveolar ridge on command. We use a sucker, placing the moistened candy behind the upper incisors and encouraging the child to go after it. A spot of peanut butter or a tiny paper wedged high between the central incisors can also be used. Can he trill his tongue when the mandible is stabilized? Test for diadochokinesis by having him utter "tuh"; can he say one per second? Is there any evidence of tongue thrust? (An open bite might alert you to this possibility.) When he swallows does he have an exaggerated lip seal? Does his tongue protrude beyond the incisors? Is there no apparent bunching in the masseter? If the answers to these last three queries are positive, then the client may be a tongue-thruster.

5. Hard palate: note the shape (is it flat? high and arched?) and width of the hard palate. Are there any scars present? Can the client produce /r/ and /l/? One public-school clinician noted that three of his cases with persistent /r/ defects had rather high and arched hard palates. He experimented with several materials (bubble gum and peanut butter were consumed too swiftly) to reduce the palatal height; finally, in cooperation with a local dentist, he made prosthetic devices of denture material. All three children began to make the elusive /r/ with their devices. The dentist gradually shaved off the structures. The cases' tongues were thus coaxed higher and higher until they were making the /r/ on their own hard palates.

6. Soft palate and velopharyngeal closure: inspect the velum for size, scars, and symmetry. Does the soft palate move back and up toward the posterior pharyngeal wall? Can you visualize lateral movement?[5]

7. Fauces: inspect the pillars for scars, the status of the palatine tonsils, and the width of the isthmus. Check the general condition of the oropharynx.

8. Others: observe the client's breathing during speech and at rest. Is there an obstruction of the nasal passages? Is the client a mouth breather? Observe the facial muscles: is a nasolabial fold flattened; does an eyelid droop (ptosis); is one side of the face smooth and devoid of normal creases? Is there anything unusual about the appearance of the individual's head?

For further information regarding the oral peripheral examination, consult the work of Van Riper (1963: 472–490) and others (Johnson, Darley, and Spriestersbach, 1963: 111–132; Darley, 1964: 91–105; Minifie, Hixon, and Williams, 1973; Darley, Aronson and Brown, 1975: 86–97). Remember, one swallow does not make a summer, and one deviancy in the oral area does not necessarily cause disordered speech.

---

[5]Individuals presenting nasal vocal quality or nasal emission will require more extensive evaluation of their velopharyngeal competency. See Chapter 9 and Project 5 at the end of this chapter.

Motor Abilities

During the oral examination the diagnostician may observe disturbances in the client's gross and fine motor abilities that suggest possible neurological dysfunction. While the diagnostic appraisal of motor dysfunction is the responsibility of the neurologist, the speech clinician should have a basis for making intelligent referrals. This can be accomplished by comparing various facets of the client's motor performance with norms corresponding to his age level.

A public-school clinician referred Steve Munroe to us with the following note:

"Steve is almost unintelligible. . . . His whole pattern of articulation seems uncontrolled and bizarre. Although he is nearly thirteen, he is only in the sixth grade and that's where the problem lies. Unless we can show, somehow, that he belongs in the orthopedically handicapped room—where he could stay through high school—they will put him in a junior high class for the trainable retarded. Why? Solely on the basis of his score on the Wechsler; although he obtained an IQ of 62, I don't think he is retarded. His articulation is so bad I'm sure he failed the verbal items because the psychometrician could not understand him; and I think his incoordination shot him down on the motor tasks. Anyway, I need help. The physician at the public medical clinic refuses to refer him for a neurological examination; he claims that Steve is clearly retarded and belongs in the trainable room."

We decided to examine Steve in two sessions. We first wanted a global impression of his motor abilities, following the format presented by Wood (1964: 64–71). Here are our notes:

1. General body description. Steve is thin and wiry, has a slightly stooped posture. He appears on the small end of normal in height and weight.
2. Locomotor. His gait is characterized by a slight shuffle, and he seems to drag his right foot slightly. His stance is not broad-based (not wider than his shoulders). Speed and range (distance or extent of excursion) seem restricted and "jerky"; they lack synergy.
3. Balance. He can stand for three seconds on one foot (left) with both arms extended and his eyes closed; he refused to attempt the task with his right foot. He tried to walk forward with one foot directly ahead of another but failed after three steps and refused to try again.
4. Manual dexterity. His copying and drawing attempts are jerky, and he must exert great effort to control a slight intentional tremor in his right arm and hand. He picked up eleven small buttons and put them in a box in seventeen seconds, using his left hand for the task after fumbling for a few seconds with his right.
5. Psychomotor. The tremor in Steve's right hand was more noticeable when we asked him to place a knitting needle through a small plastic loop suspended on a string. There was overflow of movement in the shoulder and upper chest area while he attempted this task. His speech efforts are often grotesque when he attempts to produce certain phonemes, particularly /r/ and /l/; some drooling was observed.

At the end of our first session we tape-recorded Steve reading a standard passage ("My Grandfather"). Later, using the procedures detailed in recent articles by Darley, Aronson, and Brown (1969a; 1969b), we rated the speech sample on the several dimensions provided by the authors. Our clinical hunch was confirmed; the ratings showed that Steve's performance was startlingly identical to the several clusters associated with pseudobulbar palsy (Darley, Aronson, and Brown, 1969b: 483). We were now certain that we had sufficient ammunition to insist upon a neurological referral but, knowing we had to work through the obdurate institutional physician, we wanted our case to be overwhelming. Well aware that medical practitioners are impressed by percentiles and normative comparisons, we administered the Oseretsky Test (Doll, 1964) during our second diagnostic session with Steve. This instrument evaluates motor proficiency by means of age-graded tasks and yields six measures. Here are the results we obtained:

1. General static coordination. Steve failed at the seven-year-old level (he could not balance on tiptoe, bending forward from the hips for ten seconds).

2. Dynamic coordination. He performed at the eight-year level. (This test requires the subject to touch all the finger tips of one hand successively with the thumb of the same hand, beginning with the little finger; it took him five seconds with his left hand and nine seconds with his right.)

3. General dynamic coordination. Steve passed all the items up to the ten-year level on this subtest. (Ten-year test task: given three trials to jump and clap his hands three times while in the air, Steve was successful on his third attempt.)

4. Motor speed. Steve also passed all the age-graded tasks up to the ten-year level. (He was required to make four piles with forty matchsticks in thirty-five seconds for the right hand, and in forty-five seconds for the left.) He took almost two minutes to complete the task with his right hand but finished in less than forty-five seconds with the left.

5. Simultaneous voluntary movements. Steve had trouble with this subtest, a task that requires simultaneous movements with both limbs. He got up to the eight-year level (tapping the floor rhythmically with his feet, alternating right and left, while at the same time tapping the table with his fingers in the same rhythm.) He became upset and confused, pounded on the table in anger, and refused to continue.

6. Synkinesis. This subtest requires the subject to perform muscle movements without overflow such as wrinkling the forehead without any other movements at the eight-year level. Steve was tired and refused to do any of the tasks.

We held a formal conference with the physician, reviewed our findings and suggested politely but strongly that, since Steve had never been evaluated by a neurologist, we were sure that the doctor would certainly want conclusive evidence beyond a reasonable doubt before relegating the child to the irreversible category of "trainable." Somewhat defensive at first, the physician eventually concurred and expedited the referral; he even went one step further and enlisted the professional counsel of a psychiatrist to direct the planning for a comprehensive, long-range program of rehabilitation for Steve.

Obviously not all of our clients will require such extensive investigation of their motor abilities. The point is, however, that the clinician must be capable of supporting his convictions with data. An emotional appeal—which the public-school therapist had tried unsuccessfully in the case of Steve—without carefully prepared evidence serves only to create a rather unprofessional image.

There does seem to be a parallel course of development between acquisition of language and growth of motor skills. For further information concerning the evaluation of motor abilities, see the work of Berry (1969: 205–207, 219–270) and Van Riper (1963: 481–482). Recently, Bruininks (1977) has revised the Oseretsky Test of Motor Proficiency to include a screening battery for children from the ages of four to eighteen; the revised instrument was standardized on 892 subjects and yields age equivalent scores and percentile ranks. Grinker and Sahs (1966), Chusid and McDonald (1967), and Rutter, Graham and Yule (1976) present extended discussions of the neurological examination.

Estimates of Development

Experienced clinicians recognize that in order to understand handicapped children, it is absolutely essential to have a thorough working knowledge of normal patterns of growth and behavior. What is typical or modal behavior for a four-year-old? What should he be able to do at this age level? It is possible, of course, to answer these questions in an impressionistic manner *if* the diagnostician has a clear idea of what is normal for various age levels. However, standardized scales devised on the basis of extensive observation of many children provide greater reliability and objectivity. Knobloch and Pasamanick (1974) have prepared a very useful guide for comparing behavior patterns at various age levels, based upon the exhaustive research of the Gesell Institute for Child Behavior. When preparing for a diagnostic session with a child, we review the descriptions of characteristic behaviors for that particular age level.

Several checklists and interviewing guides have been devised from the data gathered at the Gesell Institute and from other research dealing with child development. Many clinicians find the Vineland Social Maturity Scale (Doll, 1964) a useful device for assembling information on a child's maturity; the diagnostician does not observe the child directly but rather queries the parents on the youngster's ability to dress and feed himself, his social interaction, and daily activities. The items on the scale are arranged in age categories. For example, here are the six items at the three- to four-year-old level:

1. Walks down stairs one step per tread
2. Plays cooperatively at the kindergarten level
3. Buttons coat or dress
4. Helps at little household tasks
5. "Performs" for others
6. Washes hands unaided.

Although it is possible to derive a social age and social quotient on the basis of the information obtained in an interview, we often prefer to use the Vineland as a screening device, which affords a way to compare the child's development—at least as perceived by his parents—against normative expectations.

There are distinct advantages to directly observing the child's performance instead of relying upon an informer. At the present time there are several tests (actually checklists for recording behavior, which allow comparison with established norms) that permit the clinician to chart the development of a child in age-graded tasks. The *Communicative Evaluation Chart* (Anderson, Miles, and Matheny, 1963). *Utah Test of Language Development* (Mecham, Jex and Jones, 1967) and the *Sequenced Inventory of Communication Development* (Hedrick, Prather and Tobin, 1975) concentrate on assessing language development; they are easy to use and do provide the clinician with an objective means of evaluating expressive and receptive verbal language skills. The *Communicative Evaluation Chart,* and a recently developed test, the *Developmental Activities Screening Inventory* (DuBose and Langley, 1977), also include items that assess physical well-being, motor coordination, normal growth and development, and visuomotor perception.

For a practical, clinically useful tool to help detect children with serious developmental delay, we prefer the Denver Developmental Screening Test (Frankenburg and Dodds, 1969). The Denver instrument is very simple to administer, takes less than twenty minutes to finish, and in its published version, comes complete with all the forms and materials needed. It permits evaluation of the following aspects of a child's functioning: gross motor abilities, fine motor coordination, language development, and personal-social maturation (the ability to perform tasks of self-care and relate to others). Here is a portion of a report we submitted to a family physician regarding Robbie O'Neill, a three-year-old child tentatively diagnosed as autistic:

> The vertical line drawn through the four dimensions represents the child's chronological age (see Figure 3.3). We administered the items through which this line passes in each dimension. On those items Robbie passed, we placed a large letter "P" on the horizontal bar at the midpoint; "F" indicates a failure and an "R" stands for refused. In order to assist you in interpreting the scale, we quote from the Manual (Frankenburg and Dodds, 1969: 7): "Each of the test items is designated by a bar which is so located under the age scale as to indicate clearly the ages at which 25%, 50%, 75%, and 90% of the standardization population could perform the particular test item. The left end of the bar designates the age at which 25% of the standardization population could perform the item; the hatch mark at the top of the bar 50%; the left end of the shaded area 75%; and the right end of the bar the age at which 90% of the standardization population could perform the item. Normal children will generally show a fair amount of scattered successes and failures on items within one area and between the four areas. A *delay* is defined as any failure by a child on an item if he is older than the age at which 90% of the children pass that item. In other words, his vertical chronological age line is to the right of the right end of the bar representing the items he fails."
>
> Robbie appears to be well coordinated in gross motor functioning; even though he refused most of the fine motor tasks, we noted a great degree of manual dexterity (he played almost continually with baby food jars filled with small nails, transferring the nails from one to another). Note that he does not use language in a meaningful way; his parents report only "compulsive" laughter, but no speech per se. Consider also Robbie's responses on the personal-social dimension: he refuses to associate with others and is operating in a very delayed fashion.

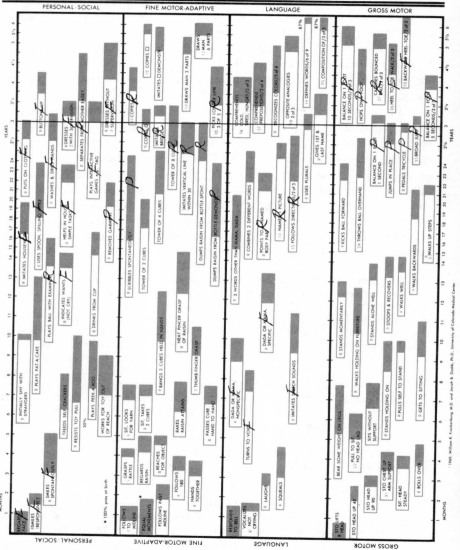

Figure 3.3 Score Sheet for Denver Developmental Screening Test. (W. Frankenburg and J. Dodds, *Denver Developmental Screening Test*. © 1969, reprinted with permission.)

76

Although the speech pathologist is concerned with developmental milestones and patterns of maturation, we quite agree with Berelson and Steiner (1964: 55): "Maturation, by definition, is always a *necessary* condition, but it is not always (strictly speaking, never) a *sufficient* condition; no child can do anything he is not biologically equipped to do, but no child can do everything he *is* biologically capable of."

Intelligence and Educational Performance

Since the development of speech and language is dependent, in part, upon the child's capacity to learn, the speech pathologist is interested in his client's intelligence; many disorders of oral communication stem from low intelligence or inability to utilize an existing level of intelligence. A client's intelligence is also an important consideration in planning therapy.

We like to obtain a general impression of a client's intelligence and, if further testing is indicated, we refer him to a qualified psychometrician. The two most comprehensive measures of intelligence are the *Stanford-Binet Intelligence Scale* (Terman and Merrill, 1960) and the *Wechsler scales* for children (1949, 1967) and adults (1955). These intruments provide a multidimensional profile of an individual's intellectual abilities. The Leiter (1948) and Raven (1948) scales assess only mechanical or performance abilities. Unless the clinician is qualified to administer these tests, he will generally rely on some screening device such as the *Goodenough Draw-A-Man Test* (1926), The *Ammons Full Range Picture Vocabulary Test* (Ammons and Ammons, 1948), the *Van Alstyne Picture Vocabulary Test* (1960), or the *Peabody Picture Vocabulary Test* (Dunn, 1965). We prefer the latter test because of its ease of scoring and interpretation and the modern stimulus pictures provided (but see precautions noted in Chapter 4). The Peabody Test is really a measure of recognition vocabulary, but it correlates highly with the more comprehensive instruments cited above (Taylor, 1963; Blatt, 1959).

We do not generally report an IQ score or percentile if the client's performance is within normal limits. If a client's performance is not within normal limits, we usually cite the age level at which he responds:

> Conrad's recognition vocabulary was evaluated with the Peabody Picture Vocabulary Test (Form A). His performance on this scale was characteristic of children two years younger; in terms of auditory recognition, then, Conrad appears to be functioning at a level of six years, or two years below his chronological age.

The Peabody Test is also useful because it allows the examiner to observe the client's behavior on a structured task and to get a feel for how he uses language. We can scrutinize his style of responding, how long he takes to complete the items (latency of response), and how he reacts to failure. Many children comment about the pictures, and the task thus provides another sample of their language output.

We should not give undue importance to one measure of intelligence. This is especially important in dealing with youngsters, since the younger the child, the less reliable is any intellectual assessment. We have also seen wide fluctuations in the tested intelligence of older children that seemed to stem from environmental events. Finally, IQ scores, like all test data, should be related to other sources of information, such as case histories, interviews, direct observation, and, when possible, school performance.

A child's school folder can be a rich source of information regarding his ability to learn and adjust. What scores did he obtain on various achievement tests? How does he go about learning? What are his attitudes toward success and failure in school? What about his abilities in problem-solving, reasoning, and identifying relationships? How does he perform in the language skills—spelling and reading in particular? What kinds of things does he perceive as worth working for in the classroom?

Motivation

Motivation is a critical variable in speech therapy, particularly at the outset of treatment and again during the carryover phase of therapy. People learn basically what they want to learn. When an individual undertakes to make a significant change in himself, questions regarding desire and drive often emerge. Is change needed? Is it possible? In what direction? To what degree? Will the work and discomfort be worth it? (Schultz and Carpenter, 1973). In order to endure the uncertainties of behavioral shift, a client must have positive expectations—hope—that a favorable outcome is likely. A person's level of motivation obviously is not constant; it will rise and ebb throughout the course of treatment. The assessment of a client's motivation, by means of testing or impressionistic observation, is then a very useful clinical procedure (Van Riper, 1973).

> What is motivation? A motive may be defined as: . . . an inner state that energizes, activates, or moves (hence, "motivation"), and that directs or channels behavior toward goals (Berelson and Steiner, 1964: 240).

Motivation arouses a person to strive, perform, to do better; it also provides direction and persistence to behavior. Motives may be classified as primary (hunger, thirst, etc.) or secondary (need for social stimulation or recognition). Maslow (1943) proposed a hierarchy of human motives ranging from physiological (sleep, hunger) to psychosocial (love, esteem) and to personal (self-actualization). In his view, deprivation of motives at the bottom of the scale will dominate the individual's behavior and prevent activity based on motives farther along the hierarchy. The speech clinician is generally interested in the relative strength of various secondary or social motives; as an agent or catalyst of change, she is concerned with how to release the potential for growth. Low motivation is commonly regarded as a poor prognostic sign; however, if the individual is highly aroused, if he manifests very high motivation, he may not be able to concentrate on the sequence of treatment. Unfortunately, a client's level of motivation is very difficult to measure directly (Korman, 1974).

One widely used means of assessing a client's motivation is to measure his level of aspiration:

> Bill said he wanted to work on his lateral lisp, but his laconic nature and scholastic underachievement belied the fact. In order to assist him in gaining insight and provide us with some examples of his typical goal-setting behavior, we administered the Cassell Test (1957). This instrument measures goal-setting behavior by means of a graphomotor task: the client draws squares around circles as swiftly as he can. A four-page booklet consisting of eight units with three rows of twenty small squares each is provided. Within a specified limit—thirty seconds—Bill attempted to draw the squares. Prior to each trial, he was requested to estimate or predict the number of squares he felt he could complete in thirty seconds. The Cassell Test yields a "D" score, which is the average of the difference between performance and subsequent estimate for all test trials. When a client consistently bids higher than his previous performance, his "D" score is positive. When he bids lower than his previous performance, his "D" score is negative. Here are Bill's scores:
>
> | Prediction | Performance |
> |:----------:|:-----------:|
> | 10 | 12 |
> | 11 | 14 |
> | 12 | 16 |
> | 12 | 16 |
> | 13 | 16 |
>
> "D" score = −3.2. Divide 5 (the number of trials) into 16 (the total discrepancy between prediction and performance).

Normally, individuals tend to have slightly positive discrepancy scores because they balance their idealistic aspirations against realistic expectations of attainment. As a group, handicapped persons, as well as persons with a long history of failure, manifest "D" scores that are lower than those obtained by normal groups. We have also noted that some handicapped individuals react to failure with very high shifts in their goal-settings; by so doing, they put the attainment of their goal out of reach and thus insulate themselves from failure. An individual's level of aspiration—the strength of his achievement motive—is influenced by several factors: the difficulty of the task; felt competence; the degree of satiation or deprivation; recent experience with success and failure; his perception of the payoff. For another means of measuring level of aspiration, see Rotter (1954).

There are other ways of assessing a client's motivation. McClelland (1972, 1973) has devised an intriguing system for determining the strength of an individual's "achievement motive" by analyzing thematic content in stories they write and by scrutinizing their doodling. A client's autobiography is another means of evaluating long-range themes regarding his motivation.

> We have also used an informal "test" of motivation in our work with young stutterers. It is based upon the observation that highly driven persons tend to feel uncomfortable if they are interrupted while completing a task and will tend to return to it as soon as they are permitted. We have used various activities—arithmetic problems, classifying and sorting objects, puzzles; when the youngster is well into

the task, we interrupt him and then record the time elapsed until he resumes the activity. Although lacking sufficient data to present norms, we have found that children with high motivation—those who strive for success—tend to return to the task more swiftly than those with low motivation—those who avoid the threat of failure. The former also do better in treatment. Persistence is essential to success in therapy as well as in life.

In a recent publication, McDaniels (1969: 139) presents a provocative formula for analyzing the potential motivation of a handicapped individual:

$$\text{MOTIVATION} = \frac{P(Os) \times U}{C}$$

Where:

$P(Os)$ = the probability of a *successful outcome* of treatment (based on the client's and clinician's judgment).

U = the meaning or value *(utility)* the client places upon the particular performance to be acquired.

C = the expense *(cost)* in money, and the physical and mental effort required.

For extended discussions of motivation, consult the work of Raph (1960) and others (Berelson and Steiner, 1964; McDaniels, 1969; McClelland and Steele, 1973; Atkinson and Raynor, 1974; Bindra, 1974; Korman, 1974; Bolles, 1975).

Audiometric Evaluation

Because of the close relationship between auditory acuity and speech and language development, we generally perform an audiometric assessment on each client. We often do this simply by combining informal, nonaudiometric testing with an audiometric screening procedure. Individuals manifesting abnormality on these tests should receive more complete audiological evaluation. For a discussion of hearing loss and assessment, consult the work of Emerick (1971) and others (O'Neill and Oyer, 1966; Sataloff, 1966; Davis and Silverman, 1970; Newby, 1972; Martin, 1975).

Socioeconomic Status

Speech clinicians do not routinely obtain a measure of socioeconomic status on each client. However, social class may have a bearing on the assessment and management of an individual's communication problem in one or more of the following ways: (1) parental attitudes toward clinical assistance may differ between classes (lower-class parents are more distrustful of authority; (2) child-rearing practices—including the amount and type of speech stimulation—seem to differ between lower and middle classes; (3) the economic position of the parents will influence the recommendations made; and (4) some types of speech differences, rather than being regarded as speech defects, may more appropriately be designated as subculture dialects.

There are several measures of social class; the scales devised by Hollingshead and Redlich (1958: 387–397) and Warner, Meeker, and Ells (1960: 139–142) are representative, and we have found them useful for conducting research or for an extensive study of a particular child:

> Social class alone may not be as important clinically as the identification of discrepancies between the elements (occupation, source of income, place of residence, amount of income) used in ranking. When there are gaps between these elements— for example, high-prestige occupation but low salary—it can provoke intense striving behavior and subsequent pressure upon children. Social mobility can produce stresses and strains that the clinician may wish to identify.

The occupation of the head of the household is the most reliable index of social status, and many clinicians find the Minnesota Scale for Parental Occupations (1950) a useful tool for ranking various jobs. We prefer, however, the North-Hatt Scale of Occupations (Reissman, 1959: 401–404); the authors present an alphabetical listing of various occupations and, on the basis of empirical research, assign a prestige or ranking score to each job.

Personality

Although the evidence suggests no systematic causal relationship between personality disturbances and speech defectiveness, clinicians recognize that many clients present varying degrees of emotional reaction to their impaired communication. Speech is perhaps man's most human attribute, and when a person cannot talk well, it affects him in a most profound way. However, a few speech impairments are a direct result of psychological conflict:

> Hugh did not seem like other stutterers we had seen: he was so calm, so relaxed, with a perpetual bittersweet smile on his face as he discussed his problem. His stuttering had started suddenly in his junior year at a religious college where he was studying to be a minister. His blocks were long, silent vigils during which he assumed a posture startlingly like one being crucified. He talked at great length, revealing sadly that now he could obviously not be a clergyman. Stuttering, he said, was a sign from the Almighty, a cross to bear. For Hugh, it seemed to us, stuttering, rather than *being* a problem, was a *solution* to a problem. The psychiatrist to whom we referred him confirmed our hunch: Hugh had made a dramatic emotional commitment during a religious revival meeting when he was an impressionable teenager. His decision had been vividly reinforced by his relatives who scrimped and saved to send him to college to be a minister. As he proceeded through school he began to realize that the church was not "his thing" but could find no face-saving way out of his commitment—until he began to stutter.

A speech clinician should not play psychologist unless he is qualified by virtue of training and experience to administer and interpret psychodiagnostic tests. He should, however, be able to recognize the difference between good mental hygiene and psychopathology. Persons who are psychologically healthy manifest most of the following characteristics:

> They are oriented by and large to reality and derive most of their satisfaction in that arena;
>
> They display adaptive or coping behavior in a sensitive way to environmental demands;
>
> They perceive the difference between socially acceptable and non-acceptable goals;
>
> They most often select socially acceptable goals for themselves;
>
> They select a variety of goals rather than just one or two;
>
> They select goals that are within their power to achieve;
>
> They tolerate a reasonable amount of frustration;
>
> They tolerate a reasonable amount of anxiety;
>
> They are able to deny immediate gratification;
>
> They establish warm relationships with others;
>
> They are reasonably consistent in their behavior;
>
> They accept the outcome of their behavior.

Not even the most well balanced individual displays all those attributes all the time. In fact, as many as one-quarter of the "normal" population have incidents that might be described as aberrant in their life histories (Sunberg and Tyler, 1962). After two decades of working with speech handicapped individuals and their relatives, it is sobering to reflect on how relatively fragile are most person's adjustments. There are signs of obvious psychopathology, however, which a diagnostician should be able to recognize (Page, 1975). Here a a few:

> Excessive readiness to react to stimuli, lability and mood swings
>
> Chronic fatigue or psychosomatic ailments
>
> Anxiety, guilt or hostility which are out of proportion to objective circumstances
>
> Phobias or obsessions which limit work or avocations
>
> Overuse of common defense mechanisms such as denial, rationalization, projection
>
> Chronic discrepancy between intent and outcome of actions

When a diagnostician identifies these characteristics of a client, he should make a referral which is humane and appropriate. It may still be difficult to determine, however, if the client possesses a primary emotional problem or a secondary, psychological reactions to the communication disorder.

It is important that, when we first set out to examine a client, we let him know that it may be necessary to look at his problem from many aspects, including psychological. We should not pop out of a box at the end of a diagnostic session and recommend that the client see a psychiatrist. Nor, in our judgment, is it clinically wise to make a psychological referral (without prior indication that a referral may be necessary) when the client is not responding to therapy. Such a referral is basically assaultive: we are saying, in effect, that if you don't respond to our treatment you must "have your head examined."

We prefer, in the case of an adult or adolescent, to help the client see his need for psychological evaluation. Generally, we do this by pointing out that the themes arising in his discussions with us are problem areas with which we are not professionally equipped to deal. The referral is then very specific—to a particular agency, or even to a particular person. Most individuals with speech disorders will not need psychiatric or psychological appraisal and treatment (Block and Goodstein, 1971), but we might have to adapt our remedial procedures to fit the needs of particular clients.

One of the most useful procedures in clinical work is the information contained in Hahn's (1961) classic article on direct, nondirect, and indirect methods in speech correction.

> We made a grave mistake with Ricky: we assumed that he could profit from the same kind of direct therapy the other children were receiving. From the start he tried to show us that he needed something different; despite our best efforts he persisted in his misarticulations. Recalling Hahn's article we decided to make a change. We assigned a senior student to work with Ricky, a student who by his appearance and manner was childlike and "simple." His job was simply to do things *with* Ricky such as making airplanes, taking him for cokes, and so on. After they had done this for a time, the senior author entered the scene and accused the student therapist, in front of Ricky, of wasting time and goofing off. The child did more work in the remaining six weeks of the school year than he had ever done; he had to achieve to protect the student, his friend.

PRECEPTS REGARDING THE CLINICAL EXAMINATION

In this chapter we have presented rather explicit methods for conducting the clinical examination. We dislike diagnostic formulae, and our purpose has not been to give out recipes, but rather to describe some way of approaching various problems without going too far astray. By way of summary, we now present a list of interrelated and overlapping precepts regarding the clinical examination.

1. We examine persons, not speech defects or speech defectives. Our primary concern is with communicators, not communication.

2. The clinical examination is conducted interpersonally; the catalyst of a diagnostic session is the person-to-person relationship between therapist and client.

3. There is an element of magic in every transaction between people. A diagnostic session can, in some instances, meliorate a problem situation by engendering hope or be deeply disappointing to a client who hopes that a test or examination will resolve his difficulty.

4. A most important requisite for conducting a clinical examination is a thorough understanding of normalcy.

5. Diagnosis is the initial phase of treatment. The very first contact with a client—the manner in which he is treated during a clinical examination—is a crucial determining factor in his response to therapy.

6. The clinical examination, or more broadly, diagnosis, is not necessarily confined to a single session.

7. Treatment is often diagnostic; we often discover the nature of a client's problem during therapy.

8. The clinical examination is performed to provide a working image of the individual; it is accomplished by interviewing, examining, and testing.

9. An important aspect in acquiring a working image of an individual is determining how he perceives himself and his situation.

10. An individual makes certain adjustments to his problem; his attempts to solve his difficulty—which may include a protective cover of defenses—may be a part of the problem but must not be confused with it.

11. Behavior is a function of the individual and the situation. We should be aware that our test results reflect not just the client's abilities but also his performance *in* the diagnostic setting.

12. Our diagnostic activities should include an assessment of a client's larger social context; the younger the individual, the more important this aspect of the evaluation becomes.

13. Tests are only tools to provide a systematic guide for our observations. They enable the clinician to scrutinize a client in a structured manner.

14. Although for the examiner the testing situation may be very familiar and routine, for the client it is a novel experience.

15. Examination and testing can be iatrogenic. It can suggest problems to the client that he had not considered.

It is remarkable that those who live around the social sciences have so quickly become comfortable in using the term deviant, as if those to whom the term is applied have enough in common that significant things can be said about them as a whole. Just as there are iatrogenic disorders caused by the work that physicians do (which gives them still more work to do), so there are categories of persons who are created by students of society and then studied by them (Goffman, 1963: 140). Do we create problem children by labelling them "tongue-thrusters," "culturally deprived," "learning disabled"?

16. Simply because a testing device is made up of a series of precisely defined tasks, administered and scored in a rigidly structured manner, this does not mean that a client's responses are similarly precise.

17. It is as important to observe *how* the client responds during a testing procedure as it is to obtain a score.

18. There is a distinct tendency for students to be caught up in diagnostic fads—the "recent article" syndrome.

19. It is very easy to reify a particular testing instrument, to endow a scale or diagnostic concept with a special form of reality independent of its creator. Some clinicians embrace a diagnostic device with militant enthusiasm and attack all intellectual queries or criticism with apostolic zeal.

20. An intellectual awareness of the nature of his problem, or the factors causing it, will not guarantee insight, acceptance, or remission by the client.

21. Impressions formed on the basis of the first careful evaluation of a client are generally accurate. There is a distinct tendency to discount or deny our findings especially, for example, if they suggest a child is mentally retarded or that an adult aphasic is not capable of further improvement.

22. A professional works when and where he is needed. The needs of the client, not the

setting in which the clinician works, determine the scope of his professional activities.

PROJECTS AND QUESTIONS

1. Sound clinical judgment is commonly regarded as an important requisite of effectiveness as a speech pathologist. How do you define "clinical judgment"? Study the following excerpt, written by a physician, and write a one-page reaction paper. Afterwards, review the Perez (1976) article.

   Clinicians can bring science to clinical judgment by better exercise of the very human capacities that appear to impair it, and by giving attention not to laboratory substances and inanimate technology, but to sick people and the human methods of evaluating sick people. [A. Feinstein, *Clinical Judgment* (Baltimore: William and Wilkins, 1967).]

2. We often ask beginning clinicians to keep a diary regarding their personal impressions of and reactions to a client, in order to help them identify possible negative attitudes toward the individual. In some instances, failure in treatment may stem from such unconscious attitudes the worker harbors toward a client. Review the following articles to determine what researchers have found with respect to attitudes of workers in the helping professions:

JANICKI, M. (1970). "Attitudes of Health Professionals toward 12 Disabilities." *Perceptual and Motor Skills*, 30: 77–78.

SALVIA, J.; G. CLARK; and J. YSSELDYKE (1973). "Teacher retention of stereotypes of exceptionality." *Exceptional Children*, 39: 651–652.

WILSON, M.; J. BEATTY; and R. FRUMPKIN (1967). "Attitudes of Future Rehabilitation Counselors toward Eight Major Disabilities." *Psychological Reports*, 21:928–941.

3. Explore the concept of experimental injury as a training activity for prospective diagnosticians. Commence by reviewing the following article:

DINNERSTEIN, A., and M. LOWENTHAL (1970). "Teaching Demonstration of Simulated Disability." *Archives of Physical Medicine and Rehabilitation*, 49: 167–169.

4. Research the topic of gerontology. Here are some references to get you started:

BRITTON, J., and J. BRITTON (1972). *Personality Changes in Aging*. New York: Springer Publishing Company.

BUTLER, R. (1975). *Why Survive?* New York: Harper and Row.

GEIST, H. (1968). *The Psychological Aspects of Retirement*. Springfield, Ill.: Charles C. Thomas.

GUBRIUM, J. (1973). *The Myth of the Golden Years*. Springfield, Ill.: Charles C. Thomas.

JARVIK, L. (1975). "Thoughts on the psychology of aging". *American Psychologist* 30: 576–583.

KAMINSKY, M. (1974). *What's Inside You It Shines Out of You*. New York: Horizon Press.

MENDELSON, M. (1976). *Tender Loving Greed*. New York: Knopf.

OYER, H., and E. OYER (1976). *Aging and Communication*. Baltimore: University Park Press.

RABINOWITZ, D., and Y. NIELSEN (1971). *Home Life: A Story of Old Age*. New York: Macmillan.

TALLAND, G. (1968). *Human Aging and Behavior*. New York: Academic Press.

TOBIN, S., and M. LIEBERMAN (1976). *Last Home for the Aged*. San Francisco: Jossey-Bass.

TOURNIER, P. (1972). *Learn to Grow Old*. New York: Harper and Row.

5. The oral peripheral examination:
   a. Look up the following terms: angle, neutroclusion, distoclusion, mesioclusion, edentulous, prognathic, cineflurography, cicatrix, deciduous teeth, palatography, uvula, bruxism.
   b. Draw a diagram of normal dentition in children and adults. Consult a standard textbook in anatomy and inspect the norms provided by Johnson, Darley, and Spriestersbach (1963: 126).
   c. Consider the three major malocclusions: employing your knowledge of motor phonetics, identify the phonemes most likely to be troublesome in each type of abnormal bite.
   d. Write an abstract of B. Weinberg (1968). "A Cephalometric Study of Normal and Defective /s/ Articulation and Variations in Incisor Dentition," *Journal of Speech and Hearing Research*, 11: 288–300.
   e. Review S. Fletcher and J. Meldrum (1968). "Lingual Function and Relative Length of the Lingual Frenulum" *Journal of Speech and Hearing Research*, 11: 382–390. What conclusions can you reach about the reported low incidence of tongue tie?
   f. What do the following articles have to say about tongue-thrusting?

American Speech and Hearing Association Joint Committee with Dentistry (1975). "Position Statement of Tongue-Thrust." *Journal of the American Speech and Hearing Association*, 17: 331–337.

HANSON, M. (1976). "Tongue thrust: A Point of View." *Journal of Speech and Hearing Disorders* 41: 172–184.

MASON, R., and W. PROFFIT (1974). "The Tongue Thrust Controversy: Background and Recommendations" *Journal of Speech and Hearing Disorders* 39: 115–132.

   g. What does McDonald say about testing for oral diadochokinesis?: McDonald, E. (1964). *Articulation Testing and Treatment: A Sensory Motor Approach*. Pittsburgh: Stanwix, p. 183. Look for norms for oral diadochokinesis in the following articles:

BLOMQUIST, B. (1950). "Diadochokinetic Movement of Nine-, Ten-, and Eleven-Year-Old Children," *Journal of Speech and Hearing Disorders*, 15: 159–164.

CANNING, B., and M. ROSE (1974). "Clinical Measurements of the Speed of Tongue and Lip Movements in British Children with Normal Speech," *British Journal of Communication Disorders*, 9: 45–50.

FLETCHER, S. (1972). "Time-by-Count Measurements of Diadochokinetic Syllable Rate," *Journal of Speech and Hearing Research* 15: 763–770.

   h. An assessment of oral stereognosis is not routinely done during a clinical examination. However, when we study children who persist in their articulation errors (after one year of therapy), we find that many have disturbances in oral tactile kinesthesia. (See Chapter 6).

6. What is the best method for separating a child from a parent: to take the child away from the mother or the mother away from the child? That is, is it better to lead the child away from the parent into the examining room with you or should both mother and child be ushered in together and then, when the child is occupied, have the mother take her leave unobtrusively?

7. Purchase a paperbound copy of the Gesell profiles of typical behaviors that appear at various chronological age levels:

ILG, F., and L. AMES (1955). *The Gesell Institute's Child Behavior from Birth to Ten*. New York: Harper and Row.

Prepare for a diagnostic session with a three and a half year old child. How would you differentiate the developmental motor, verbal and interpersonal difficulties of that epoch from real problems?

8. Familiarize yourself with the concept of symptom substitution by reviewing the following article:

IRWIN, J. (1971). "Symptom substitution." *Acta Symbolica* 2: 18–21.

9. Explore the concept of laterality: what is the relationship between speech behavior and unilateral motor lead? In what manner could the diagnostician distinguish between native hemispheric control and the impact of learning? How would you test for handedness, footedness, and which eye is dominant?

10. Generally, the diagnostician will not have difficulty recognizing psychosis. This serious psychological abnormality is characterized by severe personality decomposition and a marked distortion of and loss of contact with reality. See if you can find criteria for distinguishing alcoholism, and severe language disorders in adults.

11. Some clients appear to derive benefits from their communication disorders—attention, ready excuse for failure. In what way might a diagnostician identify these secondary gains?

BIBLIOGRAPHY

AMMONS, R., and H. AMMONS (1948). *Ammons Full-Range Picture Vocabulary Test.* Missoula, Mont.: Psychological Test Specialists.

ANASTASI, A. (1968). *Psychological Testing,* 3rd ed. New York: Macmillan.

ANDERSON, R.; M. MILES; and P. MATHENY (1963). *Communicative Evaluation Chart.* Golden, Colo.: Business Forms, Inc.

ATKINSON, J., and J. RAYNOR eds. (1974). *Motivation and Achievement.* Washington, D.C.: V. H. Winston & Sons.

BARKER, R., et al. (1953). *Adjustment to Physical Handicap and Illness: A Survey of the Social Phsycology of Physique and Disability.* New York: Social Science Research Council, Bulletin 55.

BAXLEY, G., and J. LEBLANC (1976). "The Hyperactive Child: Characteristics, Treatment and Evaluation of Research Design," in *Advances in Child Development and Behavior.* New York: Academic Press.

BERELSON, B., and G. STEINER (1964). *Human Behavior.* New York: Harcourt, Brace and World, Inc.

BERRY, M. (1969). *Language Disorders of Children.* New York: Appleton-Century-Crofts.

BINDRA, D. (1974). "A Motivational View of Learning, Performance and Behavior." *Psychological Review,* 81: 199–213.

BLATT, S. (1959). "Recall and Recognition Vocabulary." *Archives of General Psychiatry,* 1: 473–476.

BLOCH, E., and L. GOODSTEIN (1971). "Functional Speech Disorders and Personality: A Decade of Research." *Journal of Speech and Hearing Disorders,* 36: 295–314.

BLUMENFELD, J.; P. THOMPSON; and B. VOGEL (1971). *Help Them Grow.* Nashville: Abingdon Press.

BOLLES, R. (1975). *Theory of Motivation.* New York: Harper and Row.

BRUININKS, R. (1977). *Bruininks-Oseretsky Test of Motor Proficiency.* Circle Pines, Minnesota: American Guidance Service.

BURROS, O. (1972). *The Mental Measurement Yearbook,* vol. 7. Highland Park, N.J.: Gryphon Press.

BUSCAGLIA, L. (1975). *The Disabled and Their Parents: A Counseling Challenge.* Thorofare, N.J.: C.B. Slack, inc.

CASSELL, R. (1957). *The Cassell Group Level of Aspiration Test.* Beverly Hills, Calif.: Western Psychological Services.

CHUSID, J., and J. MCDONALD (1967). *Correlative Neuroanatomy and Functional Neurology,* 13th ed. Los Altos, Calif.: Lange Medical Publications.

COMFORT, A. (1976). *A Good Age.* New York: Crown.

CRONBACH, L. (1960). *Essentials of Psychological Testing,* 2nd Ed. New York: Harper & Row.

DARLEY, F. (1964). *Diagnosis and Appraisal of Communication Disorders.* Englewood Cliffs, N.J.: Prentice-Hall, Inc.

DARLEY, F.; A. ARONSON; and J. BROWN (1969a). "Differential Diagnostic Patterns of Dysarthria." *Journal of Speech and Hearing Research,* 12: 246–269.

———— (1969b). "Clusters of Deviant Speech Dimensions in the Dysarthrias." *Journal of Speech and Hearing Research,* 12: 462–496.

———— (1975) *Motor Disorders of Speech.* Philadelphia: W.B. Saunders, Co.

DAVIS, F. (1975). "Standards for Educational and Psychological Tests." in *Tests in Print II,* ed. O. Burros. Highland Park, N.J.: Gryphon Press.

DAVIS, H., and S. SILERMAN (1970). *Hearing and Deafness,* 3rd ed. New York: Holt, Rinehart & Winston, Inc.

DODSON, F. (1970). *How to Parent.* New York: The New American Library.

DOLL, E. (1964). *Vineland Social Maturity Scale.* Circle Pines, Minn.: American Guidance Service, Inc.

DREIKURS, R. (1972). *Coping with Children's Misbehavior: A Parent's Guide.* New York: Hawthorn Books, Inc.

DUBOSE, R., and M. LANGLEY (1977). *Developmental Screening Inventory.* Boston: Teaching Resources Corporation.

DUNN, L. (1965). *Expanded Manual for the Peabody Picture Vocabulary Test.* Circle Pines, Minn.: American Guidance Service.

EMERICK, L. (1971). *A Workbook in Clinical Audiometry.* Springfield, Ill.: Charles C. Thomas.

EMERICK, L., and S. HOOD (1974). *The Client-Clinician Relationship.* Springfield, Ill.: Charles C. Thomas.

FLETCHER, S. (1972). "Time-by-Count Measurement of Diadochokinetic syllable rate." *Journal of Speech and Hearing Research,* 15: 763–770.

FRANKENBURG, W., and J. DODDS (1969). *Denver Developmental Screening Test.* Denver: University of Colorado Medical Center.

GINOTT, H. (1965). *Between Parent and Child.* New York: Macmillan.

GINOTT, H. (1969). *Between Parent and Teenager.* New York: Avon.

GOFFMAN, E. (1963). *Stigma: Notes on the Management of Spoiled Identity.* Englewood Cliffs, N.J.: Prentice-Hall, Inc.

GOODENOUGH, F. L. (1926). *Measurement of Intelligence by Drawings.* Yonkers, N.Y.: World Book Company.

GRINKER, R., and A. SAHS (1966). *Neurology,* 6th ed. Springfield, Ill.: Charles C. Thomas.

HAHN, E. (1961). "Indicators for Direct, Nondirect, and Indirect Methods in Speech Correction." *Journal of Speech and Hearing Disorders,* 26: 230–236.

HEDRICK, D.; E. PRATHER; and A. TOBIN (1975). *Sequenced Inventory of Communicative Development.* Seattle: University of Washington Press.

HOLLINGSHEAD, A., and F. REDLICH (1958). *Social Class and Mental Illness.* New York: John Wiley & Sons, Inc.

HUBBELL, R. (1977). "On Facilitating Spontaneous Talking in Young Children." *Journal of Speech and Hearing Disorders,* 42: 216–231.

JOHNSON, W.; F. DARLEY; and D. SPRIESTERSBACH (1963). *Diagnostic Methods in Speech Pathology*. New York: Harper & Row.

KEENAN, J., and E. BRAZZELL (1975). *Aphasia Language Performance Scales*. Murfreesboro, Tenn.: Pinnacle Press.

KNOBLOCH, H., and PASAMANICK, B. (1974). *Developmental Diagnosis*, 3rd ed. New York: Harper & Row.

KORMAN, A. (1974). *The Psychology of Motivation*. Englewood Cliffs, N.J.: Prentice-Hall, Inc.

LEITER, R. (1948). *International Performance Scale*. Chicago: Stoelting.

LEUTENEGGER, R. (1975). *Patient Care and Rehabilitation of Communication-Impaired Adults*. Springfield, Ill.: Charles C. Thomas.

MARTIN, F. (1975). *Introduction to Audiology*. Englewood Cliffs, N.J.: Prentice-Hall, Inc.

MASLOW, A. (1943). "A Theory of Human Motivation." *Psych Review*, 50: 370–396.

McCLELLAND, D., and R. STEELE (1972). *Motivation Workshops*. New York: General Learning Press.

——— (1973). *Human Motivation: A Book of Readings*. New York: General Learning Press.

McDANIELS, J. (1969). *Physical Disability and Human Behavior*. New York: Pergamon Press.

MECHAM, M.; J. JEX; and J. JONES (1967). *The Utah Test of Language Development*. Salt Lake City: Communication Research Associates.

MINIFIE, F.; T. HIXON; and F. WILLIAMS (1973). *Normal Aspects of Speech, Hearing and Language*. Englewood Cliffs, N.J.: Prentice-Hall, Inc.

Minnesota Scale for Parental Occupations (1950). Minneapolis: Institute of Child Welfare, University of Minnesota.

NEWBY, H. (1972). *Audiology*, 3rd ed. New York: Appleton-Century-Crofts.

O'NEILL, J., and H. OYER (1966). *Applied Audiometry*. New York: Dodd, Mead & Co.

OHLSEN, M. (1974). *Guidance Services in the Modern School*. New York: Harcourt, Brace, Jovanovich.

PAGE, J. (1975). *Psychopathology*. New York: Aldine.

PEREZ, F. (1976). "Behavioral Analysis of Clinical Judgment." *Perceptual and Motor Skills*, 43: 711–718.

PERSKE, R. (1973). *New Directions for Parents of Persons Who Are Retarded*. New York: Abingdon Press.

RAPH, J. (1960). "Determinates of Motivation in Speech Therapy." *Journal of Speech and Hearing Disorders*, 25: 13–17.

RAVEN, J. (1948). *Progressive Matrices*. New York: Psychological Corporation.

REISSMAN, L. (1959). *Class in American Society*. New York: The Free Press.

ROTTER, J. (1954). *Social Learning and Clinical Psychology*. Englewood Cliffs, N.J.: Prentice-Hall, Inc.

ROWEN, B. (1973). *The Children We See*. New York: Holt, Rinehart & Winston.

RUTTER, M.; P. GRAHAM; and W. YULE (1976). *A Neuropsychiatric Study in Childhood*. Philadelphia: J.B. Lippincott.

SATALOFF, J. (1966). *Hearing Loss*. Philadelphia: J.B. Lippincott.

SCHUELL, H.; J. JENKINS; and E. JIMENEZ-PABON (1964). *Aphasia in Adults*. New York: Harper & Row.

SCHULTZ, M., and M. CARPENTER (1973). "The Bases of Speech Pathology and Audiology." *Journal of Speech and Hearing Disorders*, 38: 395–404.

SUNBERG, N., and L. TYLER (1962). *Clinical Psychology*. New York: Appleton-Century-Crofts.

TAYLOR, J. (1963). "Screening Intelligence." *Journal of Speech and Hearing Disorders*, 28: 90–91.

TERMAN, L., and M. MERRILL (1960). *Stanford-Binet Intelligence Scale: Manual for the Third Revision* (Form L-M). Boston: Houghton Mifflin Company.

VAN ALSTYNE, D. (1960). *Van Alstyne Picture Vocabulary Test*. New York: Harcourt, Brace & World.

VAN RIPER, C. (1963). *Speech Correction: Principles and Methods*, 4th ed. Englewood Cliffs, N.J.: Prentice-Hall, Inc.

—— (1972). *Speech Correction: Principles and Methods*, 5th ed. Englewood Cliffs, N.J.: Prentice-Hall, Inc.

—— (1973). *The Treatment of Stuttering*, Englewood Cliffs, N.J.: Prentice-Hall, Inc.

WARNER, W.; M. MEEKER; and K. ELLS (1960). *Social Class in America*. New York: Harper & Row.

WECHSLER, P. (1955). *Manual for the Wechsler Adult Intelligence Scale*. New York: Psychological Corporation.

—— (1949). *Manual for the Wechsler Intelligence Scale for Children*. New York: Psychological Corporation.

—— (1967). *Preschool and Primary Scale of Intelligence*. New York: Psychological Corporation.

WEINER, P., and W. HOOCK (1973). "The Standardization of Tests: Criteria and Criticism." *Journal of Speech and Hearing Research,* 16: 616–626.

WOOD, N. (1964). *Delayed Speech and Language Development*. Englewood Cliffs, N.J.: Prentice-Hall, Inc.

4

Diagnosis of Language Disorders in Children

It will be difficult to convince the student of language disorders that we are indeed at the frontier of our knowledge of this interesting and perplexing topic. The voluminous literature relating to language-disordered children leads one to believe that a great deal is known about how to test and treat language disorders. However, it has been said that less than 5 percent of what is accepted as fact today regarding language disorders will be considered valid twenty-five years from now. So rapid is the growth of knowledge and so tenuous is the nature of the theoretical framework for our understanding of language that it is somewhat presumptuous to put in print anything of an absolute nature regarding diagnosis of language disorders in children.

The vastness of the language area has led some to abandon the study in frustration. As the topic unfolds the student realizes that some background in linguistics, child development, learning theory, and speech pathology is necessary in order to adequately understand the complexities of the problem. Contradictory and conflicting points of view should be considered healthy and encouraging rather than demoralizing and frustrating. The broad scope of the language area is a challenge, not a threat, and should be met with interest and enthusiasm. Students should set small attainable goals, systematize their studies, and work for an understanding of the rationale of diagnosis as well as the technique.

THEORETICAL FRAMEWORK

Although everyone knows what language is, there is no universally accepted definition. Language work to an elementary school teacher may be "show and tell" time, whereas the learning-disabilities teacher may equate language problems with reading disability, while the speech clinician may define language disorders relative to the rules of syntax, semantics, and phonology. For purposes of this discussion, language is defined as a socially acquired, primarily aural, inductively acquired, symbol system used to communicate between and within individuals. Figure 4.1 differentiates three primary concepts which are central to the writer's definition of language. Pre- and sub-language behaviors are those factors which are necessary for the development of the language system but are not a part of the system itself.

The reader can identify in many sources instances where "language" work consists of eye-hand coordination training, teaching children how to attend to stimuli, gross motor drills, and similar activities. According to the present writing such activities would not be included as language-directed but rather as sub-language work. This differentiation is important in order to clearly understand the conflicting uses of the term language.

Language as a central-nervous-system capacity is, in essence, a system of rules or a body of knowledge. Language-dependent behaviors included in the top of Figure 4.1 are activities which are believed to depend upon the language system but are not part of the system itself. Reading and speaking, for example, are activities which use the language system. Hopefully this differentiation among sub-language, language, and language-dependent levels assists the reader in understanding the variety of perspectives found in the literature.

An appreciation of the various theoretical explanations of language should assist the reader in his scouting of the literature in three basic ways. First, the developmental nature of language acquisition will be more meaningful if it is placed in some unified context. The knowledgeable student of language is able to measure individual development based upon the factors that influence the child, the child's typical stages of language learning, and the general characteristics of the normal process. Second, the nature of language as a symbol system is only truly put into perspective from a theoretical base; without some background in theory the student is helpless to interpret conflicting information and points of view. Third, the theoretical foundations must be familiar to anyone who wishes to investigate and manipulate abnormal language behavior. An understanding of the abnormal most logically stems from a thorough appreciation of the normal.

Learning Theory

Almost unchallenged, learning theory has held the limelight as the primary source of authoritative information about language for many years. Speech pathology has drawn heavily upon learning theory both for its understanding of

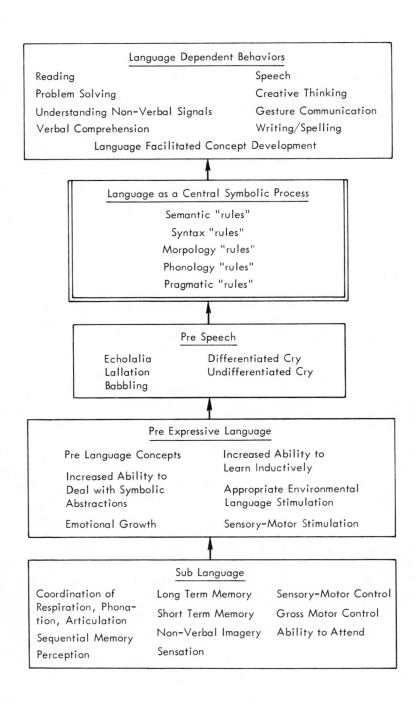

Figure 4.1 Sub-Language, Language, and Language-Dependent Areas of Behavior.

normal behavior and as a therapeutic rationale. Wingate (1971) aptly describes the dependency relationship developed between speech pathology and psychology in stuttering theory and therapy, and the same case could be made for our understanding of language. At the foundation of all learning theory is the understanding that language, as a form of human behavior, is basically learned.

Linguistic Theory

Psychology and linguistics are, of course, parallel disciplines and rarely converged until recently. This unfortunate hiatus has produced quite different views of language behavior. The currently most popular and seminal linguistic theory is probably the generative grammar theory attributed to Chomsky (1957) and his associates. Although there have been several variations and major modifications since its inception, one central theme appears paramount. Perkins (1977: 99–100) states it clearly:

> Human infants apparently begin life as cryptographers innately equipped biologically to ''crack'' society's communication code within a few years. No other hypothesis offered so far comes close to explaining a baby's extraordinary capacity to decipher speech.

The biological orientation of Lenneberg (1967), the ''sentence-centerism'' of McNeil (1970), and the ''transformational'' postulates of Chomsky all appear to rely heavily on the assumption that language facility is a basic part of human nature.

The classic battle is clearly in focus: Is language a learned behavior that requires just the right amount of motivation, stimulation, and reinforcement? Or is it an innate characteristic of the human species, in which case a child has all of the language potential at birth and only needs maturation and progressive refinement of potential to fit into his own language system? The awesome impact of this conflict has yet to be felt in any real, applicable way in the rehabilitation fields. In fact, it is curious to note that although the theories differ significantly, there have been only minimal attempts to synthesize the linguistic postulates into some practical therapeutic application. The unfortunate consequence has been that speech pathologists have followed the shifting winds of psychological theory for the past fifty years. Since linguists have displayed (until recently) little interest in clinical applications of their formulations, it is understandable that speech clinicians have relied more upon applicable psychological theory.

> Over the past thirty years there have been several shifts in emphasis in the study of linguistics. It may be helpful in understanding current perspectives to trace the contributions of the following: L. Bloomfield and descriptive linguistics, N. Chomsky and transformation grammar, C. Fillmore and case grammar, J. Piaget and cognitive development, and M. Halliday and pragmatics.

GUIDING PRINCIPLES

We now present five interrelated principles which we feel will aid the clinician in conducting a more revealing and productive diagnosis of language disorders in children. In the ensuing discussion we shall try to be consistent with these principles.

1. Language is a broad and all-encompassing category of human behavior: *Know your competency areas and remain within them.* Speaking, listening, writing, reading, thinking, problem-solving, discriminating, perceiving, recalling—all directly involve language. No one can be expected to be knowledgeable in *all* of the areas of language, but an understanding of the breadth of the language system creates a reverence for its impact upon human behavior. The well-informed diagnostician is aware that the area he is assessing has far-reaching implications.

2. Our knowledge of language, both normal and abnormal, is fragmented and incomplete: *Accept this state of affairs not as a source of frustration but as a source of motivation to learn more and add to the body of knowledge.* The student of language disorders is often demoralized by the apparently overwhelming amount of information available and the inconclusive nature of so many vital issues. No final chapters have been written on any aspect of language disorders and diagnosis.

3. No single measure (or session) is adequate to totally evaluate and understand a child's language ability: *Make your diagnosis an ongoing rather than a static undertaking.* There are two major arguments in favor of this point of view. First, a child's language behavior is continually changing, and no single measure can predict or describe the course of the change. In fact, the course of language development may be as important to diagnosis as the presenting problem. Second, the language process is so complex that it demands more than one method of diagnosis. Diagnosis must tell the clinician where the child is, how he got there, where he should be, and how to initiate work with him to move him from where he is to where he should be. Diagnosis must reflect the progress made and point out the progress not made. It must serve as a continuing source of information to be monitored.

4. Diagnosis of language facility should be made *in situ* rather than through some abstract process. *The crucial aspect of language is the ability to receive and transmit information for useful purposes in real life situations* (Clark, 1975). The importance of this point of view cannot be overestimated. Language diagnosticians have for too long been satisfied with test results which, in reality, only measured some small portion of a child's total language performance in an artifical testing situation. This is not to say that test data are of no importance; on the contrary, most of the remainder of this chapter will be devoted to a discussion of the practical application of standardized tests. We simply wish to encourage the diagnostician to look carefully at the child's total language behavior as he uses it for everyday functioning.

5. *Know the normal language developmental process.* Knowledge of the normal language-development process provides the key to language diagnosis. Comparison of child behavior with expected behaviors not only leads to determinations of the existence of language disorders but also gives clues as to where to begin the clinical process and remedial goals.

DIAGNOSIS OF ORAL LANGUAGE DISORDERS

The complexity of language diagnosis is a direct reflection of the myriad of variables that impinge on language acquisition. "A young child's success in learning to talk depends on his ability to perceive and organize his environment, the language that is a part of that environment, and the relation between the two" (Bloom, 1970: 1).

Language is a set of *systems* that have social, neurophysiological, psychological, and temporal requisites and that allow the individual to relate sound to meaning as an individualistic, internalized, representational process. We are concerned with the development of the systems that affect sound differentiation and production, syntax and grammatical acquisition, vocabulary development, conceptualization, and the transfer of these basic attributes to varying modalities through such skills as speaking, writing, reading, and understanding.

Screening Procedures

Screening children in order to identify significant language disorders is typically part of most early childhood education programs and is routine in "kindergarten roundup" programs conducted by public schools. As public laws mandate special educational services to handicapped children at younger ages, the need for efficient identification procedures increases.

In determining which screening device to employ the clinician must take the following considerations into account:

1. Efficiency: Does the test provide accurate information in a short amount of time?
2. Identification only: The task demands of the test need only relate to whether the child has a language problem or not; the purpose of this testing is not in-depth diagnosis.
3. Information readily available: Laborious scoring and interpretive demands should be avoided.
4. Inexpensive: Since large numbers of children will be evaluated, materials should be inexpensive.
5. Group administration: It would be helpful if some portions of the screening device may be group administered.
6. Standardized procedure: Uniformity of administration is just as important in screening as in diagnostic testing; therefore, clear instructions as to administration and scoring procedures are needed.

7. Available norms: Norms should be developed from a standardization population that is randomly chosen and representative of the population which will be tested. Standardization populations should also be large enough to give stability to the norms provided.
8. Validity and reliability: As with all testing procedures, the examiner expects the instrument to measure what it purports to measure and have adequate stability to insure some degree of confidence in the obtained score.

No screening device for language has yet been devised which adequately meets all of these criteria. However, a number of devices, as yet mostly in the experimental stage of development, warrant mention.

Northwestern Syntax Screening Test. The *NSST* (Lee, 1969) was developed as a screening instrument by Laura Lee and has been extensively employed by speech clinicians. Partially because the test is rather lengthy and partially because the kit provides more information than the traditional screening device, it has become widely used for diagnostic purposes beyond the author's original intention. Lee (1977) has strongly urged that the test be used for screening purposes only.

The *NSST* taps both receptive and expressive abilities and measures a variety of syntactic elements. Arndt (1977) criticizes the test for the small number of items included, makeup of the standardization sample, and lack of information regarding temporal stability. Byrne (1977) concludes her discussion of the test with the suggestion that "we should stop using the present version." (1977: 321) Lest we throw out the baby with the bath water, it may be well to continue to encourage development of instruments such as the *NSST* and develop personal norms useful within limited populations. It has been our experience that the skilled clinician can use instruments such as the NSST effectively through wise interpretation of the data and minimal reliance upon published norms. Most clinicians who employ it use it as an intermediate testing device once it has been established that a language problem exists. The end result is that the test functions as something more than just a screening device.

Utah Test of Language Development. Mecham et al. (1973) proposed the administration of a limited number of items from the *Utah Test of Language Development* as a screening instrument. Only 2½ minutes are needed to administer the items, which include reciting nursery rhymes, naming colors, repeating sentences, copying forms, and naming pictures. Extremely limited norms are available (Mecham et al., 1973) for the screening portion of the test, and the user may find it necessary to develop regional norms if this test is employed.

Preschool Language Screening Test. Fluharty (1974) devised this test for screening three-to-five-year-old children. Tasks are included which are purported to indicate the child's articulation, vocabulary, and receptive and expressive language levels. The test consists of thirty-five items divided into three sections, and requires approximately five minutes to administer. Item selection was based upon transformational theory. The test was standardized on only 203 preschool children selected from three socioeconomic levels and both black and white racial backgrounds. Although cut-off scores are presented by the author, further data collection is warranted. The Fluharty test offers the advantages of speed, careful construction using linguistic theory as a guide, and it does tap several language aspects.

Screening Test for Auditory Comprehension of Language. Carrow (1973) developed this twenty-five item screening test from the larger *Test of Auditory Comprehension of Language.* The test measures comprehension exclusively and is intended for group administration. The test was standardized on 400 middle-class children in age groups three through six. The norms are based on group results and are not applicable to one-to-one testing. The *STACL* is a valuable screening instrument for language comprehension but is usually used in conjunction with some measure of expressive skill.

Stephens Oral Language Screening Test. The SOLST (Stephens, 1977) is designed as a screening device for articulation and syntax. The test uses sentence imitation for evaluation of children from four years four months to seven years of age. A scoring procedure for syntax is employed which reflects varying degrees of response accuracy while traditional articulation screening procedures are used.

Stephens presents comparison data on the SOLST with the DSS and CELI procedures. In addition standardization data is presented for impressively large groups of children for prekindergarten, kindergarten, and first grade children. The author has done an admirable job of presenting data and has left the actual screening selection process to the examiner.

This test is quick to administer with only fifteen sentences to be repeated and,with some practice, the scoring procedure is useful diagnostically. As an efficient articulation and syntax screening tool the SOLST is worthy of consideration.

Several broader screening devices contain a language section. Investigate the following:

BLUMA, S.; M. SHEARER; A. FROHMAN; and J. HILLIARD (1976). *Portage Guide to Early Education.* Portage, Wis., CESA 12.

FRANKENBERG, W., and J. DODDS (1967). *Denver Developmental Screening Test.* Denver: University of Colorado Medical Center.

GRAY, B., and B. RYAN (1971). *Programmed Conditioning for Language Test.* Monterey, California, Accelerated Achievement Associates.

HANNA, E., and J. GARDNER (1974) *Preschool Language Screening Test.* Northridge, California, Joyce Publications.

KNOBLOCH, H.; P. PASAMANICK; and E. SHERARD (1966). *A Developmental Screening Inventory For Infants.* Pediatrics, Vol. 38, Dec.

MARDELL, C., and D. GOLDENBERG (1975). *Developmental Indicators for the Assessment of Learning* (DIAL), Highland Park, Ill., DIAL Inc.

MONSEES, E., and C. BERMAN (1968). ''Speech and language screening in a summer headstart program.'' *Journal of Speech and Hearing Disorders,* 33: 121–125.

SANFORD, A. (1974). *Learning Accomplishment Profile,* Winston-Salem, N.C., Kaplan Press.

SLINGERLAND, B. (1967). *Screening Tests for Identifying Children with Specific Language Disability,* Cambridge, Mass.: Educators Publishing Service, Inc.

THWING, E., and H. IRETON (1975). *Minnesota Child Development Inventory* (MCDI), Minneapolis, Interpretive Scoring Systems.

Determining the Existence of a Problem

With the exception of traumatic cases, every eight-year-old child with deviant language behavior was once a three-year-old with *deviating* language behavior. Language is an emerging behavior which explodes to nearly full maturity in the first three years of life and continues to be refined and developed for several years thereafter. As we look at the language of a preacademic child, we must look not only at his behavior of yesterday and today but beyond to his future potential. With a clear knowledge of what is expected of a child of a given age, it is possible to accurately identify existing or potential language difficulties in very young children; with our current understanding of the importance of these first few years, early diagnosis and therapeutic intervention are imperative.

Determining whether a child's language behavior is within normal limits is not always an easy task. Parents, teachers, physicians, and other referring sources often seek assistance without having a clear concept of the exact nature of the problem:

> Jimmy was an alert two-year-old with observing eyes and a placid disposition. He understood directions and conversations appropriately for his two years but was speechless. Jimmy's mother was concerned, but not to the point of seeking help until a year later when the child passed his third birthday without (reportedly) emitting a single meaningful word. The family physician calmly acknowledged all the information offered by Mrs. H. and then offered his professional opinion: ''Jimmy will grow out of it.'' As the child approached his fourth birthday, he spoke his first words, his first phrase, and indeed his first sentence, all at the same time. ''Mama, kitty's got a robin!'' came the shriek from the backyard. Mrs. H. knew at once that the voice was that of her son and the doctor's sage advice had come true. Jimmy's expressive language was normal by his fifth birthday.

The trouble with this account is that all too often the hopes of maturational miracles disappear as the five-year-old struggles unsuccessfully to compete in a verbally oriented kindergarten class.

The speech clinician cannot afford to be uncertain about the existence of a problem. He must have tools available to him which will aid in the determination, and he must have the knowledge to use those tools effectively. Father says his son is speaking well for his age, mother says her son doesn't talk right, the physician claims the child will grow out of it, and the speech clinician must resolve the dilemma. This, then, is the starting point in diagnosis. The information gained will lead the diagnostician logically into the other areas of evaluation or encourage him to terminate the diagnosis at that point.

Does the child have a language problem? In a sense this concern is more theoretical than real, since we are asking the diagnostician to keep the concept in his head during the total assessment instead of segmenting his diagnosis into artificial categories. The clinician looks at a child through the prism of any of the various measuring techniques, and he uses this focus to organize and classify the information received. Continuous refinement of technique will provide greater diagnostic information regarding not only the existence of the problem but at what level of competence the child is performing. Such information has direct implications for the therapy process when the clinician attempts to initiate work at the proper level of complexity.

Early students (Head, 1926; Myklebust, 1954) promulgated a three-part concept of the language process that employed the categories of reception, central integration, and expression. Myklebust's clinical applications of this early formulation to an assessment and therapeutic model were widely accepted, and the terms receptive, inner, and expressive language were still extensively used by practicing therapists. Even the most recent revision of the ITPA (Kirk, McCarthy, and Kirk, 1968) and similar measures rely heavily on the input-integration-output concept. Berry (1969) refutes the validity of this model on the basis of neurological as well as behavioral findings. Even though we acknowledge that reception and expression are not separate entities, but interrelated behaviors with strong neurological interdependencies (Schuell, Jenkins, Jimenez-Pabon, 1964), the convenience of the breakdown and the efficiency of the classical model are too great to ignore.

Language is the function of the central nervous system. As such it is not indebted to specific input or output modalities. Language assessment, therefore, should most logically deal with central processing functions and not the various receptive and expressive channels. From a practical basis, however, this would lead to a restricted form of information. Clearly, language acquisition would be impossible if auditory, visual, and haptic channels were all dysfunctioning; and language competence would be of limited value if all methods of expression were peripherally interrupted.

General language development measures. A variety of approaches are used to establish a child's general language-performance level. Some diagnosticians prefer to use survey measures which tap a number of language functions to get an overview of the child's abilities, while others use parent interview techniques, developmental scales, or measures of a variety of so-called psycholinguistic abilities. Certain of these techniques use norms and established standardized procedures, while others relate the child's performance to the normal developmental process in a comparison of performance to criterion. No matter what the technique, the purpose is to determine whether the child does present a language disorder or is functioning normally.

The selection of the diagnostic technique to be used with any given child is a function of the child, his age and general language functioning, and the diagnostician's preferences. A brief review of some of the major general language development measures follows:

Growing out of Osgood's (1957) three-dimensional model of language behavior, the *Illinois Test of Psycholinguistic Abilities* (Kirk, McCarthy, and Kirk, 1968) enjoyed a monopoly in the clinician's language-assessment armamentarium several years ago. First published in experimental form in 1961, the test swiftly filled a void in the field, and there were few reference points with which to compare it. Since that time, however, the test has come under careful scrutiny and is now considered as only one of many useful measures. The test, designed for use with children two to ten years of age, consists of twelve subtests and yields a language age and a diagnostic profile of psycholinguistic abilities. Clinical experience has shown that the *ITPA* language age correlates highly with general intellectual abilities. The following statement from Hammill and Bartel (1975) is representative of the opinion of many language clinicians.:

> Although the ITPA has been valuable in stimulating interest and research in language, its major shortcoming is the omission of subtests for linguistic abilities (syntax, phonology, or transformations) . . . The test is valuable when the examiner is concerned with such variables as memory or closure, or with receptive, associative, or expressive performance at various levels. (Hammill and Bartel, 1975: 172).

Since we have found the *ITPA* to correlate highly with intelligence, and since it does not directly tap language functioning, it is not particularly valuable as a measure to determine the existence of a language disorder. However, it is a useful device to assist in directing the remedial effort, since it provides the profile of abilities outlining the child's particular strengths and weaknesses. [For a comprehensive review of the *ITPA* and the uses of it, see Newcomer, P., and D. Hammill (1976). *Psycholinguistics In the Schools* (1976); for research confirmation of our clinical findings regarding the relationship between the ITPA language age and intelligence, see Huszinga, R., (1973).]

Two tests which are somewhat similar in purpose are the *Houston Test for Language Development* (Crabtree, 1963) and the *Utah Test of Language Development* (Mecham, M., J. Jex, and J. Jones, 1967). Both tests measure general language functioning. The Houston test measures receptive and expressive abilities in children ranging in age from 6 months to 6 years. Part of the test is based upon child observation and part upon direct interaction with the child. The test attempts to follow developmental norms; however, only superficial standardization attempts have been made. The test assists in providing a general view of the child's language skills and includes measures of syntactical complexity, intonation, vocabulary, comprehension, and self-identity. The *Houston Test for Language Development* can best be considered an early contribution to our language-diagnosis armament. Newer and more comprehensive procedures have since been developed.

The *Utah Test of Language Development* (Mecham et al., 1967) includes fifty-one items to measure receptive and expressive language in children 18 months to 14½ years. The test culminates in a language age and includes items of a concept-development nature such as knowledge of colors, money, and numbers. Since only 273 children, all identified as normal white subjects, served in the standardization population, the original norms should be interpreted with caution. Mecham, Jex, and Jones report (1973) the administration of the *UTLD* to an additional 989 children, but complete norm data on that testing has not been published.

Two prominent tests aimed at establishing the child's language functioning use the interview technique exclusively. The *Verbal Language Development Scale* (Mecham, 1958) is an extension of the communication portion of the *Vineland Social Maturity Scale* and as such provides the diagnostician with a language age-equivalent as observed by an adult. This 50-item test has not been thoroughly standardized, and little normative data is provided. More sophisticated techniques now exist to evaluate the language functioning of young children. Some examiners find the *VLDS* a helpful adjunct when conducting an interview with the parents of a language-delayed child.

Bzoch and League (1971) clearly state their preference for a separation between reception and expression in their publication of the *Receptive-Expressive Emergent Language Scale* (REEL). This measure, primarily an interview technique, provides the examiner with a receptive quotient, expressive quotient, and composite language quotient on children from birth to three years of age. As the authors state (1971: 16):

> The REEL Scale is grounded on three basic premises regarding language function. Briefly stated, these are as follows:
>
> 1. The auditory modality is the primary means of acquiring language.
>
> 2. Language is an innate (genetically based) capacity of man.
>
> 3. Speech behavior and cognitive development are inseparably interconnected.

Although the authors indicate its usefulness for differential diagnosis, the REEL appears to have greatest value in revealing language problems and determining the level of language functioning of a given child. The interview technique has inherent shortcomings, and although the authors contend that a single brief interview is adequate to accurately score the REEL, it is better to use it in conjunction with extended observation of the child.

Similarly based on the receptive-expressive dichotomy is the *Preschool Language Scale* of Zimmerman, Steiner, and Evatt (1969). The test gives an auditory comprehension age and quotient as well as a verbal ability age and quotient; it is designed for children from one and one-half years of age to seven years. Unlike the REEL, this scale requires the clinician to examine the child directly.

The scale is basically a compilation of subtests from other tests and fails to evaluate many important language areas such as components of the grammatical system, transformational forms, and morphonological items. The authors of the *Preschool Language Scale* state that each task within the scale was given an age placement on the basis of empirical evidence of the average age of attainment by preschool children; however, no normative data is provided in the test manual. The scale is in its experimental form and appears in need of further research and development.

The *Michigan Picture Language Inventory* (Lerea, 1958; Wolski, 1962) evaluates vocabulary comprehension, vocabulary expression, language-structure comprehension, and language-structure expression. Lerea's tests of grammatical structure included the following areas: nouns (singular and plural), personal and possessive pronouns, adjectives and adverbs, demonstrative articles, prepositions, and verbs and auxiliaries. This initial edition of the *MPLI* is considered by the author to be experimental, but the general assessment concept holds promise. It is anticipated, however, that it will be necessary to evaluate greater amounts of language (both input and output) than one-word stimuli and responses in order to get a true picture of a child's language structure.

The *Parsons Language Sample* (Spradlin, 1963) is comprised of seven subtests based on the Skinnerian system of language behavior. The subtests acknowledge the receptive-expressive nature of language and include tests of tacting, echoic, intraverbal (all vocal), echoic gesture, comprehension, intraverbal gesture (all nonverbal), and the test of manding which is both verbal and nonverbal. It is interesting to note that Spradlin (1967), author of the *PLS*, later made several criticisms of the test and similar instruments. His criticisms included the fact that the *PLS*, in the main, demands only single-word responses from the child, thus giving little opportunity to measure the intricacies of grammatical acquisition. Strangely, the Skinnerian model of language development has failed to generate a great deal of research in the diagnosis of language disorders. This is no doubt in part due to the fact that the behaviorists have shunned diagnosis in the traditional sense in order to concentrate more heavily on other factors.

In the *Test of Language Development*, Newcomer and Hammill (1977) attempted to put together a battery of subtests measuring expressive and receptive areas of phonology, semantics, and syntax. Although a linguistic frame of reference was maintained throughout, the authors stated they were not dictated by any single linguistic theory. The test, designed for children aged 4-0 years to 8-11 years, includes picture vocabulary, oral vocabulary, grammatic understanding, sentence imitation, grammatic completion, word discrimination, and word articulation subtests. A language age and linguistic quotient are derived based upon norminative data collected on 1,014 children from a cross section of geographic and socioeconomic levels. Scaled score equivalents for raw scores are obtainable for each subtest, allowing comparison of strengths in the various language areas. The word-discrimination and word-articulation subtests appear to be somewhat out of place in this language-oriented test, and many of the other subtests appear to be shortened versions of similar measures. No adequate procedure is included to measure extended discourse. Compared to many of the commercially available language tests, the *TOLD* shows significant improvement in standardization procedure. With due precautions, many of which are mentioned in the test manual, this test should be useful in language diagnoses.

Using items from established tests and some newly developed, Hedrick, Prather, and Tobin (1975) published the *Sequenced Inventory of Communication Development*. Intended for children aged 4 months to 48 months the inventory measures both receptive and expressive communication abilities. Although the measure results in an expressive and receptive communication age, the authors caution that this should be only considered an aid in the diagnostic process and that other measures should be used in conjunction with it. The receptive items include awareness, discrimination and understanding elements, while the expressive items include motor, vocal, verbal, imitative, initiating, and responding behaviors. The inventory includes an impressive compilation of items developmentally arranged. Although the test is somewhat cumbersome to administer at first, it provides a great deal of useful information and is of value to the clinician if used only as a ready reference to normal communication development. It should be noted that the standardization population consisted of only 252 children.

Based upon the work of Schlesinger (1971), the *Environmental Language Inventory* (MacDonald and Nickols, 1974) measures language structures relating to semantic intention. A limited number of semantic-grammatical rules are thought to be present in emerging language. Table 4-1 presents the semantic grammatical rules which provide the basis for the *ELI* design.

Table 4-1 Semantic Grammatical Rules Which Form the Basis of the Environmental Language Inventory

1. Agent-Action	(Daddy throw)
2. Action-Object	(Throw ball)
3. Agent-Object	(Mommy sock)
4. Location (Agent/Object)	(Ball chair)
5. Location (Action)	(Throw here)
6. Negation - X	(No ball)
7. Modifier + Head Attribution	(Big train)
8. Modifier + Possession	(My car)
9. Modifier + Recurrence	(More milk)
10. Introducer - X	(Hi dolly see boy)

To summarize, then, the *Environmental Language Inventory (ELI)* strategy presents an approach to diagnosis and training of language delay through rules, context, and generalization. The rules are those governing the early constructions of normally developing children. The context includes both the linguistic and non-linguistic environment of a given rule and is used to elicit that rule in the child's speech. Finally, the strategy is designed toward generalization training with its inclusion of imitative, conversational, and play tasks. The term "environmental language intervention" is used to indicate that the present strategy reflects an environmental approach to language in two ways. First, by utilizing both the linguistic and non-linguistic environment of an utterance, the strategy recognizes the semantic component of that utterance. At the same time, by using imitation, conversation, and play as the modes for diagnosis and training, the strategy extends intervention to the child's natural language development. (MacDonald and Nickols, 1974: 7)

The *ELI* takes about thirty to forty-five minutes to administer and provides the clinician with valuable information relative to a semantic-based language-intervention program. (See MacDonald et al. 1974) The procedure represents a welcome addition to the growing trend to integrate assessment of language structure and function.

Measures of specific language functions. Many tests are available which measure only a single component of language. Such indexes provide the diagnostician with information regarding a single element of language and may assist in the determination of the existence of a language disorder as well as establishing a starting point for clinical intervention. We will differentiate between receptive and expressive skills and point out measures which tap semantic, phonologic, and syntactic aspects of the system.

The comprehension of individual semantic units requires recognition of the word, relating that word to past experiences, and correct retrieval of the meaning and concepts related to the word. One way to measure a child's reception of language units is to determine the number of spoken words he understands. The *Peabody Picture Vocabulary Test* (Dunn, 1965) consists of sets of pages with four line drawings on each page. The scoring procedure results in a language age, intelligence quotient, and percentile rank. We, and other reviewers, strongly resist the use of this test as a measure of intelligence, particularly when such measures are for children with known language disorders. The test is designed for individuals aged 2 years and 3 months to 18 years and 5 months. It is among the best measures of language with regard to standardization, population, and reliability studies.

The *PPVT* is an extremely popular test. Stark (1971) found that over 70 percent of the speech clinicians responding to his survey reported using the test. Several cautions should be noted. Kresheck and Nicolosi (1973) found a possible cultural bias against Black children in the *PPVT,* and the same authors (1972) also found that forms *A* and *B* result in significantly different mental ages although they are presented as parallel forms. Blood and Greenberg (1976) reported finding significant differences between the *PPVT* and the *Test for Auditory Comprehension of Language* (Carrow, 1973). The *PPVT* resulted in significantly higher scores, and others have reported similarly elevated scores on the *PPVT* relative to measures of intelligence.

The *Full Range Picture Vocabulary Test* (Ammons and Ammons, 1958) tests receptive vocabulary for individuals aged 2 years through adulthood. This test also provides two forms, and the authors report a high reliability coefficient on test-retest studies. The test contains several pictures which are dated and has not received as wide distribution as the *PPVT*.

Since both instruments cited above use words presented with no overt or related clues (such as facial expression, context, intonation), and since children probably learn language skills form the whole (context) to the part, these assessment tools probably do not provide an accurate picture of how the child will perform in everyday speaking situations. As Berry (1969: 265) points out, ". . . they do not assess the child's ability to understand words joined in language sequences or to use them in connected speech."

> It is not uncommon to learn more about the testing process during a diagnostic session than about the child. Timmy S. taught us a great deal one morning. Following a completely fruitless testing session in which we were examining Tim's ability to understand prepositions, the child was given a chance to go out and play with the other children of the summer clinic. The test had called for the child to point to pictures that depicted the preposition spoken by the examiner. The child was unable to identify even the most elementary items, which led the examiner to conclude that he understood none of them. During the following play session, Tim demanded that he be *in front of* the line, cried when the ball went *over* the fence, told the aid that the ball was *under* the car, and urged his playmates to crawl *between* his legs during a game of leapfrog. In other words, Tim used and understood many prepositions during everyday activities but was unable to display his knowledge in a single test situation.

The *Assessment of Children's Language Comprehension* (Foster, Giddan, and Stark, 1973) begins to answer some of the shortcomings of the pure vocabulary tests by adding increasing amounts of contextual elements to the receptive task. The authors state (p. 14) that the purpose of the test is "to discover at what point there is a breakdown in performance and, most importantly, to implement teaching with relevant remedial measures." The test, intended for children 3-7, consists of four levels of difficulty, beginning with a fifty-item vocabulary test in which the child is required to identify common words. At the second level of difficulty, the child is required to correctly identify the picture (from four stimuli) when the examiner indicates not only the noun but a verb or a modifier as well. As an example, the child may be asked to point to *the man sitting*—when four pictures include a man walking, a man sitting, a cat walking, and a cat sitting. At the next level of difficulty, a preposition is added to the stimuli; and at the fourth level the child must understand the subject (with or without a modifying word), the verb, and the prepositional phrase. Norms are provided on only 311 children from mixed racial, socioeconomic, and educational backgrounds and should be considered tentative. The *ACLC*, nevertheless, provides a helpful asset in the determination of the amount of language complexity a child is able to understand, and the addition of direct remedial suggestions makes the measure somewhat unique.

The *Vocabulary Comprehension Scale* (Bangs, 1975) measures understanding of pronouns and words of position, size, quality and quantity in children 2-0 to 6-0 years. The unique aspect of this procedure is the use of an interaction/play type of setting, using cardboard objects and established interaction formats, in which the examiner determines the child's understanding of the various test elements. This format adds the dimension of realism and context to the testing situation; unfortunately, the test was standardized on only eighty children in Houston, Texas, with only ten children in each age group. The end result is that the examiner receives some idea of the child's specific knowledge of various word meanings, but can have little confidence in the comparison value of the findings. The scale should be considered experimental in nature until further data collection has been accomplished.

The *Test for Auditory Comprehension of Language* (Carrow, 1973) is probably the most popular test of its kind among language clinicians. The test was designed to assess auditory comprehension of form class and function words, morphology, grammar, and syntax for children aged 3 to 6 years 11 months. As in other tests, the items are presented verbally by the examiner, and the child responds by identifying one of three picture choices. Items in the test are sequenced by grammatical category rather than level of difficulty, so the entire test must be administered to each child. The resulting score can be interpreted through percentile ranks and comparison made with children of his age group. From a diagnostic point of view, it is also helpful that comparison can be made on each of the various item classes. Once again the size of the standardization group is rather small: only 200 children from various Black, Anglo, and Mexican-American backgrounds were tested. The *TACL* provides useful information regarding the child's comprehension of various language elements and tentative information regarding his overall language comprehension relative to other children. As with any other currently available diagnostic tool, the *TACL* cannot stand alone in determining the significance of a child's language differences.

Although formal standardized tests are a necessary part of any language diagnosis, it is almost never possible to begin a diagnostic session directly with such a procedure. We have been impressed with the need to formulate opinions of a child's functioning in the early moments of a diagnostic session, prior to the administration of formal tests, while also setting the tone for optimal cooperation and performance. A procedure of semi-structured interaction has been used in the first few minutes of each language diagnosis, which provides an adequate estimate of the child's language comprehension. Emphasis here is upon natural interaction, and neither the child nor the clinician relates to the procedure as a test. Although it is used as a checklist of the child's level of language comprehension, the clinician does not bring the paper and pencil into the room. Nor does she follow a rigid structure in order to tap every possible language element. Emphasis in this initial interaction is on natural conversation in a pressure-free setting.

> Billy entered the room where the clinician was sitting on the floor arranging items of a toy village. Following a few minutes of quiet play the following edited conversation was recorded. ''Those are all big cars, you take the biggest one and give

me the red one . . . I think the fireman should go in the house . . . May I have the
truck that's beside the house? . . . Put the small ball on the truck . . . The fire truck
can go home slowly . . . I'm going to wash the car so I'll need a bucket and a rag
. . . give them to me . . ."

Nearly half an hour of such interaction was recorded, and the clinician came
away with a good insight as to how well the child comprehended language *in
context*. The end result is more appropriate test selection and more meaningful
findings. A suggested guideline for such interaction follows.

University of Minnesota, Duluth Informal Language Evaluation Format — Receptive Language

1. Determination of general organizational abilities.
   Use no instructions other than "Let's play."
   Place two objects (that might lend themselves to imaginative play) before the
     child: table and chair or baby and crib, etc. If he shows an interest in these
     objects, add two more; if interest continues, add two more, and so on.
   Note his organizational ability; note to what extent he structures the objects in a
     meaningful and significant manner.
   a. Does he structure the objects meaningfully, in a way that seems to re-
       late them to his daily experiences?
   b. Does he seem interested in only one object at a time or even in only a part
       of one object at a time, but not in grouping objects into an organized
       whole?
   c. Does he logically relate highly concrete objects, but not those of higher
       abstraction?
   d. Does he put the objects together in a haphazard fashion, showing a lack
       of understanding of their relationships?
   e. Does he put the objects in his mouth?
   f. Does he reject the play situation entirely?
   g. Does he grasp at an object and retain it indefinitely without
       attempts to use it meaningfully?
2. Semantics — Testing for understanding of word meaning.
   Nouns
   Materials: doll, toy fruit, car, furniture, tools, food, clothes.
   Presentation: Have the child point to, touch, or give you the following objects.
     — dolls representing family members, mother-father-brother-sister
     — parts of the body,
         — begin with five major items; hair, eyes, nose, mouth, arm.
         — if these are known, test elbow, knee, shoulder, skin, palm.
     — clothing
         — have child dress a doll with clothing as it is named
     — some general categorization
         — have child hand you the object referred to: fruit, vehicle, furniture,
         tools, toy, food, clothing, etc.

Verbs

Materials: three flexible dolls

Presentation: Bend three flexible dolls into various shapes to show the following verbs and ask the child to "find the one that is sitting," etc.

sitting or sit, run or running, jumping,hit or hitting, sleeping, etc.

Pronouns

Materials: toys

Presentation: Through the use of toys and client-clinician relationship determine the child's understanding of:

he-his, she-hers, they, my, mine, yours, it. (It may be necessary to use male and female dolls for indication of he-she knowledge. Have the child point to the correct doll when clinician says, "He is sleeping," etc.

Adjectives

Materials: dolls, blocks, sandpaper, smooth plastic, sponge ball, clown faces, etc.

Presentation: have the child identify each object. Paired objects are needed which depict the following:

big/little	hard/soft
near/far	high/low
happy/sad	fat/thin
short/tall	clean/dirty
rough/smooth	etc.

Adverbs

Materials: ball, airplane, and car or truck

Presentation: Using a ball, airplane, etc. have the child follow instructions:

— roll ball slowly

— roll ball fast

— fly plane quickly

Prepositions

Materials: Objects and convenient chair, table, box

Presentation: Using objects test the following concepts: in, on, under, through, above, beside, over, between, etc.

Conjunctions

Materials: Objects or toys

Presentation: test for knowledge of the following:

and

"Give me the ball and the cup"

but

"Put the spoon in the cup but wait until I clap my hands"

"Sit in the chair but don't touch the floor?"

or

"Give me the spider or the zebra"

(choice out of three)

Action-Agent-Use

Materials: spoon, glass, car, bed, fish, etc.

Presentation: Have the child show the clinician which object—

you eat with

you drink from

you ride in

you sleep on

swims ("which one swims")

flies ("which one flies")

cries ("which one cries")

stir ("which one could stir")

cut ("which one could cut")

3. Morphological Types

Plurals

Materials: Several blocks or cars or other toys

Presentation: Place the objects in groups of two or three and by themselves and ask the child, "Show me a block," or "Show me blocks."

Past Tense

Materials: trucks

Presentation: Have one truck empty, one with dirt in it, one tipped with all the dirt dumped, and ask "Which truck dumped?"

Possessive

Materials: balls

Presentation: Have many balls all around. Pick one and say "This is your ball" and another saying "This is my ball." "Show me *Carl's* ball."

er, ist, est

Materials: Some similar objects (people, forms, plastic animals)

Presentation: —er (any two of differing size) "which one is bigger?"

—ist, —est (any three of different sizes) "which one is shortest?"

Present Progressive

Materials: dolls or trucks

Presentation: Three dolls—one standing, one sitting, one sleeping, "Which doll is sleeping?" Same thing with three trucks—one full, one empty, one in the act of dumping, "Which truck is dumping?"

Future

Materials: balloons and blocks

Presentation: Have one balloon unblown, one half blown and one very distended. "Which one will pop?"

Have a series of blocks lined up, a bunch scrambled up, some stacked up. "Which blocks will fall?"

4. Test of Sentence Type

Tests for understanding of different types of sentences.

Materials: felt board, felt pictures of common noun objects used to form sentences for testing

Presentation: Pointing to correct picture after the clinician gives the sentence.

Plan to have maybe three pictures on the board at the same time. The pictures would be changed for each portion of the test.

Active

The cat chases the mouse.

Also have picture of mouse chasing a cat and picture of both animals sleeping, etc.

Negative

This is not a dog.

Also have picture of one fish and then two dogs.

Question

Yes/no—"Is the bird in the tree?" (Move the bird, ask the question over)

| which | Which one is food? |
| where | Where is the tree? |

tag—This is an apple, isn't it?

Conjunction

The boy is sleeping and the girl is jumping the rope.

Relative

The man, who is walking the dog, has a hat on.

Passive

The mouse is being chased by the cat.

5. Concepts

Materials:

blocks of different colors; at least one larger than others in all dimensions; one larger in only one dimension (wider)

two paper bags

"whole-part" picture or object, i.e., pie, cake, apple, etc.

one or two balls

dolls or pictures of family members (mother, father, brother, sister)

Presentation:

self-body—"Simon-Says" type of game

family relationship—identify dolls or pictures

same-different—two blocks and one ball together, point to same or "hand me the two that are the same."

color—blocks of different colors, identify: "Hand me a red block."

number—blocks, "give me _____ blocks (1, 2, 3, etc.)

spatial relationships—top-bottom; near-far. Top-bottom, three blocks in a pile, "Hand me the top blocks, middle, bottom." Near, far, two blocks one nearer the child than the other. (Can use any comparable term, i.e., close to you, far from you). "Hand me the block that's near you."

size—big, little (Blocks of different sizes or balls) "Give me the big block."

wide-narrow—two blocks, one wider in only one dimension. "Give me the wide block."

nothing-something—two paper bags, one with something in it, one with nothing in it. "This bag has something, this bag has nothing." Have the child hand the bag indicated (related to number?)

whole-part—(Picture or object) "Hand me the whole one, or hand me the part."

If some degree of cooperation has been obtained, two further procedures are employed. Both are attempts to formally evaluate the child's use of language for communicative purposes; in other words, to relate language structure with communication function. In the first procedure, a doll is used as a "listener." The child is told that the doll cannot see (with some children we have simply blindfolded the doll) but is very eager to know what is happening in the room. The request is made for the child to tell the doll about the activities. The clinician then attempts to perform actions which could be described through the constructions indicated in Table 4-2.

Table 4-2 Examples of Semantic Relations Acted Out As Prompts for Child's Descriptions

Semantic Relations	*Possible Responses
Notice-Greeting	Hi Dolly
Recurrence	More water
Nonexistence	Allgone fire
Attribution	Big shoe
Possessive	Monkey's tail
Locative	Man car (man is in the car)
Locative	Drive street (car is "driving" in the street)
Agent-Action	Horse run
Agent-Object	Car train (the car hit the train)
Action-Object	Pet dog

*The possible responses are put in two-word form although obviously the child's responses will reflect his level of expressive language.

In the concluding play situation preceding formal testing, some attempt is made to determine the communicative functions of the child's language. Much of the information for this section must come from parent report; however, it is possible with many children to engage in an activity which allows maximal testing of the desired elements. We have found that activities which involve construction of an object or repair of a broken object work well with some children. Using Halliday's (1977) function of language system as a general guide, we attempt to elicit the functions listed in Table 4-3.

Formal attempts to test semantic functions and pragmatics of language usage are in the formulative stages of development.

A somewhat similar although more structured procedure is described by Bellugi-Klima (1971). In this assessment of the child's comprehension of syntac-

Table 4-3 Examples of Language Functions Elicited During Informal Play Session.

Function	Possible Responses
Instrumental	Give me the wheel
Regulatory	Do this
Interactional	Let's do this
Personal	Look it works
	That's good
Heuristic	How should we do this
Imaginative	Hello-Green horse
Informative	I do this at home

tic structures is measured on the basis of his ability to manipulate objects and toys following stimulus sentences produced by the examiner. The child is requested to act out such sentences as, "The boy picked up a shoe." "Who isn't sleeping?" "The geese are flying away." Three levels of difficulty are identified based upon developmental studies. The levels include:

Level One
  1. Subject-verb-object relationship-active sentence
  2. Singular-plural nouns
  3. Possessives
Level Two
  1. Negative/affirmative statements
  2. Negative/affirmative questions
  3. Singular/plural noun and verb inflections
  4. Adjective modifiers
Level Three
  1. Negative affix
  2. Reflexization
  3. Comparatives
  4. Passives
  5. Self-embedded

McNeill (1970) describes an interesting approach to the study of comprehension conducted by Slobin and Welsh (unpublished) in which the researchers used imitation to measure comprehension. As McNeill (1970: 13–14) points out, "They exploit the fact that a successful reformulation in imitation depends on a successful comprehension of the sentence imitated." The point of interest regarding comprehension is not verbatim repetition but rather preservation of meaning. In this case it is possible for the diagnostician to construct a series of sentences of varying complexity and incorporate varying types of grammatical classes.

Unlike sentence-imitation tasks requiring exact repetition of the stimulus sentence, these measures sometimes call for a reformulation of the sentence. Fokes (unpublished) has devised a number of sentences which require rephrasing by the child. She included seventeen sentence types in her test in the following order;

do-negative, passive, be-negative, model aux., tax questions, adversatives, disjoint, comparatives, complex aux. verbs, affix negative, negative indefinite NP, negative indefinites VP, temporal connections, causal connectives, conditional, deletions and conjoin, exceptions.

The *Wiig-Semel Test of Linguistic Concepts* (Wiig and Semel, 1973) measures the understanding of fifty linguistic concepts; ten each represent comparatives, passive sentence types, temporal-sequential relationships, spatial, and familial relationships. The test sentences have from five to seven words, and the child need only respond with yes/no responses for the majority of items. The test was standardized on 210 grade-school children randomly selected.

The preceding review of tests of receptive language is intended to assist the diagnostician in the selection of tests. The discussion is not intended to be exhaustive nor is it an in-depth critique of each test. For a more extensive review of most of the tests, see the *Buros Mental Measurement Yearbook* (eighth edition in press).

No test can be considered the best test of auditory comprehension. The clinician must match what is available with what her present needs are and with the known characteristics of the child. Very often the diagnostician is already aware that the child presents a significant language disorder prior to administration of a formal test. In such instances the purpose of testing is not so much to compare the child with norms but to compare the child's performance relative to the various stages of normal language development. The battery of tests selected should directly reflect these issues.

A variety of procedures are used to measure expressive verbal language. As with tests of reception, however, there is a general lack of adequately standardized procedures, and the diagnostician must continue to qualify test findings and employ substantial amounts of clinical judgment. We have chosen to discuss five levels of expressive verbal-language development (see Table 4-4); however, several alternative paradigms are available (See Wigg and Semel, 1976, Chapter 9).

In word-finding tasks the child is presented with stimuli and expected to respond with a specific verbal response. Retrieval and production of the appropriate word is demanded. The vocal subtests of the *Parsons Language Sample* (Spradlin, 1963) are designed to measure the child's vocal responses under verbal operants called Tacts, Echoic, and Intraverbal. In the tact subtest the child names 28 objects or pictures in response to the examiner's question, "What is it?" In the echoic test the child repeats 10 words, sentences, and sets of digits. In the intraverbal subtest the child's responses are basically of a sentence completion nature.

Table 4-4   Measures of Expressive Verbal Language

Word Finding	Vocal Sub-tests of P.L.S.
	Vocabular Usage Test
Verbal Opposites	Opposite Analogies Subtest of MSCA
	Verbal Opposites Subtests of DTLA
Verbal Definitions	Word Naming Subtest of S-B, I.S.
	Verbal Expression Subtest of ITPA
	Free Association Subtest of DTLA and WISC
	Oral Vocabulary of TOLD
Morphological Rules	Berko Test of English Morphology
	Berry-Talbott Test of Grammar
Grammatical-Syntax	Mean Length of Utterance
	Length-Complexity Index
	Language Sampling, Analysis, and Training
	Developmental Sentence Types
	Developmental Sentence Scoring

At least two attempts have been made to turn the *Peabody Picture Vocabulary Test* into a test of expressive vocabulary. (Nation, 1972; Love, 1964). The *Vocabulary Usage Test* (Nation, 1972) is designed for children 34-63 months of age and measures expressive vocabulary, primarily through use of sentence-completion task using the test plates from the *PPVT*. Very tentative norms have been established from a sample of twenty-five children. Love's procedures use the first fifty-five words from the *PPVT* for children 18-60 months. A vocabulary definition test involving thirty-nine of the words from the same source is described as suitable for children about five years of age. Both of these measures are essentially experimental in nature.

The Visual Confrontation Naming subtest of the *Boston Diagnostic Aphasia Examination* (Goodglass & Kaplan, 1972) is designed to measure retrieval of verbal labels in response to pictures, and may be useful with older children and adolescents (Wigg and Semel, 1975).

The retrieval of verbal opposites is measured in the subtests of a number of language scales. The opposite-analogies subtest of the *McCarthy Scales of Children's Abilities* (McCarthy, 1970) and the verbal-opposites subtest of the *Detroit Tests of Learning Aptitude* (Baker & Leland, 1959) require recall and production of verbal opposites. A related task is included in the *Stanford-Binet Intelligence Scale* (Terman & Merrill, 1960) in the opposite-analogies subtests presented at several age levels. Failure to respond appropriately on such tests may indicate that the child does not have adequate vocabulary for the test and simply does not know the words, or that the child does not understand the opposite relationship, or that the child is unable to recall the word from memory. Since so many possibilities exist in explanation of failure in such tests, the tests are seldom or never administered alone and most often are only used to corroborate other findings.

The term ''verbal definitions'' refers to the ability to retrieve and formulate specific responses to identified stimuli. This expressive skill is clearly related to memory and organizational skills as well as to expressive-language requirements. The *Stanford-Binet Intelligence Scale*, the *Illinois Test of Psycholinguistic Ability*, the *Detroit Tests of Learning Aptitude*, the *Wechsler Intelligence Scale for Children*, the *Test of Language Development*, and other general measures all have subtests which evaluate verbal definitions. We have found that many clinical uses can be made of the *ITPA's* subtest, since it leads directly to a format for remediation based upon the number of attributes the child is expected to describe (i.e., label, color, shape, composition, functions, etc.).

Berko's (1958) now-classic test of the child's use of morphological rules is of interest for its ingenious technique and excellent potential. Berko tested the child's ability to produce the plural and possessive forms of nouns, the third-person singular of verbs, past tense of verbs, comparative forms of adjectives, and others. The test included drawings of hypothetical creatures engaged in various activities and ordinary creatures engaged in hypothetical activities. The most often described example is a creature introduced as follows: "Here is a wug. Here are two others, there are two _____." The attempt is to elicit the plural "wugs." Similar techniques could be devised for testing several grammatical skills. Unfortunately, the Berko test was never commercially available, although several adaptations of it have been developed for private use.

The *Berry-Talbott Test of Grammar* (1966) provides a set of pictures and examples similar to the Berko test for measuring morphological rules. The test cannot be considered fully standardized; however, it is useful as a rough screening device.

Two primary techniques are used to measure expressive grammatical abilities. *Spontaneous language sampling* and *elicited imitation* provide most clinicians with this type of information. Since both techniques have distinct assets and liabilities, many clinicians employ both in a comprehensive language evaluation.

Spontaneous Language Sampling is a rigorous and time-consuming procedure. The clinician can expect to spend at least one hour collecting data and several hours in transcription and interpretation. The procedure involves collecting a language sample, transcribing the session, making grammatical analysis of the child's conversation, making a determination of the child's language level, and concluding with some statement of appropriate clinical goals and procedures. The adequacy of a language-sampling technique is to a large extent dependent upon the representativeness of the sample obtained with regard to quantity, quality, and variety of language as well as being dependent on the employment of a carefully devised procedure for evaluation of the language corpus.

Although there is no universally accepted procedure for eliciting a language sample, this may be an instance where the clinician has greater freedom to employ judgment based upon what is known of the child. Since the goal is to elicit "typical" behavior from the child, this may not be done in a stereotyped fashion with every child. Some children respond better to questions, while others respond to open conversation, etc. Table 4-5 provides the guidelines we find helpful in collecting a language sample.

Table 4-5 Guidelines for Taking a Language Sample

1. Two language samples should be collected at separate times.

2. Allow appropriate time to establish a positive relationship with the child prior to initiating the recording.

3. Use unobtrusive tape recording procedures. It is best not to write while interacting with the child.

4. Type the transcript from the recording as soon as possible following the session, so that your memory of the child's responses can assist.

5. Keep your talking to a minimum. It may be helpful to restate what the child has said if intelligibility was poor.

6. Avoid questions which call for yes or no answers. Attempt to use questions which expand the conversation, such as "which" and "what" questions. Children tend to reply with stereotyped answers to "why" and "when" questions.

7. Record approximately a half-hour sample gaining a 50–100 sentence sample. (Fifteen minutes each session)

8. *Know the child's interests, if possible, and use these in a natural conversational setting, using toys and real objects as focal points. It may not be necessary to use toys and objects if the child will respond to natural conversation regarding her family, school, playmates, favorite activities, etc. (Longhurst and File, 1977).

9. Always identify the record, stating time of day, parents' estimate of how normal the sample was, date, place, unique conditions, prompts used, etc.

*Although it may not always be practical, Labov's (1970) method may provide the richest language corpus: he suggests that children be left alone with a guinea pig and told to talk to the pig so it won't get lonely.

Once the sampling is completed and transcribed, a decision must be made as to what parts of the sample can be used for analysis. Lee's suggestions (1974) are widely incorporated. She suggests that the corpus consist of fifty complete, different, consecutive, intelligible, non-echolalic sentences. A general definition of each requirement is as follows:

(a) *Complete*—noun and verb must be present in subject-predicate relationship.

(b) *Different*—no repetitions of sentences are allowed so that overused stereotypes do not skew the results.

(c) *Consecutive*—sentences must be consecutive so that inclination to only include high scoring sentences is avoided.

(d) *Intelligible*—unintelligible statements are not included in the corpus, therefore minimizing guessing.

(e) *Nonecholalic*—echoic utterances are not counted since interest is in self-formulated sentences.

The system devised by Crystal et al. (1976) does not restrict the corpus selection in any way; therefore, every statement must be transcribed and accounted for. Such an inclusive method may result in richer data.

Analysis of the language sample may begin with several traditionally popular techniques. Mean length of utterance (MLU) is a common measurement first used by researchers such as McCarthy (1930) and Templin (1957) and more recently refined by Brown (1973) and his co-workers. Brown uses MLU as an index of grammatical development, based upon the premise that increased length of utterance parallels an increase in grammatical complexity. This basic premise has been debated in the literature for years, but we agree with Brown that MLU plus age data provide a fairly reliable *estimate* of language level; however, several shortcomings of the procedure commend its use only as a preliminary measure (Shriner, 1969). Brown's guidelines for calculating MLU are as follows (Brown, 1973):

1. Start with the second page of the transcription unless that page involves a recitation of some kind. In this latter case start with the first recitation-free stretch. Count the first 100 utterances satisfying the following rules.

2. Only fully transcribed utterances are used; none with blanks. Portions of utterances, entered in parentheses to indicate doubtful transcription, are used.

3. Include all exact utterance repetitions (marked with a plus sign in records). Stuttering is marked as repeated efforts at a single word; cound the word once in the most complete form produced. In the few cases where a word is produced for emphasis or the like *(no, no, no)* count each occurrence.

4. Do not count such fillers as *mm* or *oh*, but do count *no, yeah*, and *hi*.

5. All compound words (two or more free morphemes), proper names, and ritualized reduplications count as single words. Examples: *birthday, rackety-boom, choo-choo, quack-quack, night-night, pocketbook, see saw.* Justification is that no evidence that the constituent morphemes function as such for these children.

6. Count as one morpheme all irregular pasts of the verb *(got, did, went, saw).* Justification is that there is not evidence that the child relates these to present forms.

7. Count as one morpheme all diminutives *(doggie, mommie)* because these children at least do not seem to use the suffix productively. Diminutives are the standard forms used by the child.

8. Count as separate morphemes all auxiliaries *(is, have, will, can, must, would).* Also all catenatives: *gonna, wanna, hafta.* These latter counted as single morphemes rather than as *going to* or *want to* because evidence is that they function so for the children. Count as separate morphemes all inflections, for example, possessive {s}, plural {s}, third person singular {s}, regular past {d}, progressive {in}.

9. The range count follows the above rules but is always calculated for the total transcription rather than for 100 utterances.
   (from Brown, 1973: 54)

Although determination of MLU has diagnostic value in determining the level of language performance of the child, it is probably even more valuable in assisting the remedial effort. Once it has been determined at which of Brown's five linguistic levels the child is performing, we have found that, along with information gained from other testing, it is helpful to use this linguistic level to determine which language constructions the child would logically be working toward.

Johnson, Darley, and Spriestersbach (1963) describe a variety of other measures which are possible from a spontaneous language sample. Such measures as *mean of the five longest responses, number of one-word responses, number of different words, and type/token ratio*, and others have been used in diagnosis, but we have found that such measures are of limited value; They appear to be of greatest value for research undertakings.

Many attempts have been made to incorporate measures of sentence length with grammatical complexity (McCarthy, 1930; Templin, 1957; Miner, 1969). Miner's *Length Complexity Index* combines both sentence length and sentence complexity using phrase structure rules. Weighted scores are assigned to each construction type. Although the procedure results in some clinically useful information, we have found it to be demanding and somewhat time consuming.

The *Language Sampling, Analysis and Training* (Tyack and Gottsleben, 1974) provides increased standardization of procedure and leads to rather specific clinical-planning suggestions. Specific instructions for collecting the language sample, 100 sentences, are followed by procedures for measuring language production. We have found the procedure to be exhaustive (and exhausting); it is probably only of value to clinicians who have had specific training in the technique.

Perhaps the most widely employed procedures for evaluation of grammatical elements of verbal expression are the *Developmental Sentence Analysis* procedures described by Lee and Canter (1971) and Lee (1974). The procedures use spontaneous-language samples to measure selected grammatical-form categories. Two procedures are described. The Developmental Sentence Types is used for children whose language is primarily at the pre-sentence level. Lee presents procedures for classifying the fragmentary statements, and although no overall score is obtained the clinician can determine the variety of constructions the child employs. The Developmental Sentence Scoring procedure measures the use of eight grammatical forms which are weighted according to developmental progression. The score which results from the *DSS* includes points obtained from the presence of the constructions as well as points for correct sentence use. Normative data from 160 children 3-6 to 11 years is provided (Lee, 1974).

The Developmental Sentence Scoring procedures have been criticized by Crystal et al. (1976), who claim that Lee's selection of grammatical features is unrepresentative of the syntactic system as a whole. They also state that the procedures which result in a score are of "uncertain" value due to the complexity of expressive language. These and other criticisms notwithstanding, we find that the DSS procedures are clinically useful in establishing the child's level of verbal expression and charting growth.

Whether the clinician selects a formal procedure as described above or performs an informal assessment of the spontaneous verbal language of the child, spontaneous-language sampling must be an important part of every language diagnosis. The task is demanding, tedious, and time consuming, and often results in only fragmentary information. Nevertheless, it is an imperative procedure if the clinician wishes to obtain as complete a picture as possible of the child's language ability.

Elicited imitation tasks are a second way to measure grammatical elements of verbal expressive language. Elicited imitation tasks are based upon the premise that a child will imitate, within certain limitations, those grammatical structures which are within his competence. In other words, the child filters the statements through his own grammatical rule system and reduces or alters his reproduction to match his own rules. (McNeill, 1970)

> Jason, a child with normal language development performed the following imitations on an elicited imitation task:
>
> *Stimulus:* Mama is going home.
>   *Jason:* Mama go.
> *Stimulus:* The big ball is mine.
>   *Jason:* My big ball.
>
> How old is Jason?

When compared with normal language development data, the child's imitation provides data regarding his level of language development as well as providing the clinician with data regarding the types and consistency of errors made.

Schwartz and Daly (1976: 34) indicate three major advantages of imitation testing:

(1) The sample to be obtained is explicitly specified and can be judged accurately;

(2) it is efficient and easy to administer and score; and

(3) examiners can be trained easily.

Although first impressions would be that the elicited imitation task is easier for the child, Slobin & Welsh (1973) indicate that it may be a more demanding task, since context and communicative intent are not present. The result may represent a more conservative estimate of the child's language skill than does spontaneous-language sampling. (Schwartz and Daly, 1976).

Obviously, in elicited imitation the clinician is able to control the language constructions the child is to attempt. This is a distinctly more efficient procedure than the spontaneous-language sample, which may or may not result in a representative sample of many syntactical constructions.

Certain factors limit the usefulness of the elicited-imitation tests. It would appear evident that the use of such tests with a known echoic child would not be indicated, since such children probably perform better on imitative tasks than in spontaneous speech. Second, imitation tests must sample a variety of grammatical constructions, ones which are typically difficult for language-disordered children (Schwartz and Daly, 1976; Carrow, 1974). Third, the imitation task should include stimuli which are not so short that they can be easily retained in short-term memory nor so long that they exceed the child's comprehension capabilities.

The *Carrow Elicited Language Inventory* (1974) is the most widely used test of its kind. The test consists of fifty-one sentences and one phrase, ranging in length from two to ten words, which Carrow indicates assist in identifying specific language structures in error and quantifying the overall language status through numerical score. The test includes a tape recording of the child's imitation; the transcription of the child's responses is on a form where grammatical features are classified and error types indicated.

The primary standardization group for the CELI was 475 white middle-class children ranging in age from 3 to 7-11 years. Mean scores for age groups plus information regarding type subcategory scores are presented along with selected percentile rankings.

The CELI provides an elaborate scoring procedure which is readily adaptable to the clinical decision making process and provides a good deal of useful diagnostic information. In general, however, elicited imitation testing should not, in our opinion, be used as a substitute for a language-sample analysis, but as a supplement to that procedure.

SUMMARY

The rush to accountability which has characterized the last twenty years has increased our reliance upon objective, data-producing instruments even in those domains where such techniques are inappropriate. The vulnerability of quantifying procedures for language diagnosis has only recently been identified (Muma, 1973). Muma points out that quantifying language-test procedures assist in resolving the question of disorder versus normal behavior, whereas descriptive approaches are more helpful in directing the remedial effort. Although the purported purpose for standardized and structured tests is to make the procedure more uniform and fair for all children, in reality these measures may bias in favor of children who do well under such conditions and penalize those who do not.

Determining if a child's language development is normal or abnormal requires more than the administration of a test or a test battery. Each of the measures described in this chapter has the potential to add information to the diagnostic quest or divert the diagnostician from making an accurate determination. Each is based upon a set of assumptions—assumptions about testing, about test construction, and most importantly about language, what it is and how it is evaluated. The appropriate use of any test requires that the diagnostician understand the theory and rationale for the test construction and judiciously select those measures which correspond with her goals and objectives for testing. Siegel (1975: 215) points out that "a test is a device for sampling some of a child's behavior not a microscope that penetrates the child's mind." The ultimate question goes beyond test results and focuses on the child's ability to use language to receive and transmit information for some functional purpose in real life settings (Clark, 1975). So many language assessment tools fractionalize the language function and separate the elements of communication that the relationship between performance on them and real life performance can only be surmised. The diagnostic challenge is to synthesize the fragments of test data into a composite picture of the child's total language capability. Ultimately the diagnostician uses information from a variety of sources in the decision-making process, and both formal and informal procedures play important roles.

Knowledge of the level of language functioning is not itself sufficient information to determine the existence of a language disorder. Comparison must be made of this language level and the child's level of cognitive functioning, since language maturation is closely related to cognitive development. Generally, it is considered appropriate to compare a child's language sophistication with his mental-age level as determined through some non-verbally based intelligence measure. If a significant gap exists between language level and mental age, the clinician can have greater confidence in her determinations.

> Nearly every language clinician has faced a parent or a group of parents whose primary posture regarding their child's language and learning problem is: "If he could only talk, I'm sure he would be OK!" Although it is true that language skill enhances general learning rate, we agree with Piaget and his followers that cognitive growth and perceptions of environmental events precede the language structures used to label and describe those events.

Further complicating the decision process, however, is the fact that rate of language development is notoriously variable while stage or sequence of acquisition is stable. Scores and percentile levels reveal little about the quality of the language performance, which may be crucial in the ultimate resolution; descriptive information about the types of language constructions within the child's repertoire provide little information, taken alone, about the child's relative language development. Once again we are confronted with the postulate that data and diagnosis are not equatable terms.

PROJECTS AND QUESTIONS

1. "Language disorders" are said to be the major problem for many children with learning disabilities. How does the special learning disabilities teacher define language?
2. Categorize as input, integrative, and output all those behaviors which you feel are dependent upon language.
3. Compare the chapters on normal language development presented in the 1954 and 1970 editions of Carmichael's *Manual of Child Psychology*. Do the differences reflect the changes in the types of information needed for understanding language functioning?
4. Although the linguists claim that "stage is more stable than age" (or that the acquisition path to language maturation is essentially invariant from child to child) there are a variety of ways to catalog normal language development. Compare the descriptions of:

BROWN, R. (1973. *A First Language: The Early Stages.* Cambridge, Mass.: Harvard University Press.

WOOD, B. (1976). *Children and Communication: Verbal and Nonverbal Language Development.* Englewood Cliffs, N.J.: Prentice-Hall, Inc.

CRYSTAL D.; P. FLETCHER, and M. GARMAN (1976). *The Grammatical Analysis of Language Disability.* New York: American Elsevier Publishing Company, Inc.

5. What are the major differences among the terms language test, language scale, and language inventory?
6. Even though the *Peabody Picture Vocabulary Test* has been severely criticized it remains a widely used tool. What are some of the reasons for its popularity?
7. Read the following articles before making a final determination of the value of elicited-imitation testing and spontaneous-language sampling:

PRUTTING, C.; T. GALLAGHER; and A. MULAC (1975). "The expressive portion of the NSST compared to a spontaneous speech sample." *Journal of Speech and Hearing Disorders,* 40: 40–48.

SCHWARTZ, A., and D. DALY (1976). "Some Explicit Guidelines for Constructing and Scoring Elicited Imitation Tasks." *Language Speech and Hearing Services in Schools,* 7: 33–40.

MUMA, J. (1973). "Language Assessment: Some underlying assumptions." *ASHA,* 15: 331–338.

8. A large number of clinicians are abandoning attempts to determine the etiology of language problems in favor of intensive study of current performance levels, useful reward systems, and task analysis. Formulate your own personal philosophy on the importance of etiology.
9. Summarize the cogent arguments presented by the psychologists in defense of the concept that language is a learned function.
10. Develop a twenty-stage task analysis of the skills necessary to generate a spoken sentence. Relate it to diagnosis.
11. Consult *ASHA* Monograph No. 14, and define what the authors mean by a "functional analysis" of speech and language.
12. What implication does the work of Shriner and Sherman (1967) have on your selection of appropriate language measures?

BIBLIOGRAPHY

AMMONS, R., and H. AMMONS (1958). *The Full-Range Picture Vocabulary Test.* Missoula, Mont.: Psychological Test Specialists.

ARNDT, W. (1977). "A Psychometric Evaluation of the Northwestern Syntax Screening Test." *Journal of Speech and Hearing Disorders,* 42: 316–319.

AYRES, A. (1964). *Southern California Motor Accuracy Test.* Los Angeles: Western Psychological Services.

BAKER, H., and B. LELAND (1959). *Detroit Tests of Learning Aptitude.* Indianapolis: Bobbs-Merrill.

BANGS, T. (1961). "Evaluating Children with Language Delay." *Journal of Speech and Hearing Disorders,* 26: 6–18.

BANGS, T. (1975). *The Vocabulary Comprehension Scale.* Austin, Texas: Learning Concepts.

BELLUGI-KLIMA, U. (1971). "Some Language Comprehension Tests." in *Language Training In Early Childhood Education,* ed. C. Lavatelli. Urbana, Ill.: University of Illinois Press.

BERKO, J. (1958). "The Child's Learning of English Morphology." *Word,* 14: 150–177.

BERRY, M. (1969). *Language Disorders of Children.* New York: Appleton-Century-Crofts.

BERRY, M., and R. TALBOTT (1966). *Exploratory Test of Grammar.* Rockford, Ill.

BLOOD, G., and B. GREENBERG (1976). "Receptive Language Testing." A paper presented at the American Speech and Hearing Association Convention. Houston, Texas.

BLOOM, L. (1970). *Language Development: Form and Function in Emerging Grammars.* Cambridge, Mass.: M.I.T. Press.

BLOOMFIELD, L. (1933). *Language.* New York: Holt, Rinehart & Winston, Inc.

BOEHM, A. (1971). *Boehm Test of Basic Concepts.* New York: Psychological Corporation.

BROWN, R. (1973). *A First Language.* Cambridge, Mass.: Harvard University Press.

BROWN, R. and J. BERKO (1960). "Word Association and the Acquisition of Grammar." *Child Development,* 31: 1–14.

BROWN, R., and C. FRAZER (1963). "The Acquisition of Syntax." in *Verbal Behavior and Learning: Problems and Process,* eds. C. Cofer and B. Musgrave, Pp. 158–201. New York: McGraw-Hill.

BYRNE, M. (1977). "A Clinician Looks at the Northwestern Syntax Screening Test." *Journal of Speech and Hearing Disorders,* 42: 320–322.

BZOCH, K., and R. LEAGUE (1971). *Assessing Language Skills in Infancy.* Gainesville, Fla.: Tree of Life Press.

CARROW, E. (1973). *Screening Test for Auditory Comprehension of Language.* Lamar, Texas: Learning Concepts.

CARROW, E. (1973). *Test for Auditory Comprehension of Language.* Austin, Texas: Learning Concepts.

CARROW, E. (1974). *Carrow Elicited Language Inventory.* Austin, Texas: Learning Concepts.

CHOMSKY, C. (1969). *The Acquisition of Syntax in Children from 5 to 10.* Cambridge, Mass.: M.I.T. Press.

CHOMSKY, N. (1965). *Aspects of the Theory of Syntax.* Cambridge, Mass.: M.I.T. Press.

——— (1957). *Syntactic Structure.* The Hague: Mouton.

CLARK, J., "Theoretical and Technical Considerations in Oral Proficiency Testing." in *Testing Language Proficiency.* ed. R. Jones and B. Spolsky, Arlington, Va.: Center for Applied Linguistics, 1975.

CRABTREE, M. (1963). *The Houston Test for Language Development.* Houston: Houston Test Co.

CRYSTAL, D.; P. FLETCHER; and M. GARMAN (1976). *The Grammatical Analysis of Language Disability.* New York: American Elsevier.

DARLEY, F., and H. WINITZ (1961). "Age of First Word: Review of Research." *Journal of Speech and Hearing Disorders,* 26: 272–290.

DUNN, L. (1965). *Peabody Picture Vocabulary Test.* Minneapolis: American Guidance Service.

FISHER, H., and J. LOGEMANN (1971). *The Fisher-Logemann Test of Articulation Competence.* Boston: Houghton Mifflin.

FLUHARTY, N. (1974). "The Design and Standardization of a Speech and Language Screening Test for Use with Preschool Children." *Journal of Speech and Hearing Disorders,* 39: 75–88.

FOSTER, R.; J. GIDDAN; and J. STARK (1973). *Assessment of Children's Language Comprehension* (Preliminary Manual). Palo Alto, Calif.: Consulting Psychologists Press, Inc.

FRANKENBURG, W.; J. DODDS; and A. FANDAL (1970). *Denver Developmental Screening Test.* Denver, Colo.: University of Colorado Medical Center.

FROSTIG, M.; D. LEFEVER; P. MASLOW; and R. WHITTLESLEY (1964). *Marianne Frostig Developmental Test of Visual Perception.* Palo Alto, Calif.: Consulting Psychologists Press.

GILLINGHAM, A., and B. STILLMAN (1970). *Remedial Training for Children with Specific Disability in Reading, Spelling, and Penmanship.* Cambridge, Mass.: Educators Publishing Service.

GOODGLASS, H., and E. KAPLAN (1972). *Boston Diagnostic Aphasia Examination.* Philadelphia: Lea & Febiger.

HATTEN, J., and P. HATTEN (1971). "A Foster Home Approach to Speech Therapy." *Journal of Speech and Hearing Disorders,* 36:257–263.

HALLIDAY, M. (1977). *Learning How to Mean: Explorations in the Development of Language.* New York: Elsevier North-Holland, Inc.

HAMMILL, D., and N. BARTEL (1975). *Teaching Children with Learning and Behavior Problems.* Boston: Allyn & Bacon, Inc.

HEAD, H. (1926). *Aphasia and Kindred Disorders of Speech.* New York: Macmillan.

HEDRICK, D.; E. PRATHER; and A. TOBIN (1975). *Sequenced Inventory of Communication Development.* Seattle and London: University of Washington Press.

HUIZINGA, R. (1973). "The Relationship of the ITPA to the Stanford-Binet Form L-M and the WISC," *Journal of Learning Disabilities,* 6: 53–58.

JOHNSON, W.; F. DARLEY; and D. SPRIESTERSBACH (1963). *Diagnostic Methods in Speech Pathology.* New York: Harper & Row.

KENDALL, D. (1966). "Language and Communication Problems in Children," in *Speech Pathology,* ed R. Reiber and R. Brubaker. Amsterdam: North-Holland Publishing Company.

KEPHART, N. (1960). *The Slow Learner in the Classroom.* Columbus, Ohio: Charles E. Merrill, Inc.

KIRK, S., and J. McCARTHY (1961). "The Illinois Test of Psycholinguistic Abilities—An Approach to Differential Diagnosis." *American Journal of Mental Deficiency,* 66: 399–412.

———— and W. KIRK (1968). *Illinois Test of Psycholinguistic Abilities.* Urbana: University of Illinois Press.

KRESLECK, J., and L. NICOLOSI (1973). "A Comparison of Black and White Children's Scores on the Peabody Picture Vocabulary Test." *Language, Speech and Hearing Services in the Schools,* 4: 37–40.

LABOV, W. (1970). "Finding Out About Children's Language." Speech delivered to the Hawaiian Council of Teachers of English, Honolulu (Cited in Longhurst and File, 1977).

LEE, L. (1974). *Developmental Sentence Analysis.* Evanston: Northwestern University Press.

———— (1977). "Reply to Arndt and Byrne," *Journal of Speech and Hearing Disorders,* 42: 323–327.

———— (1969). *The Northwestern Syntax Screening Test.* Evanston, Ill.: Northwestern University Press.

———— and S. CANTER (1971). "Developmental Sentence Scoring: A Clinical Procedure for Estimating Syntax Development in Children's Spontaneous Speech." *Journal of Speech and Hearing Disorders,* 36: 311–330.

LENNEBERG, E. (1967). *Biological Foundations of Language.* New York: John Wiley & Sons, Inc.

LEREA, L. (1958). "Assessing Language Development." *Journal of Speech and Hearing Research,* 1: 75–85.

LONGHURST, T., and J. FILE (1977). "A Comparison of Developmental Sentence Scores from Head Start Children Collected in Four Conditions." *Language Speech and Hearing Services in Schools,* 8: 54–64.

LOVE, R. (1964). "Oral Language Behavior of Older Cerebral Palsied Children." *Journal of Speech and Hearing Research,* 7: 349–362.

MACDONALD, J.; J. BLOTT; K. GORDON; B. SPIEGEL; and M. HARTMANN (1974). "An Experimental Parent-Assisted Language Program for Preschool Retarded Children." *Journal of Speech and Hearing Disorders,* 39: 395–415.

———— and M. NICKOLS (1974). *Environmental Language Inventory.* Columbus, Ohio: The Nisonger Center.

MCCARTHY, D. (1970). *McCarthy Scales of Children's Abilities.* New York: Psychological Corporation.

———— (1930), "The Language Development of the Preschool Child." *Child Welfare Monograph No. 4.* Minneapolis: University of Minnesota Press.

MCNEILL, D. (1970a). *The Acquisition of Language.* New York: Harper & Row.

MECHAM, M. (1958). *Verbal Language Development Scale.* Beverly Hills, Calif.: Western Psychological Services.

MECHAM, M.; J. JONES; and J. JEX (1973). "Use of the Utah Test of Language Development for Screening Language Disabilities." *Journal of Learning Disabilities,* 6: 524–527.

———— (1967). *Utah Test of Language Development.* Salt Lake City: Communication Research Associates.

MENYUK, P. (1964). "Comparison of Grammar of Children with Functionally Deviant and Normal Speech." *Journal of Speech and Hearing Research,* 7: 109–121.

MINER, L. (1969). "Scoring Procedures for the Length Complexity Index: A Preliminary Report." *Journal of Communication Disorders,* 2: 224–240.

MUMA, K. (1973). "Language Assessment: Some Underlying Assumptions." *Asha,* 15: 331–338.

MYKLEBUST, H. (1954). *Auditory Disorders in Children.* New York: Grune and Stratton.

NATION, J. (1972). "A Vocabulary Usage Test." *Journal of Psycholinguistic Research,* 1: 221–231.

NEWCOMER, P., and D. HAMMILL (1976). *Psycholinguistics in the Schools.* Columbus, Ohio: Charles E. Merrill.

NEWCOMER, P., and D. HAMMILL (1977). *Test of Language Development.* Austin, Texas: Empiric Press.

NICOLOSI, L., and J. KRESLECK (1972). "Variability in Test Scores Between Form A and Form B on the Peabody Picture Vocabulary Test." *Language Speech and Hearing Services in the Schools,* 3: 44–47.

OSGOOD, C. (1957a). "A Behavioristic Analysis of Perception and Language as Cognitive Phenomena," in *Contemporary Approaches to Cognition.* Pp. 75–118. Cambridge, Mass.: Harvard University Press.

PERKINS, W. (1977). *Speech Pathology: An Applied Behavioral Science.* St. Louis, Mo.: C. V. Mosby Co.

PIAGET, J. (1952). *The Language and Thought of the Child.* London: Routledge and Kegan Paul.

SCHLESINGER, I. (1971). "Production of Utterances and Language Acquisition," in The *Ontogenesis of Grammar,* ed. D. Slobin. New York: Academic Press.

SCHUELL, H.; J. JENKINS; and E. JIMENEZ-PABON (1964). *Aphasia in Adults.* New York: Harper & Row.

Schwartz, A., and D. Daly (1976). "Some Explicit Guidelines for Constructing and Scoring Elicited Imitation Tasks." *Language Speech and Hearing Services in Schools*, 7: 33–40.

Shriner, T. (1969). "A Review of Mean Length of Response As a Measure of Expressive Language Development in Children." *Journal of Speech and Hearing Disorders*, 14: 61–67.

Siegel, G. (1975). "The Use of Language Tests." *Language Speech and Hearing Services in Schools*, 6: 211–217.

Skinner, B. F. (1957). *Verbal Behavior*. New York: Appleton-Century-Crofts.

Slobin, D., and C. Welsh (1973). "Elicited Imitation as a Research Tool in Developmental Psycholinguistics," in *Studies in Child Language Development*, ed. C. Ferguson and D. Slobin. New York: Holt, Rinehart & Winston.

Spradlin, J. (1963). "Assessment of Speech and Language of Retarded Children: The Parsons Language Sample." *Journal of Speech and Hearing Disorders, Monograph Supplement*, 10: 3–31.

———— (1967), "Procedures for Evaluating Processes Associated with Receptive and Expressive Language." In *Language and Mental Retardation*, eds. R. Schiefelbusch, R. Copeland, and J. Smith. New York: Holt, Rinehart & Winston.

Staats, A. (1968). *Learning, Language, and Cognition*. New York: Holt, Rinehart & Winston.

Stark, J. (1971). "Current Practices in Language," *Asha*, 13: 217–220.

Stark, J. (1969). "Early Language Development and Use." *Journal of Communication Disorders*, 2: 48–56.

Stephens, I. (1977). *Stephens Oral Language Screening Test*. Peninsula, Ohio: Interim Publishers.

Templin, M. (1957). *Certain Language Skills in Children*. Minneapolis: University of Minnesota Press.

Terman, L., and M. Merrill (1960). *Stanford-Binet Intelligence Scale*. Boston: Houghton Mifflin Co.

Tyack, D., and R. Gottsleben (1974). *Language Sampling, Analysis, and Training*. Palo Alto, California: Consulting Psychologists Press.

Wechsler, D. (1949). *Manual for the WISC*. New York: Psychological Corporation.

Wiig, E., and E. Semel (1973). "Comprehension of Linguistic Concepts Requiring Logical Operations." *Journal of Speech and Hearing Research*, 16: 627–636.

Wiig, E., and E. Semel (1976). *Language Disabilities in Children and Adolescents*. Columbus, Ohio: Charles E. Merrill.

Wingate, M. (1971). "The Fear of Stuttering." *Journal of the American Speech and Hearing Association*, 13: 3–5.

Wolski, W. (1962). *The Michigan Picture Language Inventory*. Ann Arbor: University of Michigan Press.

Zimmerman, I.; V. Steiner; and R. Evatt (1969). *Preschool Language Scale*. Columbus, Ohio: Charles E. Merrill.

Language Disorders In Children: Determining the Etiology and Directing the Clinical Effort

DETERMINING THE ETIOLOGY

Once it has been determined that the child under investigation has some sort of language deviation, we must determine exactly *why* this language deficit exists.

West (1957: 596) defines differential diagnosis as "a discriminating diagnosis aimed at distinguishing a given case of disorder from one or more other disorders presenting confusingly similar symptom pictures." The need for information on the etiology of a language disorder is not always clearly evident; in fact, some clinical approaches make no such demands upon the examiner.

1. Differential diagnosis gives broad direction to the therapy effort. If a child is determined to be hard-of-hearing, the ensuing therapy should, logically, take that fact into account. Without such information it would be possible to direct therapy to specific deficit areas, but the efficacy of the entire effort would be blunted.

2. Differential diagnosis may aid in the prognosis, or prediction of the rate and range of growth of the child. Knowledge of the etiological category may provide the clinician with some information about the typical group characteristics of growth patterns and the rehabilitative growth possible. Although the clinician should not apply group norms to the individual, such general patterns may prove helpful.

3. Such diagnostic information may help eliminate any agents that may yet be active. Perpetuating etiological factors should be identified and, if possible, eradicated.

4. Differential diagnosis may help to prevent the recurrence of the syndrome of behavior in other members of the client's family. If the etiological factor is such that

it may occur again to affect younger children, the family should be informed and helped in taking preventive steps.

5. Differential diagnosis serves as a clinical agent for the environment in yet another way. Parents, when seeking help for their children's problems, find comfort in knowing *why* a particular problem occurs. Such information generally lessens guilt feelings and aids in the general environmental milieu.

6. Every diagnostician should seek such information for its own sake. It will add to his basic knowledge of disorder types and help him in future diagnostic ventures.

The accumulation of evidence which leads to a particular diagnosis may take any one of a number of avenues.

1. The language pattern is typical of a specific etiological group:

Certain etiologies result in a predictable language pattern. David, an emotionally disturbed child living in a residential treatment center, engaged in the following conversation with his speech clinician:

Clinician: What would you like to do today?
   David: The First National is the number one bank. It's your yes bank in Duluth.
Clinician: David, I think we should go to work.
   David: Un-do it with the Un-Cola.

David's tangential responses, almost always in the form of a commercial, reflected his emotional disturbance. Tangent and non-associated conversations are typical of such children.

Aram and Nation (1975), however, question the concept that children of various etiological groups present characteristic language variations by which the group can be defined. They suggest classification according to linguistic differences. Their research on a heterogeneous group of forty-seven language-disordered children concluded that except for age and spurious findings for race (1975, p. 239), "the patterns of language behavior identified here were not related to any of the nonlinguistic measures studies." With the current level of sophistication of language analysis, it is probably appropriate to caution the clinician against making differential diagnostic decisions based upon language pattern alone. However, it is not unreasonable to assume that, as refinements take place in language evaluation, distinct and subtle patterns will become evident linking language behavior to etiological category.

2. A significant event in the child's past implicates a specific cause.

Events which might logically lead to a particular diagnosis such as known anoxia at birth or physical trauma from an auto accident often provide sufficient evidence.

3. The general pattern of the case history events leads to a certain etiological factor.

The following isolated bits of information from the case history lead the clinician to conclude that Cheryl's language disorder was related to a general learning disability:

    a. Cheryl's mother was educated in a class for the mentally retarded.

    b. Cheryl walked unaided at 42 months of age.

    c. Cheryl spoke her first word at 2 years but she only used the word for two weeks and then "lost it."

    d. Cheryl was not toilet trained until five years of age.

Although these factors taken alone would not be sufficient to verify the diagnosis, they do assist in the confirmation from other findings.

    4. Concommitent factors are present which are known to cause language delay.

When a certain factor, such as mental retardation, emotional disturbance, or environmental deprivation is known to exist, the task of differential diagnosis is eased. The tendency to terminate the search once an obvious factor has been uncovered should be resisted, however, since multiple factors are present in many or most instances.

    5. The causal factor may be determined by direct assessment.

The identification of many causes, such as hearing loss, are generally identified through direct testing.

    6. The response, or lack of response, to a particular remedial approach may provide a diagnostic clue.

The term "trial therapy" has been used to denote a period of time during which a particular clinical approach is tried in order to determine if it is effective. The assumption is that if you match the proper approach to the needs of the child, progress is maximized. If a child's articulation errors are related to his lack of knowledge of the rules of the phoneme system, then work on auditory discrimination may be ineffective. The lack of progress in an "ear training" program should lead the clinician to alter approach and look for other explanations of the cause of the problem.

    7. Some constellation of the above factors may lead to the diagnosis. In most instances the diagnosis made will probably be based upon a number of factors.

What are the potential factors that might interfere with language acquisition? Unfortunately the answer is not as clear-cut as it was once thought to be; and, in part, we must rely on the definition of language offered earlier. If we assume that language acquisition consists of a broad spectrum of skills that include vocabulary-building, phonemic development, grammatical development, concept formation, problem-solving, and so forth, then it appears that the factors traditionally supposed to interfere with language development may indeed be active. If, however, we consider language development to be the learning of the abstract rules that govern language behavior, then the research findings are much less certain.

This sounds very much like we are making a distinction between language competence (the underlying understanding of the language system) and language performance (the actual language behavior as exhibited through speaking, and writing); in fact, this may be the case. Part of the reason that the original question of which factors influence language acquisition is so difficult to answer straight-forwardly is that much of the research on language acquisition has failed to make the distinction between speech ability and underlying linguistic competence. Adding further to our dilemma is the always-present influence of bias. Those who theorize that language is primarily a learned behavior tend to find many factors that have an impact on language acquisition, whereas scholars who propose that language competence is largely an innate human skill tend to find that the traditional factors of sex, intelligence, and socioeconomic status have little impact on acquisition. Since we are looking at language acquisition as it is displayed in speech behavior, we shall discuss differential diagnosis from a rather traditional stance.

Mental Retardation. Although there remains substantial controversy re-garding the relationship of language and cognition, we assume that, to a large extent, the level of cognitive development determines the level of language sophistication. It is tempting to digress into a discussion of Piaget's theories of cognitive development and describe the current controversy over the "stages" concept of intellectual development; however, we will forego that and simply caution that much of what is currently postulated regarding cognitive development and language is theoretical in nature.

Language development is highly dependent upon the level of cognitive development. Although many other factors are also operational, the complexity of the thought process and the cognitive operations play a vital role in language. Many theorists, following Piaget's lead, point out that the child's semantic intent is related to his cognitive understanding, and the meanings of early words and sentences are dependent upon the concepts established in the early stages of development (Brown 1973; Wells 1974). As Bowerman (1976) implies, the child actively pursues linguistic forms and structures which adequately represent his knowledge. The child will not attempt to convey negation or plurality or posses-sion until those concepts have meaning. Two factors appear to be central to this theme. First, meaning, or semantic intent, is central to the child's communication attempts; thus the study of the child's semantic system may be of great importance in clinical language work. Second, the child's language reflects his attempts to represent concepts he already has but which are represented in some non-language (i.e., sensory-motor, etc.) form.

If the sensory avenues are intact, the mentally retarded child will receive the sensory information necessary to develop language. However, deficits in perception or organization of those stimuli, in memory, and in the ability to grasp linguistic abstractions result in language delay. These children tend to have greater difficulty learning inductively, and the transfer of learning from specific to general cases is diminished.

Behavioral clues to mental retardation may include articulation deviations, attentional deficits, lack of clearly established handedness, general development delay across several behaviors, and additional congenital differences. Mentally retarded children tend to develop language at a slower pace than normal children, and the ultimate product is less complex and more stereotyped. It is generally assumed that the child's language learning will continue until puberty, with the mental age reached at that point determining the level of language sophistication (Lenneberg, 1969).

Grossman (1973) classifies mental retardation relative to the following categories of etiology, and provides a comprehensive discussion of each:

Infections and Intoxications
Trauma or Physical Agent
Metabolism or Nutrition
Gross Brain Disease (Postnatal)
Unknown Prenatal Influence
Chromosomal Abnormality
Gestational Disorders
Following Psychiatric Disorder
Environmental Influence
Other Conditions

Although the measurement of intellectual functioning is seldom the province of the speech clinician, she is often called upon to make referrals and draw conclusions from test data. Most of the traditional measures used by psychometrists to measure intelligence are not applicable to children with language disorders. Speech performance, either from a production or reception standpoint, strongly influences the results of nearly every major measure of intelligence; thus the language-deficient children are placed at an immediate disadvantage. Measures such as the *Leiter International Performance Scale* (Arthur, 1952) are free of language interference. The speech clinician has the duty to warn psychologists and educators against overinterpreting intelligence measures that deal harshly with language-deficient children.

Emotional Disturbance. There is little question that the emotional stability of a child affects the quality and quantity of his verbal behavior. However, there is some question as to whether the emotional state significantly affects the child's ability to learn the language system. The net result of severe emotional disturbance is often bizarre speech behavior that ranges from mutism to complex and continuous verbiage. Once again, the task of analysis does not fall to the speech clinician; however, it is important for the diagnostician to keep in mind that how a child talks may reflect as much about his psyche as what he says.[1]

Leaving the formalized testing to the psychometrician, the speech clinician may look for the following characteristics that indicate the need for psychological evaluation.

1. Infantile language patterns that are not consistent with the overall potential of the child.

2. Language patterns that change significantly in both quality and quantity from one environment to another.

3. The persistence of echolalic and monologue speech to the exclusion of socialized speech behavior beyond the fourth year.

4. Atypical patterns of tonal quality, along with restricted or bizarre characteristics of emotional expression—generally, a lack of crying and laughing or strange patterns thereof.

5. Conversations filled with "tangential" remarks and responses. Eisenson (1963) explains tangential responses as replies which speak to an incidental aspect of a statement but disregard the meaning.

6. Speaking too much or too little in a given circumstance is a warning signal. Child-rearing practices no longer stress that children should be seen but not heard, and the mute child should be earnestly encouraged to communicate in the testing situation. If, on the other hand, a child is exceedingly verbal to the point of obsession, this too may be diagnostically significant:

   Sally had been variously diagnosed as retarded, cerebral palsied, and aphasic, but whatever the diagnosis, she was, at age thirteen, still without speech and was using a language board to communicate. Upon entering the examining room with the student clinician, she began pointing to the word "Helen" on her board and then to the word "visit." Once the student commented that it was nice that Sally was going to visit Helen (her aunt), Sally pointed to the phrase "I like you" and spelled out "we are good friends." Within five minutes of the initiation of the diagnostic session, Sally had told about the new curtains in her bedroom, her father's operation for back trouble, and how much she loves her mother. Following the session the student was incensed when it was suggested that Sally had some emotional problems in conjunction with her speech and language difficulties. The idea that she said too much and volunteered too much unrequested and unimportant information never occurred to the student, who was completely taken by this "friendly" and "outgoing" child.

7. Language is an extension of the thought process, and therefore the diagnostician must look at the logic and organization displayed.

8. A disinterest in people or communication, together with a preoccupation with mechanical objects, is typical of this group.

   This child may learn unrelated words from watching television and may appear to use speech primarily for self-stimulation.

---

[1]Rousey and Moriarty (1965) suggest that the psyche has a profound impact on articulatory accuracy. What implication might this have for language evaluation?

Such lists could, of course, be endless, but they do serve as a baseline for further elaboration. A word of warning is in order about the interpretation of behavior, however. It is essential that the examiner make a careful analysis of the child's total environment before drawing conclusions about the significance of his behavior. Not only are there cultural and subcultural differences in modes of behavior, but family environments also have significant variances.

> Bert was totally confounding the student clinician with his apparent euphoria and inability to understand any questions put to him. When asked if he walked to the clinic, Bert would pose a taut, wry, little smile and nod in affirmation. Later he was asked if he got to the clinic in a car, and he gave the same kind of response. In fact, the student got a similar smile and nod to the same question substituting a train, cab, bicycle, and kitchen sink. Things clarified greatly when the mother was interviewed, and her face froze in a meaningless smile as she resisted any meaningful interaction with sterile and superficial answers.

Echolalia deserves special mention since it represents a primary means of language use in autistic children. Baltaxe (1971) defined echolalia as a meaningless repetition of words in word groups just spoken by another person. The echolalia may be immediate or delayed and may or may not have communicative value. When the clinician determines that a child is excessive in the use of echoic responses, she should determine if the echolalia has communication value for the child, if it is grammatical or represents the child's reductions of the adult model, and whether the echoic behavior presents itself immediately or after a time delay.

The discussion of pragmatic language disorders found later in this chapter is related in a very specific way to the language behaviors found in disturbed children.

Minimal Brain Dysfunction. The term "brain damage" is often used to refer to children with minimal brain dysfunction; however, there are so many valid arguments against the use of the term "brain damage" as an etiological category for language disturbance that it is amazing that it is still in use. It is a testimony to the early works of scholars such as Strauss and Lehtinen (1947), who were so effective in describing a syndrome of behavior, that the term became solidly accepted. We perceive and remember best those characteristics that have labels, so it is often convenient, if misleading, for the brain to group many variables into a single category. Our argument against the use of the term "brain damage" centers around three aspects: (1) impact on the environment, (2) the impurity of the diagnostic category, and (3) the lack of usefulness as an aid to therapy.

The impact of the term "brain damage" on the parent can be devastating. Feelings of guilt arise, along with the implication that some sort of actual physical damage has taken place to an otherwise normal organism. Nearly every parent can recall some severe fall or imagined trauma to his child which could have caused the problem and might have been prevented. Parents tend to hear the term as a sort of static characteristic that dooms their child to a life of inadequacy; the label has an unchanging, permanent, hopeless ring to it. Many parents also equate the term with mental retardation, since brain functioning is obviously associated with intellectual potential. The studies of Siegel and Harkins (1963) show what can happen to adult-child interaction when the adult assumes that the child is mentally retarded; the change in the quality and quantity of verbal stimulation may be significant. Lastly, there is a tangential environmental effect in the frequently prescribed medication for brain-damaged children. Not infrequently the use of medication places the onus of control of the child on some outside authority—in this case the prescribed medication. We have observed several instances in which both child and parent believed no control was possible without medication.

> Paul was an active four-year-old when he was diagnosed by the neurologist as brain damaged. A then-popular medication was prescribed and used for six years. When Paul was ten years old, however, his parents felt that further problems were evident, and they returned him for additional testing. The diagnosis was reconfirmed and a new medication prescribed. The neurologist informed the child that the new pills were "memory pills" and must be taken every morning before school. Not long thereafter, Paul returned home from school admonishing his mother for forgetting to give him his pill that morning. "I must have forgotten to take it, mom; I forgot all sorts of stuff today and got in lots of trouble," he said. The idea that the pill was all that was keeping the child functioning was instilled in his and his parent's thinking.

The term "brain damage" is not a pure diagnostic category. Cerebral-palsied children are brain damaged, epileptic children have brain differences, some emotionally disturbed children, some deaf, and some retarded children have brain damage; the aphasoid child is brain damaged, as is the child with central dysarthria, whether or not he fits into one of the other categories. If brain damage implies brain difference, we are all "brain damaged" to some degree.

The use of the designation "brain damage" as an aid to future therapy has not been fruitful. The term is not descriptive as once thought, and no single rehabilitative technique has come forth to help this type of child. The continuing search for specific treatment methods to fit specific causes keeps alive, however, our search for the causes, and without this pursuit the answers that must ultimately come will be lost.

The ability of the central nervous system to deal with symbolic abstractions is critical to language development. If the attribute is lost or diminished due to agenesis or trauma, the resultant disorder is termed "childhood aphasia" or "aphasoid syndrome." Whatever the label, the possibility that the child without language or speech development is aphasic should be investigated.

Differentiating the aphasic child from other etiological groups is an exhausting, time-consuming, and often frustrating undertaking. Since it is inherent in the concept of aphasia that the child have some central nervous system differences, the possibility is very real that this child may also have a degree of retardation, hearing loss, and eventual secondary emotional reactions. Seldom, if ever, is it possible to arrive at a diagnosis of aphasia in one session, and once again we must stress the need for ongoing diagnosis. The eventual need for diagnostic treatment and the possibility of gaining diagnostic information from observing the results of treatment must not be overlooked.

Since it takes the combined efforts of several disciplines to arrive at a satisfactory diagnosis of aphasia, it may well, and often does, fall upon the shoulders of the speech clinician to collate and integrate the various diagnostic findings and draw some conclusions from them. In light of this Wood states:

> First, the classification of aphasia in children assumes that the major factor separating this disorder from all other speech and language problems is the disturbance in symbolic language formulation. . . . The deaf child does not develop speech normally, but his lack of speech production is related directly to his inability to hear sound. Yet deaf children may have integrated symbolic language in all language functions that do not require sound. The mentally retarded child functions at a retarded symbolic level, but symbolic formulation is not the only area of his deficiency. Thus, the mentally retarded child is expected to develop symbolic language in proportion to his mental age. The emotionally disturbed child may reject sound and may not talk, but his problem, again, is not relegated to a primary disturbance in symbolic formulation. Diagnostically, these differentiations are of extreme importance. Second, some of the more overt symptoms of aphasia may resemble the symptoms of other childhood problems, but the total problem constellations are distinctly different. . . . Third, the classification of aphasia cannot be used merely because all other possible diagnostic classifications have been excluded (1964: 32–33).

To further complicate our task of diagnosis, most authorities differentiate between children with primarily motor, or expressive, disabilities and children with primarily sensory, or receptive, disabilities; and although these two subcategories overlap a great deal, there are some distinguishing patterns of behavior. It should be noted, however, that when the disability is linked either to a single input or output modality and does not appear to interfere with the central language process, it is technically not aphasia but rather apraxia, agraphia, or agnosia (Wepman et al., 1960).

From our own clinical observations and the writings of others, we feel that two primary areas of difficulty epitomize the aphasia condition in children. First, there is a general and marked difficulty in processing auditory information. This difficulty is primarily exhibited in verbal communication but may also show up on tests of hearing acuity. Most "aphasic" children will be found to have normal peripheral hearing, but the results of traditional tests are often equivocal. Their responses to spoken language are inconsistent, but generally improve when the signal is slowed down and distractions are eliminated.

The second characteristic is less easily defined. Aphasic children, in our experience, have greater difficulty learning inductively; that is, these children appear to have greater than normal problems learning the rules of language from the disparate examples of those rules presented to them by their environment. This later problem may be directly related to the first, since the auditory problems may not allow for a consistency of patterning needed to generalize the regularities of the spoken samples of language being heard. The problem may be more pervasive, however, in organizational skills in general. The end result is that clinical intervention programs which emphasize organization, structure, reduced pace, and repetition are often effective.

Since any single characteristic may well indicate more than one etiological category, it is often necessary to look for a constellation of factors that indicate aphasia. The following may provide a starting point:

1. The case-history information may suggest possible brain cell damage—i.e., anoxia, trauma, or hemorrhage.

2. Neurological examination findings may suggest possible brain damage—i.e., EEG abnormalities, infantile reflex patterns, or motor incoordination. Landau, Goldstein, and Kleffner (1960) found that aphasic children have a higher percentage of EEG abnormalities than the normal population, but it should be remembered that the absence of abnormal EEG or any other neurological signs must not rule out aphasia.

3. Intelligence scores on verbal and nonverbal tests may vary significantly, with the nonverbal being higher.

4. Shows an interest in people and seeks to interact with them and participate in social activities. (This may diminish somewhat as the child grows older.)

5. The aphasic child is significantly behind his age group in ability to classify and group things into some sort of organized pattern. He is generally unable to see the similarities among members of a given class or category, and thus is unable to deal well in abstractions. This is admittedly an oversimplification, and the reader is warned that there is a wide spectrum of behavior to be judged.

6. The aphasic child has difficulty imitating articulatory movements and recalling sequences and patterns. This is generally typical of the motor aphasic child.

7. With great stimulation and time-consuming effort the aphasic child is able to learn and produce articulatory patterns, but appears unable to generalize this skill to new words without repeating the laborious task of drill once again.

8. After learning articulatory movements for a given word, this child may need an unusual amount of help in transferring this skill to other settings.

9. The aphasic child's comprehension of speech is poor, and it is not improved with amplification. Some authorities claim that actual decrements in understanding are typical of aphasic children under amplification. These comprehension difficulties may be manifest in poor auditory discrimination for individual speech sounds or be so extensive as to make the comprehension of speech difficult or impossible. Obviously discrimination ability is partly dependent upon reception of the speech signal, but the actual task of comparing and judging the similarities and differences is a function of the central nervous system.

10. The child shows confusion or is delayed in establishing laterality, but not always.

11. The child commonly has difficulty in establishing a flow of speech, which results in awkward grammatical constructions, numerous hesitations, false starts and repetitions, and altered timing patterns. The term "cluttering" is often used to identify this speech pattern.

12. The child usually has difficulty perceiving forms or patterns. He finds it difficult to select the significant auditory, visual, or tactile pattern from the surroundings. This "figure-ground" difficulty often appears related to a tendency to fix on some aspect of the stimulus without perceiving that aspect as a part of a gestalt.

13. Hardy (1962) speaks of the child's inability to process successive stimuli rapidly. These children tend to be able to handle fewer bits of information than normal children, and this is exhibited in poor recall ability for serially presented stimuli.
14. Hardy also discusses the capacity of the child to "track" verbal stimuli. He defines tracking as "a matter of being able to process an indefinite variety of incoming information, employing all the attributes of the sensorium, and to relate this to previous and presently pertinent experience" (42). The ability to use what is remembered of past experiences by recalling them and applying them to present stimuli is sometimes deficient in these children.

Many workers disagree with the use of the term "congenital aphasia" as an etiological category. Lenneberg (1964) articulates the argument clearly, citing evidence that the cortex has a large degree of functional equipotentiality during the first three years of life. He states further:

> Whatever function becomes localized in adult life can become established in early childhood in spite of the presence of fixed cortical and subcortical lesions, and it seems immaterial where these lesions are located. The entire left hemisphere may be incapacitated during the first two years and remain so thereafter without interfering with the establishment of language at the usual age. However, a similar lesion would result in irreversible language loss if it occurred during or after the middle of the second decade. Neither trauma nor surgical lesions, nor focal infections, nor agenesis (including the corpus callosum) regardless of cortical locality will prevent acquisition of language as long as the insult occurs at early enough an age, is confined to a single hemisphere, and does not reduce the individual to a state of idiocy. . . . Thus there is clearly no justification for speaking of congenital motor aphasia (168–169).

Neuromotor incoordination. In order for articulate speech to be produced, it is imperative that the brain be capable of organizing neural impulses before sending them to the speech structure, that the neural pathways be capable of transmitting these organized impulses to the musculature, and that the musculature itself be capable of receiving the stimuli and responding appropriately. If the child is unable to produce such coordinated action, articulate speech will suffer. This implies, however, that such circumstances will probably result only in an expressive language deficit. This is probably not the case. As Berry (1969) points out, we perceive speech-sound sequences only after the neuromusculature patterns of articulation have been established. If this is indeed true, then the child's receptive and internal language skills are no doubt linked to his production skills and will suffer some sort of limitation if the organized production of speech is deficient.

In addition to this alleged association between motor speech and language acquisition, there is another relationship which must be mentioned. Several workers, Kephart (1960), for example, have postulated a hierarchical relationship between lower-level functions, i.e., perceptual-motor behavior, and higher cognitive functions. If this hierarchy of development does exist, motor coordination takes on even greater significance for language acquisition. Lenneberg (1964), on the other hand, speaks of the congenitally inarticulate child as a youngster who has an excellent comprehension of language and a fully developed language system, but who cannot control the speech musculature to produce articulate speech patterns.

The control of the speech musculature is, in part, a function of nerve-muscle patterns that lead from the brain; it is also a function of the nerve-brain–nerve-muscle patterns. That is to say, coordinated muscle control is indebted to the feedback of information from the tactile, kinesthetic, proprioceptive sensors informing the brain where the structures are and where they are going. In certain types of expressive language impairments, it may be necessary to differentiate between neuromotor and sensory-motor breakdowns. Liberman gives priority to the kinesthetic feedback information over the auditory in the control and comprehension of language. He states:

> We believe that a speaker (and listener) learns to connect speech sounds with their appropriate articulations and that the sensory feedback from these movements (or, more likely, the corresponding neurological processes) comes to mediate between the acoustic stimulus and its perception (1957: 117–123).

Environmental Deprivation. The importance of the quantity and quality of the interaction of the child with his communication models has been disputed for some time. However, the trend appears to be toward ascribing greater importance to language models than was suspected in the 1950s and 1960s.

Children are continuously provided with language models as well as information regarding the content and structural adequacy of their language. Broen (1972) concluded from her investigations into parent-child communication that parents adjust their language to the level of the child. With younger children parents tend to talk slower, using more pauses, smaller vocabularies, and repetitions of a limited number of sentence types. This line of thinking, currently being pursued by many researchers, is an interesting reversal of certain concepts ascribed to the transformational theorists. Could it be that children aren't so much natural language learners as parents are natural language teachers? If the importance of parent-child language interaction is as great as it currently appears to be, the following diagnostic endeavors may prove fruitful in determining the cause and directing the clinical process.

1. Determine who the major language models are for the child—their age, relationship to the child, and amount of time typically spent with the child.
2. Through comprehensive case history and interviewing, determine the amount and quality of language stimulation in the child's first three years of life. Some researchers (Ajuriaguerra, et al., 1976) have reported an inordinately high incidence of emotionally and language-disturbed children among children who suffered separation from parents or serious illnesses at the time of onset of language.
3. Undertake extensive observation of the parent-child interaction, preferably in the home setting, and take note of the following:
   a. Amount of language stimulation present
   b. Rate of speech of models
   c. Sentence complexity and types presented by models

d. Vocabulary use
e. Parental expansions
f. Clarity of the model (signal clarity, linguistic clarity)
g. Parental response to content of child's speech
h. Parental response to structure of child's speech
i. Opportunity for the child to talk

We are only beginning to scientifically measure the impact of parent-child interaction on language development. The clinician will want to keep abreast of new findings and alter diagnostic approaches accordingly.

Auditory acuity. Among the most obvious physical factors influencing language acquisition is hearing acuity. Deaf and severely hard-of-hearing children do not learn to perform in the language realm as well or as rapidly as do hearing children. Once again, however, we must be sobered by the fact that these children have to a large extent the basic symbolic resources of the hearing child and thus are quite capable of acquiring language if adequate stimulation can only be channeled into the central nervous system through some alternate route. Lenneberg (1967) makes a strong case for this. However, if we examine a five-year-old deaf child who has not had the opportunity to receive the language system due to his auditory deficit and the shortcomings of his environment, he does indeed suffer from language incompetence as well as diminished language performance. Whether you consider the problem to be due to the child's impairment or to the environment has little effect upon the final disposition of the case. Every child with language delay must undergo extensive hearing evaluations. For a complete discussion of audiological evaluations see Newby (1972) and others (O'Neill and Oyer, 1966; Davis and Silverman, 1970).

Differential diagnosis of children with language disorders requires careful analysis of historical information, intuitive observation of the child and his environment, skillful test administration and interpretation, and a thorough knowledge of normal and abnormal behavior. It is totally unreasonable to expect anyone to have all of the skills and knowledge necessary to make this diagnosis unilaterally. It is imperative that diagnosis be done by a team. The lack of interdisciplinary cooperation has resulted in far too many children being diagnosed by numerous "specialists," each viewing the child through his own professional biases, and each reaching different conclusions.

DIRECTING THE CLINICAL EFFORT

As clinical approaches differ, so in fact do the uses clinicians make of the information provided from diagnosis. Some favor enhancing the strengths of the child; others prefer to direct their therapy efforts toward the weaknesses; many simply take the diagnostic information as an indication of where the child stands at a given point in time and use that as a starting point for treatment.

In addition to searching for the strengths and weaknesses of the client, this last goal of diagnosis may also aid the clinician by (1) determining the severity of the problem, (2) setting a baseline for remediation, (3) giving direction to grouping and scheduling considerations, (4) measuring progress, and (5) making a prognosis. Only by carefully interrelating the data from the various diagnostic sources is it possible to obtain the information necessary for effective work.

Six areas need to be investigated in order to establish and maintain appropriate clinical procedures.

1. Sub-language skills
2. Level of cognitive development
3. Semantic elements of language
4. Syntactic elements of language
5. Phonological elements of language
6. Pragmatic elements of language

Sub-language Skills

The evaluation of sub-language skills involves the measurement of performance in a number of domains. Some of these skills have a proven relationship with language development, while with others the research is inconclusive. Some of what we do in this area is based on conjecture and logic rather than on research findings.

These skills are evaluated to direct the clinician toward areas which might need clinical attention prior to or during the work on the language system itself. Figure 5.1, a checklist adapted from the work of Stremel-Campbell (1977) and others, may be helpful in structuring observation of the child's early sub-language abilities.

The auditory modality is known to be the primary language-learning channel. For this reason many clinicians evaluate a number of auditory sensory and perceptual areas. Unfortunately, standardization is lacking with most procedures; the picture is further complicated because many of the tests, although meant to evaluate sub-language skills, use language forms as test elements.

Auditory acuity. Tests of auditory acuity have been discussed elsewhere in this and other texts. The child who is unable to properly receive and transmit the acoustic signal to his central nervous system is a candidate for therapeutic procedures such as lip-reading, auditory training, speech therapy, and language development.

Behavior	Source of Information		Consistency				Comments
	Observation	Parent Report	Consistently Displayed	Inconsistently Displayed	Never Displayed	Unknown	
is ambulatory							
establishes eye contact							
attends to people							
follows moving object with eye							
maintains attention (60 seconds)							
can be reinforced							
reaches for object							
moves body for object							
localizes sound							
recognizes familiar faces							
recognizes familiar voices							
engages in sound play							
imitates motor movements							
matches objects							

Checklist of Sub-Language Skills

Figure 5.1 Checklist of Sub-Language Skills

Behavior	Source of Information		Consistency				Comments
sequences two objects							
sequences four objects							
groups objects re. intrinsic qualities							
matches re. function							
meaningful play with toys							
intersecting play with others							
imitates speech sounds							
matches pictures							
matches objects/pictures							
matches shapes							
matches size							
matches color							
	Observation	Parent Report	Consistently Displayed	Inconsistently Displayed	Never-Displayed	Unknown	

Checklist of Sub-Language Skills (cont.)

Figure 5.1 Checklist, cont'd.

Auditory attention. Auditory attention has been variously defined but, in essence, refers to the ability to focus on a given message as a significant stimulus. Chalfant and Scheffelin state:

> Inattentiveness to auditory stimuli might be related to: (a) Low level or absence of hearing acuity; (b) distractibility involving competitive visual or auditory stimuli; (c) hyperactive behavior; (d) severe emotional disturbance; (e) severe mental retardation; or (f) inability to obtain meaning from auditory stimuli (1969: 11).

There are no well-developed techniques for evaluating a child's attention to auditory stimuli. The examiner must rely on observations of the child to determine if he shows awareness of sound by turning his head, changing his facial expression, or moving toward or away from the sound source. If a child is capable of receiving the sound signal but incapable of attending to that stimulus long enough for it to become meaningful, there will be severe impact on language development.

Auditory localization. Auditory localization is the ability to locate the direction of the significant sound in a perceptual field. In the more elementary form, localization refers simply to identifying the direction of any given sound; but its more complex form involves selecting a significant sound from a field of competing sounds. Informal tests of sound localization would be easy to develop and should add significant data to the diagnosis, since this ability no doubt helps the child to relate sounds to objects and persons and to develop the perceptual skills of discrimination.

Berelson and Steiner (1964: 88) define perception as "the more complex process by which people select, organize, and interpret sensory stimulation into a meaningful and coherent picture of the world." Inherent in the concept of perception is the recognition of the constancies in a particular stimulus that allow the individual to distinguish that stimulus from all competing stimuli and to separate the significant sound from the background sounds. The following test areas are included under auditory perception:

Figure-ground differentiation. The ability to select and identify the relevant auditory stimuli from increasingly complex and competing background sounds is tested. It is quite possible to construct a test of figure-ground differentiation by using tape-recorded materials of varying amplitude, interest, and similarity with the stimulus signals. The Goldman-Fristoe-Woodcock Test of Auditory Discrimination (1970) is comprised of three portions: a training portion, a test of auditory discrimination in quiet conditions, and a test of auditory discrimination where a background noise of 9 db. less intense than the signal has been superimposed over the stimulus. The background noise consists of semi-intelligible noise recorded in a busy school cafeteria. The test includes a prerecorded test tape and a book of stimulus pictures. Norms are provided for individuals aged from three years, eight months, to over seventy years.

Auditory closure. Auditory closure is the ability to integrate the various separate units of a stimulus into a whole. In order for a listener to understand spoken language, he must be capable of making sense out of the sequentially presented sounds, syllables, words, phrases, and sentences. The skills of figure-ground differentiation, memory, and discrimination must in some way be coordinated to provide the listener with the meaning of the total message. Berry (1969) argues strongly that the perception of speech is syncratic in nature. That is, the child comprehends the whole of a given language stimulus before he can differentiate and analyze the parts. Whatever the order of development, however, it is important to identify this ability. Since our definition of closure stresses the ability to integrate separate units of a stimulus, we must test two somewhat different skills. These skills are sometimes labeled auditory blending (or synthesis) and auditory closure; however, we feel that they both belong under the heading of closure. Speech-sound synthesis is tested by having the child repeat words which have been spoken to him with each sound separated by slight time intervals. The sound blending subtest of the ITPA is an example of this type of measure. Van Riper (1972) presents a test of speech-sound synthesis as it pertains to articulation acquisition. The language diagnostician should follow up this type of testing with an analysis of the child's ability to synthesize larger samples of language such as sentences and paragraphs. Tests of closure which evaluate the child's ability to fill in missing parts in recreating the whole of the message evaluate a somewhat different but closely related skill. The auditory closure subtest of the ITPA measures this skill. In this test, words such as airplane are pronounced "air-pla-" and telephone is "tele-one." The child's task is to identify the word spoken, and the assumed skill involved is achieving closure from an incomplete stimulus. Sentence completion tasks which involve filling in blanks deal with closure at the contextual level. The Auditory-Vocal Association Test of the ITPA and the Intraverbal Test of the Parsons Language Sample use such techniques. Berry (1969) has devised an exploratory measure of linguistic closure for children from four to eight years of age.

Auditory discrimination. Berry (1969) uses the term discrimination synonymously with perception. An individual's ability to identify differences in auditory signals has long been thought to be crucial to speech and language development. Speech clinicians have persistently relied on "ear training" in therapy because they strongly believe that the ear must discriminate before the mouth can articulate.

Tests of auditory discrimination have been developed by Templin (1957); Wepman (1958); Mecham, Jex, and Jones (1969); Goldman, Fristoe, and Woodcock (1970); Berry (1969); Prather et al. (1971); Lindamood and Lindamood (1971); and others. However, no formal test adequately measures the actual discriminating task required for language production. For accurate speech production, and potentially for adequate language-learning, the child must be able to instantly judge the accuracy of his own speech output by comparing the heard auditory signal with some internal criterion of correctness. In actuality this judgment must be made instantly and intrapersonally; yet most tests follow significant time lapse between stimulus and response, and are interpersonal in nature.

Memory. The relationship between language and memory is complex and much controversy yet remains. However, four primary memory elements appear to have a bearing on language behavior. Short-term memory of sentence elements, long-term storage of language rules, sequential memory, and memory for the prosody and supra-segmental elements of language will be briefly discussed.

In order to understand a spoken sentence, the listener must be able to retain the various elements of the sentence long enough to interrelate them. Obviously the memory demands in the sentence (a) "Daddy swims" are significantly less than in sentence (b) "My daddy, the big man in the green swimming suit, knows how to swim." But for both sentences the listener must retain knowledge of who the agent was, and retain it long enough to link it with the action. The problem with testing short-term memory is that so many other language facets enter in as extraneous task demands.

The clinician may devise a series of sentences with varying amounts of distraction between the major semantic elements, and determine the child's ability to answer simple questions such as, "who swims?" Elements to be evaluated could include agents, actions, attributes, and all of the other semantic elements of early child language.

Measurement of long-term memory for storage of grammatical rules is usually accomplished through tests of language comprehension (as discussed in Chapter 4). Unfortunately it is impossible to determine if failure on such tasks reflects poor long-term memory or some other factor.

An informal procedure to determine the child's knowledge of rules involves the use of error-identification procedures. Here the child is presented with two sentence samples and asked which is correct.

> In order to test the child's knowledge of some of the rules of subject/verb agreement, the clinician placed a puppet on each hand and told the child that each puppet was going to tell him something, but only one puppet was able to tell his message correctly. The child was asked to point to the puppet "who knows how to talk." The following sentences are examples of those presented:
>
> *Puppet A:* The boy walk to school.
> *Puppet B:* The boy walks to school.
> *Puppet A:* The horses runs fast.
> *Puppet B:* The horses run fast.

Berko's test of English morphology (1958) gets at the child's knowledge of the rules of the language in a similar manner.

Auditory sequential memory is generally tested by presenting the child with a sequence of stimuli and requesting that he repeat the sequence. The Auditory

Sequential Memory Test of the *ITPA*, the repeating digits subtest of the *Stanford-Binet Intelligence Scale* and the Digit Span subtest of the *WISC* all use digits for stimuli. In the Stanford-Binet test the digits are presented at a rate of one per second and the approximate norms are as follows (Terman and Merrill, 1960):

Age	Digit Recall
2½	2
3	3
4½	4
7	5
10	6
Adult	7

The recall of unrelated words is measured in the Auditory Attention Span for Unrelated Words subtest of the *Detroit Tests of Learning Aptitude* (Baker & Leland, 1959). In this test words are presented at a one-per-second rate and the child is requested to repeat the words in presented order. Symbolic factors and comprehension complicate the interpretation of memory tasks using words, but it is assumed that this is more closely related to language functioning.

As the recall task begins to involve language units larger than the word, skills of syntax and verbal patterning become increasingly important. Although used for experimental purposes, the sentence-imitation tests devised by Slobin and Welsh (1967) as cited by McNeill (1970) present interesting information. These researchers investigated the child's ability to comprehend sentences through his ability to preserve meaning in repetition. Verbatim repetition of presented sentences was not expected. In this case, a correct response would be for the child to maintain the meaning of the sentence in his repetition. The skills involved imply syntactic development, comprehension, recall, and expression.

It is common to use directions as a method for measuring a child's ability to handle increasingly complex sentence forms. This measure of comprehension and recall demands no verbal response since the child is simply requested to perform a series of tasks: "point to the pencil, put the penny in the cup, and give me the crayon." Such tasks can be very simple or complicated, so the examiner is able to adapt the level of difficulty to the child.

The *Stanford-Binet Intelligence Scale* also measures memory for sentences at selected age levels. These tests demand verbatim recall of sentences. Several of the elicited-imitation tests (mentioned in Chapter 4) measure short-term memory, but have as their primary goal evaluation of the language skills relative to the stimulus sentences.

The recall of the content of stories is widely used to evaluate adult aphasics. Once again, linguistic comprehension is involved as well as longer-term retention and recall. Generally this testing takes the form of a narrative story followed by a question and answer period. It is also possible to ask the child to retell the story and establish some sort of criterion for judging those responses.

Berry (1969) suggests certain qualitative judgments which might be made of the child's responses, and it is obvious that certain techniques also lend themselves to quantitative measurement of the child's recall ability. It is possible to vary such attributes as the length of the story, content complexity, nature of the questions, and length of time between the story and the questions, in order to fit the measurement of the child.

> Chauncey was four when we first saw him for evaluation. The student clinician assigned to the diagnosis had written a short story about three ducks who didn't like to swim until late one spring day when their high and dry playground was flooded by heavy rains. Upon completion of the story, Chauncey was asked to recall the story. He stated: "Duckie not swim . . . play. Duckie all wet . . . swim fast." The student's accurate conclusion was that Chauncey had adequate recall for content although grammatical complexity was delayed.

In our use of stories for measurement of recall, we have attempted to determine if the child is able to recall the following major elements of the presentation: 1) significant details regarding names in the story, 2) sequence of the story, 3) main idea, 4) major actions within the story, and 5) outcomes of the story.

Matching, grouping, and categorizing are all sub-language skills thought to be related to ultimate language learning. It would appear that the ability to group similar perceptual experiences into single units would aid the language learner to organize his world. Without the ability to see similarities in slightly differing events, the world would be an unmanageable maze of new and unrelated stimuli with little or no organization or meaning.

The matching of identical objects, object-to-picture matching, and matching of shapes, sizes, colors, and functions presents the clinician with a hierarchy of difficulty to present to the child. The *Leiter International Performance Scale* (1952) uses matching and other visual perceptual tasks in the determination of intellectual level. Elements of matching are included in the Visual Reception subtest of the *ITPA*, the *Developmental Test of Visual Perception* and the *Stanford-Binet Intelligence Scale;* however, the clinician is encouraged to devise her own testing battery ordering the difficulty of the task and the subtlety of the discrimination.

The abstraction process consists of leaving out details and attending to the similarities among perceptual experiences. As the child perceives differences and similarities in stimuli in his environment, he is increasingly capable of grouping these experiences into categories. This capability is the essence of concept development. Verbal concepts are formed when the child begins to respond to different words with the same or similar internal mediational behaviors (Kendler and Karasik, 1958). The exact relationship between concept formation and language has not been satisfactorily described; however, it is safe to assume that many language skills involve concept development—for instance, abstracting the qualities of certain words that make them nouns. The process is complicated, as Staats indicates:

> The process of concept formation is seen as one which involves complicated principles of learning, communication, and mediated generalization. The relationship

between the language process and the environmental process is complex. The language processes arise from a response to the environment but then in turn affect responses to other aspects of the environment (1968:143).

As the child is exposed to a greater variety of experiences that isolate perceptual invariants, increasingly complex concepts become available. For this reason the testing of concept development becomes a theoretically limitless task. The relationship between language and concept formation is apparent in that language serves to store and transmit concepts; and the ability to manipulate symbolically experiential variables allows man to develop and refine concepts with ever-increasing complexity. Whorf (1956) points out, however, that language systems not only enhance concept formation but also define and limit them. To this extent, language both facilitates and restricts conceptualization.

Many of the diagnostic tests of language function are in effect measures of concept development—i.e., intelligence and achievement tests. The child's ability to solve problems, reason, recall, organize, plan, and deal in abstractions is all firmly based in language.

The author of the field research edition of the Basic Concept Inventory (Engelmann, 1967: 5) states: "The Basic Concept Inventory is a broad checklist of basic concepts that are involved in new learning situations in the first grade." Intended for culturally disadvantaged slow learners, the emotionally disturbed, and the mentally retarded, the test is based on the premise that learning involves concepts and knowledge of the child's ability to conceptualize is strategic to educational (and presumably remedial) undertakings.

The Boehm Test of Basic Concepts (1971) is a very useful measure to identify those children who have difficulty with concepts that are important for academic achievement. The fifty-item test measures the child's concepts of space, quantity, time, and miscellaneous items and can be given to groups of children. The test has value for children from five to eight years of age. As with many such measures, this test taps the child's vocabulary as well as his conceptualization and familiarity with the pictured items; it has met with wide acceptance and has a distinct value in directing the remedial effort.

Level of Cognitive Development

Although formal standardized intelligence tests provide an indication of the child's readiness for language development, they do not provide a great deal of assistance in planning the remedial effort. Measures of mental maturity based upon Piaget's concepts will, on the other hand, provide a clear indication of the types of language structures and functions the child is ready to master. Since it is assumed that the child will only learn those language structures and functions which he already understands at some non-language level, the logical end result of evaluation of the cognitive function is to provide a picture of the child's knowledge base. Clinical intervention could then attempt to assist the child to discover the language link to communicate his non-language knowledge.

Some attempts have been made to construct tests of cognitive functioning based upon Piaget's theory; however, there is general agreement that standardized testing which results in scores and IQs is contrary to some of the precepts of the theory.[2] A basic principle involved is that performance must be interpreted only in relation to the context and the materials used to elicit such performance. Muma (1978) attempts to spell out the relationship between cognitive functioning and language assessment in a fashion which leads directly to clinical planning.

Semantic Elements of Language

Although the diagnostic procedures described in Chapter 4 were directed at determination of the existence of the language problem, the information gained could profitably be applied to clinical planning. Of primary interest to the clinician in planning language sessions is knowledge of which semantic grammatical rules the child understands and uses. MacDonald and Nickols (1974) used imitation, conversation, and planned procedures to evaluate the ten semantic elements identified on page 104.

Table 5-1 presents an adaptation of Brown's (1970) presentation of meaning categories, grammatical structures and child utterances. This represents an additional procedure for evaluation of early language development.

Table 5-1 Meaning Categories in Early Child Utterances

Meaning	Structures	Examples
Nomination	that + N	that ball
	it + N	it shoe
Notice	hi + N	hi car
Recurrence	more + N	more milk
	verb + again	play 'gin
Nonexistence	no + N	no doggie
	all gone + N	all gone candy
Attributive	Adj + N	big train
Possessive	N + N	mommy hat
Locative	N + N	ball chair
Locative	Verb + N	sit chair
Agent-Action	N + V	Eve read
Agent-Object	N + N	mommy sock
Action-Object	V + N	read book

SOURCE: R. Brown, *Psycholinguistics* (New York: Free Press, 1970).

[2]Descriptions of measurement procedures based upon Piaget's concepts may be found in the following readings: I. Uzgiris and J. Hunt, (1975). *Assessment in Infancy*. Chicago: University of Illinois Press. A. Mehrabian and M. Williams, (1971). "Piagetian Measures of Cognitive Development for Children up to Age Two." *Journal of Psycholinguistic Research*, 1: 113–26. B. Friedlander, G. Sterritt, and G. Kirk, (1975). *Exceptional Infant Assessment and Intervention*, Vol. 3 New York: Brunner-Mazel. D. Burk, (1973). *Piagetian Attainment Kit*. Minneapolis: Paul S. Amidon and Associates, Inc.

The language sample gathered during the diagnostic session is generally analyzed relative to the syntactic constructions present; however, it is possible to enrich this information by determining which semantic relationships are being expressed in the child's speech. Knowledge of the child's semantic-rule base directs the clinician to areas which need further development.

Syntactic Elements of Language

The procedures available to measure the syntactic performance of a child have been outlined in Chapter 4. Knowledge of the child's syntax structure has primarily two functions in directing the clinical effort. First, this knowledge will aid the clinician to enter the process at the level most beneficial for the child; and second, through continuous reassessment procedures, this knowledge should help to inform the clinician of the impact of a given procedure on the child's development.

Phonological Elements of Language

Articulation testing will be thoroughly discussed in Chapter 6. Articulation production is not separate from language functioning and language systems. The examination of articulation production must include a careful analysis of the linguistic systems that guide the sound productions of the child and of how well the child has learned or mislearned those systems. Just as there is a grammatical system that the child learns and incorporates in his production of syntactically accurate sentences, there is a plan that guides the learning of the sound system of speech. Articulation testing thus becomes more than a tabulatory process for identifying which sounds are in error; rather, it directs the remedial effort by identifying a broader breakdown in the idiosyncratic system that guides articulation performance. For too long speech clinicians have seen articulation testing as simply a procedure for identifying the existence of the problem, and now they must begin to organize and evaluate the data to help in other ways.

Pragmatic Elements of Language

The assessment of semantic, syntactic, and phonological elements of language along with determination of the child's cognitive functioning have dominated language diagnostic procedures in the past. Currently, however, the evaluation of the communicative intent of the speaker is coming under greater scrutiny. Dore (1973) suggests that the child's cognitive organization has a bearing on the relational notions underlying language, and the child's affective characteristics and means of obtaining desired results relates to the uses the child makes of language. Language development is seen as a merging of underlying knowledge of language structure and the functional uses language has for the child. Leonard

(1976) proposes an organizational paradigm for language development based upon the precepts of case grammar and pragmatics.

For language diagnostic purposes the investigation of the child's pragmatic system assists in the development of an overall clinical plan. Knowing the purposes to which the child puts language, the clinician may introduce new purposes not yet in the child's repertoire, emphasizing the potential influences of language and promoting the functional uses of language for everyday purposes. Halliday's (1975) list of early uses of language is presented in Table 5-2.

Table 5-2 Early Uses of Language

Instrumental	The use of language to satisfy one's own material needs (I want the ball)
Regulatory	The use of language to exert control over others (Close the door)
Interactional	The use of language to establish and maintain contact with people who are important (Hi, Daddy)
Personal	The use of language to express one's own individuality, self-awareness, uniqueness (I like candy)
Heuristic	The use of language to explore the objective environment (What's that?)
Imaginative	The use of language to create an environment of one's own (I'm a bunny rabbit)
Informative	The use of language to give information to someone who did not have the information (Eric is sick today)

Source: M. Halliday, *Learning How to Mean: Explorations in the Development of Language* (New York: Elsevier North-Holland, Inc. 1975).

Undoubtedly, there is a developmental order to acquisiton of the various language uses. Stremel-Campbell (1977) presented the following checklist of regulatory functions of language.

Demonstrates inappropriate behavior

Gestures with prompt

Gestures without prompt

Gets object and gives it to adult with prompt

Gets object and gives it to adult without prompt

Uses speech utterance with prompt

Uses speech utterance without prompt

Uses other modality with prompt

Uses other modality without prompt

The clinician could develop a similar procedure for evaluation of each of the uses of language.

Nation and Aram (1977: 332) suggest that the diagnostician conclude by asking himself four yes/no questions. "Can the client change his disordered behavior? Is therapeutic intervention necessary to do so? Are referrals necessary? Is service available?" Once these questions have been answered the clinician begins to plan specific management alternatives.

The nature of clinical intervention with the language-handicapped child is greatly dependent upon the diagnostic information accumulated. The clinician should now make an attempt to alter those etiological factors which are present; in many instances, referral is indicated to accomplish this. The selection of appropriate clinical objectives is based upon a knowledge of the sequential task ladder of normal language development and information regarding the child's current status with regard to the rules of semantics, syntax, phonology, and pragmatics. Knowing the child's level of cognitive functioning and how he orders his world will assist the clinician to select the appropriate level of intervention.

PROJECTS AND QUESTIONS

1. Childhood aphasia has been described in a number of ways. What might be the differences among acquired aphasia, congenital aphasia, and developmental aphasia?
2. What is "auditory agnosia" and how might it be related to language disorders?
3. The clinical approach to language-disordered children has progressed from humanism to behaviorism to mentalism. What diagnostic developments have paralleled this development?
4. Compare the works of J. Piaget and B. Skinner with regard to language acquisition.
5. What single diagnostic procedure do you consider most important to determine the level of receptive language in a child?
6. What single diagnostic procedure do you consider most important to determine the level of expressive language in a child?
7. Establish a diagnostic procedure to assist a clinician in determining when to abandon oral language training and begin a non-oral approach.
8. With a child whose speech attempts are entirely composed of unintelligible jargon, what diagnostic clues may assist the clinician in determining whether to work on articulation or language?
9. Briefly list the psychological, physical, environmental, and intellectual requisites for language. Contrast your list with the point of view presented by DeVito (1970).
10. What impact has behavior modification theory had on the use of the *ITPA?*

BIBLIOGRAPHY

ARAM, D., and J. NATION (1975). "Patterns of Language Behavior in Children with Developmental Language Disorders." *Journal of Speech and Hearing Research,* 18: 229–241.

ARTHUR, G. (1952). *The Arthur Adaptation of the Leiter International Performance Scale.* Washington, D.C.: Psychological Service Center Press.

BAKER, H., and B. LELAND (1959). *Detroit Tests of Learning Aptitude.* Indianapolis: Bobbs-Merrill.

BALTAXE, C. (1971). "Differential Language Development In Normal and Autistic Children." Paper presented at the Convention of the American Speech and Hearing Association, Chicago.

BERELSON, B., and G. STEINER (1964). *Human Behavior: An Inventory of Scientific Findings.* New York: Harcourt, Brace & World, Inc.

BERKO, J. (1958). "The Child's Learning of English Morphology." *Word,* 14: 150–177.

BERRY, M. (1969). *Language Disorders of Children.* New York: Appleton-Century-Crofts.

BOEHM, A. (1971). *Boehm Test of Basic Concepts.* New York: Psychological Corporation.

BOWERMAN, M. (1976). "Semantic Factors in the Acquisition of Rules for Word Use and Sentence Construction," in *Normal and Deficient Child Language,* ed. D. Morehead and A. Morehead, Baltimore: University Park Press.

BROEN, P. (1972). "The Verbal Environment of the Language-Learning Child." *ASHA* Monograph No. 17. Washington, D.C.: American Speech and Hearing Association.

BROWN, R. (1970). *Psycholinguistics.* New York: Free Press.

——— (1973). *A First Language.* Cambridge, Mass.: Harvard University Press.

BURK, D. (1973). *Piagetian Attainment Kit.* Minneapolis: Paul S. Amidon and Associates, Inc.

CHALFANT, J., and M. SCHEFFELIN (1969). *Central Processing Dysfunctions in Children: A Review of Research.* Bethesda, Md.: U.S. Department of Health, Education, and Welfare.

DAVIS, H., and R. SILVERMAN (1970), *Hearing and Deafness.* New York: Holt, Reinhart & Winston.

DE AJURIAGUERRA, J.; F. GUIGNARD; A. JAEGGI; F. KOEHER; M. MAQUARD; A. PAUNIER; D. QUINODOZ; and E. SIOTIS (1963). "Organisation Psychologique et Troubles du Development du language," in *Problemes de Psychololinguistique.* Paris: Universitaires de France Press.

DEVITO, J. (1970). *The Psychology of Speech and Language.* New York: Random House, Inc.

DORE, J. (1973). "The Development of Speech Arts." Ph.D. Dissertation. New York: City University of New York.

EISENSON, J.; J. AUER; and J. IRWIN (1963). *The Psychology of Communication.* New York: Appleton-Century-Crofts.

ENGELMANN, S. (1967). *The Basic Concept Inventory.* Chicago, Follett Educational Corporation.

FRIEDLANDER, B.; G. STERRITT; and G. KIRK (1975). *Exceptional Infant Assessment and Intervention,* Vol. 3, New York: Brunner-Mazel.

FROSTIG, M.; D. LEFEVER; P. MASLOW; and R. WHITTLESLEY (1964). *Marianne Frostig Developmental Test of Visual Perception.* Palo Alto, Calif.: Consulting Psychologists Press.

GOLDMAN, R.; M. FRISTOE; and R. WOODCOCK (1970). *Goldman-Fristoe-Woodcock Test of Auditory Discrimination.* Circle Pines, Minn.: American Guidance Service, Inc.

GROSSMAN, H. ed. (1973). *Manual on Terminology and Classification in Mental Retardation.* Baltimore: Garamond/Pridemark Press.

HALLIDAY, M. (1975). *Learning How to Mean.* New York: Elsevier North-Holland, Inc.

HARDY, W. (1962). "The Causes of Childhood Aphasia," in *Childhood Aphasia,* Proceedings of the Institute on Childhood Aphasia, ed. R. West. San Francisco: Society for Crippled Children and Adults.

KENDLER, H., and A. KARASIK (1958). "Concept Formation as a Function of Competition Between Response Produced Cues." *Journal of Experimental Psychology,* 55: 278–283.

KEPHART, N. (1960). *The Slow Learner in the Classroom*. Columbus, Ohio: Charles E. Merrill, Inc.

KIRK, S.; J. MCCARTHY; and W. KIRK (1968). *Illinois Test of Psycholinguistic Abilities*. Urbana: University of Illinois Press.

LANDAU, R.; R. GOLDSTEIN; and F. KLEFFNER (1960). "Congenital Aphasia. A Clinicopathologic Study." *Neurology*, 10: 915–921.

LENNEBERG, E. (1967). *Biological Foundations of Language*. New York: John Wiley & Sons.

———, ed. (1964). "Language Disorders in Childhood." *Harvard Education Review*, 34: 152–177.

——— (1969). "On Explaining Language," *Science*, 164: 635–643.

LEONARD, L. (1976). *Meaning in Child Language*. New York: Grune & Stratton.

LINDAMOOD, C., and P. LINDAMOOD (1971). *Lindamood Auditory Conceptualization Test*. Boston: Teaching Resources.

MACDONALD J., and M. NICKOLS (1974). *Environmental Language Inventory*. Columbus: The Ohio State University.

MCNEILL, D. (1970a). *The Acquisition of Language*. New York: Harper & Row.

——— (1970b). "The Development of Language." in *Carmichael's Manual of Child Psychology*, ed. P. Mussen. New York: John Wiley & Sons.

MECHAM, M.; J. JEX; and J. JONES (1969). *Test of Listening Accuracy in Children*. Provo, Utah: Brigham Young University Press.

MEHRABIAN, A., and M. WILLIAMS (1971). "Piagetian Measures of Cognitive Development for Children Up to Age 2." *Journal of Psycholinguistic Research*, 1: 113–126.

METRAUX, R. (1942). "Auditory Memory Span for Speech Sounds of Speech-Defective Children Compared with Normal Children." *Journal of Speech Disorders*, 7: 33–36.

MUMA, J.(1978). *Language Handbook: Concepts, Assessment, Intervention*. Englewood Cliffs, N.J.: Prentice-Hall.

NATION, J., and D. ARAM (1977). *Diagnosis of Speech and Language Disorders*. Saint Louis: C. V. Mosby Company.

NEWBY, H. (1972). *Audiology*. New York: Appleton-Century-Crofts.

O'NEILL, J., and H. OYER (1966). *Applied Audiometry*. New York: Dodd, Mead & Co.

PRATHER, E.; A. MINER; M. ADDICOTT; and L. SUNDERLAND (1971). *Washington Speech Sound Discrimination Test*. Danville, Ill.: The Interstate Printers & Publishers, Inc.

ROUSEY, C., and A. MORIARTY (1965). *Diagnostic Implications of Speech Sounds: The Reflections of Development Conflict and Trauma*. Springfield, Ill.: Charles C. Thomas.

SIEGEL, G., and H. HARKINS (1963). "Verbal Behavior of Adults in Two Conditions with Institutionalized Retarded Children." *Journal of Speech and Hearing Disorders. Monograph Supplement*, 10: 39–46.

STRAUSS, A., and L. LEHTINEN (1947). *Psychopathology and Education of the Brain-Injured Child*. New York: Grune & Stratton.

STREMEL-CAMPBELL, K. (1977). Convention Presentation. Minneapolis: Minnesota Speech and Hearing Association.

TEMPLIN, M. (1957). *Certain Language Skills in Children*. Minneapolis: University of Minnesota Press.

TERMAN, L., and M. MERRILL (1960). *Stanford-Binet Intelligence Scale*. Boston: Houghton Mifflin Co.

UZGIRIS, I., and J. HUNT (1975). *Assessment In Infancy*. Chicago: University of Illinois Press.

VAN RIPER, C. (1972). *Speech Correction: Principles and Methods*. Englewood Cliffs, N.J.: Prentice-Hall, Inc.

WELLS, G. (1974). "Learning to Code Experience Through Language." *Journal of Child Language*, 1: 243–269.

WEPMAN, J. (1958). *Auditory Discrimination Test*. Chicago: Language Research Association.

——, and H. HASS (1969). "Surface Structure, Deep Structure, and Transformations: A Model for Syntactic Development. *Journal of Speech and Hearing Disorders*, 34: 303–312.

——; L. JONES; R. BOCK; and D. VAN PELT (1960). "Studies in Aphasia: Background and Theoretical Formulations." *Journal of Speech and Hearing Disorders*, 25: 323–332.

WEST, R.; M. ANSBERRY; and A. CARR (1957). *The Rehabilitation of Speech*. New York: Harper & Row.

WHORF, B. (1956). *Language, Thought, and Reality*. New York: John Wiley & Sons, Inc.

WINITZ, H. (1969). *Articulatory Acquisition and Behavior*. New York: Appleton-Century-Crofts.

WOOD, N. (1964). *Delayed Speech and Language Development*. Englewood Cliffs, N.J.: Prentice-Hall, Inc.

6

Articulation Disorders

When compared to language, voice, or fluency problems, lisping or /r/ defects may seem relatively minor, even trivial, to the diagnostician. While it is *generally* true that speech sound errors are not debilitating (it is possible to point to celebrities in sports, movies, even television news reporting who have obvious articulatory "errors") many of our most difficult cases have been children and adults with misarticulation. Only a few clients were so limited in sound production that they were unable to converse; it was impossible to determine how much or in what way many of our milder cases were personally, socially or vocationally handicapped. We do know, however, that persons with articulation defects have been our most frequent clients.

Disturbances of speech-sound production—misarticulations—are probably the most common type of speech disorder. Most surveys (Hull, 1969; Gillespie and Cooper, 1973; Peckham, 1973; Cooper, Parris and Wells, 1974; Neal, 1976) show that the majority of children making up public-school caseloads present "functional" articulation disorders—i.e., there is no readily apparent basis for their sound errors (Powers, 1971a). In addition, individuals with neuromuscular impairment (such as paralysis of the facial muscles), orofacial deformity (such as cleft palate), or hearing loss also have difficulty producing speech sounds accurately.[1] The clinician, therefore, should have a thorough understanding of articulation and the disorders of articulation.

Articulation may be defined as an incredibly swift and complicated process whereby the lips, jaws, palate, and tongue modify or impede the breath stream to produce a repertoire of standard speech sounds. In other words, an individual performs a series of "valving" movements with his oral apparatus (physiological activity) producing audible events (acoustic signals) which have a shared significance (perception) for a community of speakers (Noll, 1970). Thus, an articulation error, or disorder, is a nonstandard production of one or more speech sounds.

There are three basic types of articulatory defects: *omissions* of sounds ("kool" for "school"), *substitution* of one standard sound for another ("thoup" for "soup"), and *distortions* (substitution of a nonstandard for a standard sound). Some writers list *additions* (the intrusion of an unwanted sound) as another type of articulatory disorder; in our experience, additions are generally results of emphasis ("*puh*lease close that door!") or idiosyncratic pronunciations ("I need some fil*um* to take photographs of the ath*uh*letes by the el*um* trees"). Persons generally misarticulate consonants more frequently than vowels.

Although we are wary of etiological classifications because of the many exceptions and the overlapping among categories, we find the following system useful diagnostically (Carrell, 1968). Articulation disorders can be placed in six categories, five major and one minor. 1) *Dyslalia*, or "habit" disorders of articulation which have no obvious physiological basis; there is considerable overlap between this type of disorder and each of the other categories; 2) *dysaudia*, sound error problems which stem from loss of hearing, particularly sensorineural impairment of moderate to significant proportions; 3) *dysglossia*, disorders resulting from structural defects in the oral area or malfunctioning of the oral mechanism, such as tongue thrusting; 4) *dyspraxia*, disturbance of the capacity to program the production of speech sounds due to impairment of the central nervous system; 5) *dysarthria*, difficulty in the motor control of speech due to faulty innervation (either peripheral or central nervous systems); and, the minor category, 6) *psycholalia*, disorders of sound production which are symptomatic of underlying emotional problems.

Laymen tend to confuse mispronunciation and slips of the tongue with articulation defects. Mispronunciations differ from articulation errors: the former involve "inadequate" or "unusual" utterances of words or phrases, whereas misarticulation is characterized by deviant production of specific speech sounds. Mispronunciations can usually be corrected readily by ear, but articulation errors do not yield so swiftly to correction.

For a more extended treatment of articulation disorders, consult the work of

---

[1]Might it be possible that the make-up of many public-school caseloads is an artifact of the type of screening tests employed? If the case-detection procedure consists solely of tasks which assess the adequacy of articulation, then only misarticulators will be identified.

Winitz (1969) and others (Powers, 1971a; Edwards and Anderson, 1972; Irwin, 1972; Daniloff, 1973; Wolfe and Goulding, 1973; Sommers and Kane, 1974; Weston and Leonard, 1976).

TESTING FOR ARTICULATION DISORDERS

The remainder of the chapter will deal with the various facets of assembling and utilizing information on clients presenting articulation errors. The discussion is divided into three segments: (a) case-detection screening (identifying the speech defectives in a large population); (b) predictive screening (determining which children will mature into good speech without therapeutic intervention); and (c) diagnostic articulation testing (determining the nature of the problem, planning and predicting the outcome of treatment).

Case-Detection Screening

Commonly, public-school speech clinicians conduct surveys to identify those individuals with speech defects. The purpose of screening is to select children with significant communication problems by assessing a total population with a brief but discriminating testing procedure.[2] The objective, then, is *detection*, not *description* of persons with defective speech.

A screening test must be swift, yet discerning. The examiner must be able to detect individuals with impaired speech while rapidly passing over all the normal speakers. Although brief, the detection process should provide a sufficient sample of each person's oral communication to permit critical judgment not just of his articulation but also his voice, rate, and language abilities. Since screening procedures and materials differ with various age groups, we shall describe methods for target populations: preschool and early elementary children (kindergarten through third grade), later elementary children (fourth through eighth grade), and older groups. See also the work of Black (1964), Irwin (1965), and Van Hattum (1969) for descriptions of screening programs used in school settings.

Preschool and early elementary children. There are essentially four ways to obtain a speech sample from a young child:

1. Observe him during free play, perhaps with other children. This procedure is very effective, but time-consuming.
2. Ask him questions. This involves too much talking on the part of the examiner, and some children are reluctant to answer questions (see Chapter 3).

---

[2]Some speech clinicians rely on teacher- and self-referrals rather than a screening program. The reader will want to review our definition of a speech defect. In what sense could the screening process be iatrogenic? See Project 1 at the end of this chapter.

3. Have him repeat words or phrases. This, too, requires unnecessary talking on the part of the clinician, and the examiner's model tends to influence the child's speech and thus does not provide a typical sample. Also, children rapidly tire of being parrots.
4. Have the child name colors, count, and identify pictures or objects. This is the most common method used; it is easy, takes very little time, and children seem to respond well to the tasks.

An experienced public-school speech clinician described her screening program in this way:

> I put all my screening materials in a plain manila file folder; on the inside I have pasted pictures of a shoe, scissors, a giraffe, an elephant, a fish, a zebra, a chair, a feather, a small bird, a can of soup and a leaf. All the pictures are colorful and realistic. I also have small circles of various colors, black, red, blue, orange, yellow and green. Finally, I have large printed numbers one through ten for the children to count. You can see that I get a pretty good sample of the speech sounds this way, particularly those sounds that are most frequently defective. I also like to hear a child's contextual speech, so I ask a few questions; sometimes they want to talk about the pictures. My favorite queries are: "Tell me about your favorite television program" and "How would I get to your house from here?" If I am in a real big rush and just need a quick sample, I have children repeat Van Riper's (1972: 195) screening sentence. I use a simple form containing the child's name, grade, teacher, and a designation of "pass" or "fail". I always try to get back to the teachers and administrators as fast as I can with the results. In one corner of my screening folder I have a chart of consonant sound maturation norms—it's very useful for talking with teachers and parents about how a particular child compares to others of his age.

Most of the published diagnostic inventories cited later in this chapter include portions designed to serve as screening tests for children. For example, the first fifty items of the Templin-Darley Tests of Articulation (1970) are a useful screening device; the authors provide tables of norms which permit comparison of an individual child's score with others of the same age level. The *Triota Ten Word Test* devised by Irwin (1972) takes only one minute to administer and yields a composite error score by age. There are several other tests designed specifically as screening instruments (Monsees and Berman, 1968; Riley, 1971; Rogers, 1972; Fluharty, 1974).

Later elementary children. We generally use reading passages or sentences loaded with the most frequently defective speech sounds for screening children in grades four through eight. The vocabulary, of course, should be appropriate to the child's reading level. Here is a reading passage we devised for screening a group of sixth-, seventh-, and eighth-grade pupils:

> Marquette is the largest city in the Upper Peninsula of Michigan. Located on the south shore of Lake Superior, Marquette is a major shipping port. Long ore boats pass in the deep blue waters each day during the summer; the ships must go through the locks at the Soo to reach ports in the south. Pine trees march up from every shore. In winter the snow is deep and it is very cold. Fishing, though, is good all year long.

We find that children respond better to reading passages based upon their home area; it tends to personalize the routine nature of the screening procedure. The clinician may also choose from among several published reading passages for later elementary children (Avant and Hutton, 1962; Eisenson and Ogilvie, 1963: 185–186; Irwin, 1965: 391).

To obtain a sample of spontaneous speech, we again rely on questions: favorite hobbies, sports, and interests. Verbal puzzles and riddles are also effective but take more time. Actually, we find that later elementary children are often rather engaging conversationalists; they are sufficiently mature to enjoy relating to a new adult, but not old enough to resent being scrutinized. Indeed, they are often intrigued with the screening test and want to know how they have done. We usually try to provide a brief explanation, especially if we note articulation errors:

> Glen, a new fifth grader, distorted the /l/ and /r/ sounds. He put the copy of the reading passage down on the table, looked expectantly at the clinician, and asked how he had done. We told him that he seemed to say two sounds differently from most people and asked him if anyone else had ever mentioned it to him. He thought a moment and then revealed that some children in his last school had called him "Elmer Fudd." He added that his teachers sometimes admonished him to speak more clearly. We told Glen that we would see him later in the week and that together we would look at those troublesome sounds. The complete transaction took less than two minutes, but as we found out when therapy commenced, it had provided closure and reassurance for the child.

Older groups. Reading passages, sentences loaded with consonant sounds most frequently defective, and conversations are commonly used to obtain speech samples in screening programs for older individuals. The clinician can construct a reading passage of his own or use any of the several published versions which include "My Grandfather" (Van Riper, 1963: 484); "Arthur the Young Rat" (Johnson, Darley, and Spriestersbach, 1963: 233); "The Rainbow Passage" (Fairbanks, 1960: 127); and "Directions" (Anderson, 1973: 45).

Many universities require that students enrolled in teacher education be screened for speech disorders. Here is a typical reading passage and selected sentences employed in such a screening program:

Reading Passage

I think I will hitch my wagon to a star, said Johnny Reed. I will show the world I can succeed. It takes more than luck to be a hero. I must try to make haste slowly. However, I will always be full of zip and vigor. Some days it is an effort to stay in the same place. I do not choose to run like that.

Sentences

Snow covered ski slopes.
The early bird gets the worm.
Duluth is the largest port city on Lake Superior.
The feather came off the hat.
She had a face that launched a thousand ships.
Each page of the soldier's journal is exciting.
Take the path to the left for Laughing Whitefish Falls.
We have chosen the road less traveled.

In addition to the oral reading, some questions are asked to elicit a sample of spontaneous speech. Queries such as, ''What are you majoring in and how did you select that field?'' or ''If I were to come to your home area as a tourist, what are some things I might want to see?'' are good starters. Two forms are used: all students screened return a small green sheet containing their name, advisor, and a pass-fail designation to the education department. The examiners use another form (Figure 6.1) only for students who manifest a significant speech impairment.

The value of a screening program is contingent upon the follow-up. It is an infringement of a student's rights, not to mention a waste of the clinician's energy, to conduct elaborate screening programs unless we are prepared to work with those individuals identified as speech defective. Consult the publication by Peins and Pettas (1963) for an outline of a screening program and a follow-up speech improvement course on the college level.

Problems in screening. We have encountered several problems in conducting screening programs. Here are a few of the most salient challenges to the clinician:

1. THE ROUTINE NATURE OF THE TASK. Screening a large number of individuals makes it extremely difficult for the clinician to establish a genuine relationship with each person being evaluated. However, it takes little time or energy to personalize the procedure; you never know whether the individual being screened might be your next client. Personal comments about a particular item of clothing or the individual's place of residence, a smile, or some small bit of humor can be helpful. When the testing is completed, many individuals want to know the results; it seems only common courtesy to tell them. In our experience, if the clinician is enjoying his job and shows it, if he treats each individual not as a subject but as an interesting and unique person, then he not only makes the child or adult feel better, he also makes the redundant task more palatable (Siegel, 1967).

Avoid stereotyped interactions with the individuals being screened; vary the wording of your questions to reduce monotony. Actually, brief screening encounters can be an excellent source of interviewing practice.

2. THE TRAFFIC PROBLEM. Try to be considerate when you have scores of children milling around, irritated teachers casting baleful glances, and administrators impatient for therapy to commence. In order to screen large groups, it is necessary to make provisions for getting people in and out of the testing site as swiftly and quietly as possible. In public schools, we have used older children as guides and monitors; it is often helpful to have an extra room or space adjacent to the testing site as a waiting room. We feel that screening tests should be done individually and privately. However, some clinicians maintain that they get more authentic speech samples by bringing in several individuals at a time to provide an audience for each person being screened.

SPEECH SCREENING FORM

Name: _____   Local Address: _____

Date: _____   Academic Advisor: _____

Voice Analysis:

Pitch _____

Loudness _____

Quality _____

Articulation Analysis:

1. r _____

2. l _____

3. th _____

4. th _____

5. s _____

6. z _____

7. sh _____

8. ch _____

9. j _____

10. Overall diction or pronunciation: _____

Rate Analysis:

Stuttering _____

Comments _____

_____

Department of Speech Pathology
and Audiology

Figure 6.1   Form Used in University Screening Program.

3. FEAR AND RESISTANCE. Young children are sometimes threatened by the prospect of speech screening. We find it helpful to go into kindergarten and first-grade classrooms before the screening and show the children exactly what we plan to do. Even some college students are apprehensive about the "speech test," and it is necessary to reduce their uncertainty by appropriate explanations.

4. DEFINITION OF A SPEECH DEFECT. In the past, many speech clinicians were overzealous in identifying speech disorders; even minor speech differences were characterized as problems, and the possessor was urged to enroll in treatment. Obviously, we cannot determine whether the individual has a speech defect on the basis of a brief screening interview; all we can specify is: *does he have a speech difference?* Although we have discussed speech screening in terms of articulatory defectiveness, the clinician also listens for disturbances in voice, rate, and for gross language impairment.

Predictive Screening

A significant number of children entering kindergarten and first grade will not have acquired all the normal complement of consonant sounds (Pendergast, et al., 1966). This places the therapist in a dilemma: at least half of these children will mature into normal articulation without therapeutic intervention—but which ones? Some of the children's speech differences are merely the results of late maturation and do not require treatment, but how do you separate the normal speakers from the potentially permanent lispers? Some clinicians simply delay treatment until the fourth or fifth grade (Roe and Milisen, 1942). However, if therapy is postponed for those who genuinely need assistance, it is possible that their speech errors will become habituated and more resistant to treatment; in addition, the child may be educationally and socially penalized if his speech pattern draws undue attention. A few therapists select certain children and not others, operating on an *ad hoc* basis. They then find it difficult to explain their selection process to teachers, parents, and administrators.

The opposite extreme is to work with all first-grade children who present articulation errors. But teaching a person, particularly a child, some skill before he is maturationally ready for it can do more harm than good: it is possible to engender a problem by therapeutic intrusion. An initial goal of treatment is to convince the child he has a problem, and if we push for improvement *before he is ready* we may create a self-concept which includes, "I have trouble with speech, I cannot say the /s/ sound."

To work with every kindergartener or first grader with a frontal lisp is no solution at all; it is far too wasteful of thereapeutic time and energy. A particularly effective local clinician has solved the problem. Here is her report:

When I first took the position as speech clinician in this school system, I discovered there were many early elementary children with mild-to-moderate speech differences which, if they persisted, could be potential problems. So, I started a three-pronged program: (1) First, I initiated a preschool screening and parent education project. I see all four-year-olds as part of a prekindergarten check and evaluate them for articulation, voice, rhythm, and language problems. Then, with a few selected children having difficulty, I perform demonstration therapy before the parents. I follow this up with parent education and counseling, gradually turning over the job to the mothers and fathers. (2) We also have a program of speech improvement for all children in kindergarten and first grade. There was some resistance from the teachers at the outset, but when they began to see the results, not only in speech and language development but also in reading readiness skills, speech improvement was made a part of the school curriculum. That has really helped. In 1959 when I first started, there were nineteen kindergarten children with articulation errors out of a total enrollment of sixty-two; last year we had only four. (3) The thing that helped us most, though was using the Predictive Screening Test of Articulation (Van Riper and Erickson, 1968). I test all first graders during the first ten weeks of class. The test is easy and brief (ten minutes or less), and the results give me a basis for picking those children who need me most. Since we have a high incidence of speech defectiveness in this region, I use a cut-off score of 35. I feel less willy-nilly and more professional when I explain to teachers, parents, and administrators why I am working with Heino and not Susie!

Many clinicians now use the Predictive Screening Test of Articulation to identify children with potentially persistent problems. The purpose of the instrument is stated succinctly by Van Riper and Erickson (1968: 1):

> We wish to emphasize that the basic purpose for which the Predictive Screening Test to Articulation has been devised is to differentiate children who will master their misarticulations without speech therapy from those who, without therapy, may persist in their errors. More specifically, the PSTA may be used to identify, among primary-school children who have functional misarticulations at the first-grade level, those children who will—and those who will not—have acquired normal mature articulation by the time they reach the third-grade level.

The Predictive Screening Test of Articulation consists of forty-seven items which were empirically shown to be predictive of articulatory maturation.[3] Most of the items assess the child's degree of stimulability: he is asked to repeat sounds, nonsense syllables, words, and a sentence after the examiner (see Figure 6.2). Item forty-five is meant to determine if he can move his tongue independent of his lower jaw, while number forty-six evaluates the child's ability to detect errors in the examiner's speech. The final task assesses whether the child can follow the examiner in a handclapping rhythm.

Van Riper and Erickson recommend a cut-off score of 34; they predict that children getting 34 or more items correct are likely to mature into good articulation:

> A cut-off score of 34 minimizes both types of error; those due to children predicted as being able to overcome their errors without therapy but who actually do not (false

---

[3]The Predictive Screening Test of Articulation is available at cost ($.50) from the Continuing Education Office, Western Michigan University, Kalamazoo, Michigan, 49001.

PREDICTIVE SCREENING TEST OF ARTICULATION (PSTA)

RESPONSE SHEET

Child's Name Lynn E.   Birth date 1/19/64 Total Score 36

Grade   1   School   Fisher   Examiner   Emerick

City   Marquette   State   Michigan   Date   9/15/70

Record the child's response to each item of the PSTA by
circling the 1 if his response is correct or by circling the
2 if his response is incorrect (or if no response is made).
Compute the child's total score by counting the number of
items where 1 has been circled. Enter this score in the
appropriate space at the top of the response sheet.

Item	Response Corr.	Incor.	Item	Response Corr.	Incor.
Part I					
1. RABBIT	1	(2)	11. SHEEP	(1)	2
2. SOAP	(1)	2	12. DISHES	(1)	2
3. LEAF	(1)	2	13. CHAIR	(1)	2
4. ZIPPER	(1)	2	14. MATCHES	(1)	2
			15. WATCH	(1)	2
Part II			16. JAR	(1)	2
5. MUSIC	(1)	2	17. ENGINE	(1)	2
6. VALENTINE	(1)	2			
7. TEETH	(1)	2	**Part III**		
8. SMOOTH	(1)	2	18. PRESENTS	1	(2)
9. ARROW	1	(2)	19. BREAD	1	(2)
10. BATHTUB	(1)	2	20. CRAYONS	1	(2)

Figure 6.2 PSTA Response Sheet Showing Test Results for a First-Grade Child

	Item	Response Corr.	Incor.		Item	Response Corr.	Incor.
						Part IV	
21.	GRASS	1	②	39.	Sentence	①	2
22.	FROG	1	②				
23.	THREE	1	②			**Part V**	
24.	CLOWN	①	2	40.	(s)	①	2
25.	FLOWER	①	2	41.	(θ)	①	2
26.	SMOKE	①	2				
27.	SNAKE	①	2			**Part VI**	
28.	SPIDER	①	2	42.	SEESEESEE	①	2
29.	STAIRS	①	2	43.	ZOOZOOZOO	①	2
30.	SKY	①	2	44.	PUHTUHKUH	①	2
31.	SWEEPING	①	2				
32.	PLANT	①	2			**Part VII**	
33.	SHREDDED WHEAT	1	②	45.	LA-LA-LA	①	2
						Part VIII	
34.	TREE	1	②	46.	Recognition	①	2
35.	DRESS	1	②				
36.	SLED	①	2			**Part IX**	
37.	SPLASH	①	2				
38.	STRING	1	②	47.	Clapping Rhythm	①	2

Tongue movement w/o jaw movement.

of correct sound error

Figure 6.2 Continued.

167

negative errors), and those due to children predicted as still having errors on third-grade entrance who instead will be error free (false positive errors) (1968: 4).

In practice, the final selection of a cut-off score may vary with the needs and orientation of the clinician as well as the nature of his program. A clinician who wished to exclude from theraphy, for example, only those children virtually certain to demonstrate spontaneous acquisition of normal articulation by the third grade might well prefer to use a relatively high cut-off score. A clinician who is able to include only a limited number of first-grade children in his caseload, on the other hand, may wish to employ a cut-off score which is so low that there is virtually no chance that he will be devoting therapy time to a child who may not have required his attention. In any event, the clinician should regard the recommended cut-off score of 34 as a tentative one until he has demonstrated it to be an optimal cut-off score in his own situation (1968: 5).

The senior author tested his six-year-old daughter two weeks after she started first grade (Figure 6.2). She had eleven incorrect items—all involving the /r/ and /w/ sounds—resulting in a total score of 36. By the end of the first grade she was using both phonemes inconsistently, and at the time of this writing she had completed second grade and possesses normal articulation.

The Predictive Screening Test of Articulation is very helpful and in most instances it is sufficient basis for identifying those first-grade children who need help. For use with younger children, the clinician should consider the *Denver Articulation Screening Exam* (Drumwright 1971; Drumwright et al. 1973); this test is designed to discriminate between significant developmental delay and normal variations in the acquisition of sounds in young (2½ to 6 years), disadvantaged children. A screening test for kindergarten children (McDonald, 1968) is also available.

Clinical decisions, however, are not determined by test scores alone, and the worker is abrogating his responsibilities if he does not use his professional judgment in selecting children for therapy. For example, some kinds of articulatory disorders—lateralized sibilants, omissions, vocalic /r/ distortions—rarely yield to maturation. Further, there are some situations in which the clinician may decide to work with a child (and those in his environment) even though the best predictive indices suggest that the child does not need therapy. Parents may be upset with the child's speech, or the child himself may be concerned about the way he talks, or he may present learning problems.

A significant amount of research has been directed toward the topic of prediction. The reader will want to consult the extensive review of the literature by Winitz (1969: 254–269) and Project 2 at the end of this chapter.

Diagnostic Articulation Testing

In order to plan treatment, it is not enough to know if an individual has an articulation error. If we are to ascertain the individual's needs and plan for immediate treatment, we must do more than identify cases. Basically, we are concerned with four areas:

> *What* sounds are in error? How many are produced in a defective manner? What type of errors does he have—omissions, substitutions, distortions? Where do the articulatory breakdowns occur in words—initially, medially, finally? Do the errors occur in all forms of utterance or only in rapid, connected speech?
>
> *How* does the client misarticulate? That is, what are the specific muscle movement patterns that produce the errors? Are there any obvious dysfunctions?
>
> *How* does his articulatory performance *vary,* and under what conditions does it vary? Does he improve when given a vivid visual and acoustic model to imitate? Does he have certain words or phonetic contexts in which he utters his defective sound correctly, or closely approximating normalcy?
>
> *Why* does he misarticulate? Are his deficiencies related to problems in discrimination, retention span, neuromuscular abilities, adequate speech models, stimulation, and motivation for good speech? If so, do these deficiencies perpetuate the articulation errors?

In other words, the diagnostician attempts to carefully describe the client's problem, identify if possible the precipitating and perpetuating factors, and synthesize all these data into a plan of therapy (Carrell, 1968). First let us consider how we go about obtaining a sample of the client's speech. The initial task in diagnostic articulation evaluation is to evoke a sample of the client's speech. We must obtain a large enough sample—single-word utterance, oral reading, connected discourse—in order to accurately infer his typical articulatory performance.

We inspect a speaker's use of the forty or more phonemes of English speech. Phonemes are abstract sound units (the smallest elements of speech) which convey meaning; they are composed of a number of audible characteristics, the production of which varies slightly from utterance to utterance. A phoneme is also a sound family: there are lots of ways to say /s/—soup, blast, kiss—but they still all belong to the family of the /s/ phoneme. These variations are called phones. We don't usually notice any difference until a speaker varies his production too widely and substitutes, for example, a sharp, piercing whistle for the /s/.

The most common way of making a phonemic inventory is to have the client name objects or pictures, read sentences and prose passages loaded with particular sounds, and speak extemporaneously. Each speech sound should be elicited at least once in every position. We prefer a method of testing articulation that permits spontaneous responses from the client. The research suggests that clients are influenced by the examiner's articulation in a "say after me" model (Winitz 1969; Shanks, Sharpe, and Jackson 1970; Kresheck and Socolofsky 1972; Paynter and Bumpas 1977). The following will illustrate the procedure of administering an articulation inventory:

> Terry, a six-year-old child from a rural area, was seen recently for speech evaluation. Although somewhat uncertain and apprehensive when she entered the examining room, she rapidly warmed to the situation as the clinician sat calmly beside her

commenting on the pictures in an appealing book for children. Then the clinician brought out a large hard-cover notebook and opened it at random, revealing colorful pictures in plastic sheets.

Clinician: This is my book; I made it myself, Terry. Aren't these pictures interesting? I bet you know all these things, don't you? Would you like to see all of them? Okay, let's go through the pictures one at a time, and I'll keep track on this piece of paper with Mr. Pencil here. Here's the first one. . . .

The clinician moved through the homemade articulation inventory, starting with items having sounds which children acquire early—/p/, /b/, /t/—and then progressing to pictures evoking more difficult phonemes generally learned at age six or seven (Sander, 1972). On each page of the inventory were three pictures which contained the sound being tested in initial (beginning), medial (middle), and final (end) positions. Pictures had been chosen that were simple, common, colorful, current, real, and reasonably self-explanatory. On the back of each page the clinician had printed the sound being tested and brief comments or questions about the illustrations. The following transcript taken from a tape recording made during the diagnostic session reveals the flavor of the interaction between child and clinician.

Terry: Oh, I know, thatth a thanta tawth (Santa Claus); he tomth at twithmith time and bwingth wotth of toyth. . . .
Clinician: Right! Say, you are really good at naming these pictures. What's this one?
Terry: A bathkit, wooks wike an Eathto bathkit. Do you think there ith an Eathto bunny? My bwotho, Joey, he thath there ithn't any Eathto bunny.
Clinician: Is that right? Well, I don't know. Look, we have one more picture on this page . . . you drink from a . . .
Terry: Dwath, thatth a pwetty wed dwath.

Notice from this brief sample (the clinician was assessing the child's production of /s/) how the examiner guides Terry through the task. Praise and encouragement are offered. Sometimes the clinician may simply point to a picture and say, "What's this called?" or he may use an open-end sentence, "You drink from a _____" to evoke a response. It is more effective for the examiner to vary his prompters. Observe also that the child was doing more than uttering single words; in fact, we almost always get a sample of connected speech during the administration of the articulation inventory. With older clients, of course, our procedures differ:

Billy was a high-school senior when he came to us for help with what he called "my damn lisp." In our initial conversation with him, we noted that most of his sibilant sounds were distorted by lateral emission. Turning on a recorder, we had Bill perform the following tasks. First he read aloud these sentences, slowly and then swiftly:

Snow covered ski slopes.
His business was doing absolutely zero.
We each chomped on cheap chocolates.
She had a face that launched a thousand ships.
They took the soldiers before Judge Brown.

Indeed the /s/, /z/, /ch/, /sh/, and /dz/ were all distorted by lateral emission. We wanted a larger sample, however, so we had him read a passage from the school newspaper that he was carrying. Finally, we asked him to retell in his own words one of the ''This Happened To Me'' features taken from *Outdoor Life* magazine. This led to the discovery that hunting was a common interest and precipitated a rather lengthy discussion of the topic.

It is far easier to describe articulation testing than it is to administer an articulation test. A student's first attempt is generally a confusing situation: she must listen carefully, attend to visual cues, record the child's responses appropriately—all the while maintaining a positive client-clinician relationship! Weston and Leonard (1976) caution the examiner to be alert to confounding variability in the child's responses, in her own perception, and in the articulation inventory itself. We recommend that the beginning diagnostician listen for only one sound at a time. If it is possible to do without annoying the child, have him repeat the test words a number of times. Tape-record, or better yet, videotape the session so that you can go back over the client's responses and check your reliability. With experience, you will be able to save time by testing more than one sound simultaneously (Fristoe and Goldman, 1968); however, a recent investigation (Mullen and Whitehead, 1977) showed that the Goldman-Fristoe Test of Articulation (1969) actually took *longer* to administer than a conventional inventory because the children misidentified many of the test pictures.

Many clinicians prefer to construct their own articulation inventory; we encourage our students to do so. Even if you decide never to use it, the experience of thinking in terms of phonemes tends to give focus to your clinical listening skills. Besides, there is often an intangible appeal to a homemade articulation test, an appeal that might make the difference in some diagnostic sessions. As Noll (1970) points out, an articulation inventory is not really a test anyway, but simply a set of stimulus pictures designed to evoke a particular word response from a child. The test, in a diagnostic sense, refers to the evaluation process of the listener, not to the picture items. In other words, the clinician is the diagnostic instrument.

These are however, several published articulation tests to choose from: Cypreansen, Wiley, and Laase, 1959; Bryngelson and Glaspey, 1962; Edmonson, 1960; Hejna, 1963; Pendergast et al., 1969; Goldman and Fristoe, 1969; Fudula, 1970; Templin and Darley, 1970; Mecham, Jex and Jones, 1970; Ingram, 1971; Ham, 1971; Fisher and Logemann, 1971; Anderson and Newby, 1973; Bzoch, 1974; Haws, 1975. Most of these inventories include stimulus pictures for testing children, and structured sentences for older clients to read; filmstrips (Goldman and Fristoe, 1967) could also be employed. Several provide norms against which a child may be rated, and one (Fudula, 1970) features a method for scaling the degree of articulatory defectiveness. The *Ohio Tests of Articulation and Perception of Sounds* (Irwin, 1973) is a particularly well validated and useful instrument. It features four articulation subtests: conventional naming of pictures; saying phrases for a sample of contextual speech; uttering nonsense words, also in context; and repeating nonsense words after the examiner.

Clinicians who have a behavioristic orientation offer an alternative to traditional articulation testing (Mowrer, Baker, Schutz 1968; Turton, 1973). A behavioral assessment consists of a preliminary baseline of articulatory behavior: the clinician obtains a specific speech sample (for example, sounds, words, phrases, which allow for the target sound in all phonetic contexts) by employing the *Sound Production Task* (Elbert, Shelton, Arndt 1967), The *McDonald Deep Test* (1964) or other stimulus materials (Diedrich, 1971; *Swirl Speech Articulation Kits,* 1973). The cardinal features of a behavioral evaluation are *quantification and precision recording;* these features permit careful charting of a client's progress during treatment. Garrett's (1973: 107) procedure for obtaining a "properant score" is illustrative:

> A properant is made by tape-recording at least a five minute sample of the subjects speech which includes a minimum of 40 attempts at the target phoneme. The clinician then plots the number of acceptable productions of the target phoneme in proportion to the total number of times the phoneme was attempted. A properant of 1.00 would indicate perfect articulation of the phoneme; a properant of 0.00 would indicate a total absence of acceptable productions of the phoneme.

For detailed discussions of articulation testing see the work of Van Riper and Irwin (1958: 48–65) and others (Johnson, Darley, and Spriestersbach, 1963: 80–99; Irwin, 1965: 82–83; Winitz, 1969: 237–273; Powers, 1971b: 881–884; Van Riper, 1972: 186–198).

Making sense of the test results. It is not difficult to administer an articulation inventory. However, evaluating a client with an articulation disorder involves more than simply recording data into neat columns. In order to plan treatment, it is necessary to analyze the information: one must identify the types of errors, discover the location of the error in the communication context, discern if patterns exist, and scrutinize the variability of the client's performance. But before inspecting the parts so closely, we need to look at the whole.

Before making a detailed analysis of the client's articulation, we like to record our general impressions of his total communicative performance. Here is an example from the clinical notes of a graduate student:

> I don't know how Lloyd ever made it through high school. His speech is unintelligible unless you know the word he is saying. When he first came in and tried to tell me his name, I couldn't understand him; he had to take off his freshman beanie and show me the name tag. I made a recording of Lloyd reading "the Bamboo Passage," and here (in phonetics) is how he read the first sentence: "Ωkɪn æt e ck vb æmbo ɪt ɪz ad u ilib æt ɪz ili e mɛnd3 vb e æs æmli." He omits almost all initial consonants, distorts the /l/ and /r/, and has several substitutions—he even substitutes /m/ for /p/.
> At first I thought he had a motor problem—he seemed to struggle a bit—but the more I watched and listened to him, it seemed like he was trying to put in those missing sounds but didn't know how. Maybe he is apraxic? I asked him to speed up, though, and his articulation got worse! He refused to try again. Anyway, I have never seen a case like this before, not an adult anyway. I have examined a couple of

children, both around five years old, who had infantile articulation patterns. You know, Lloyd did sound a little bit like those kids.

I reviewed Lloyd's video tape and noticed several other things about his speech: (1) he keeps his jaws clenched tight when he talks—perhaps this is why he sounds nasal to me; (2) his whole posture is rigid and his face masklike—maybe he adopted this style of speaking as a coverup; (3) his rate is rather slow and his voice is flat and expressionless, but this, too, could be secondary to the severe articulation problem.

I think I'm beginning to get the feel for estimating severity. I read the article by Jordon (1960) and I found and made thermofax copies of the crude scales published by Powers (1971b) and Milisen et al. (1954). I don't completely understand the Wood Index (1949) or the Arizona Articulation Proficiency Scale (Fundala, 1970), but it seems like a numerical measure of severity would be handy sometimes. Can we talk about it at our conference?

Prior to meeting with the student, we put this note in her clinic mailbox:

Your clinical analysis of Lloyd's articulation was well done; you have a good beginning on a difficult topic. Here are some additional materials for review before we meet:

1. Serious attempts at devising empirically derived scales of the severity of articulatory defectiveness were undertaken by Sherman and Cullinan (1960) and Prather (1960).

2. Some clinicians assign a numerical value to the kinds of errors, omission=3, substitution=2, and distortion=1.

3. We usually try to make an estimate of the client's intelligibility—in the form of a percentage—but it is an imprecise judgment. Intelligibility obviously relates to the speech standards of the community in which the client lives. We might make an audio recording of Lloyd and ask a number of persons to rate his intelligibility. To be more precise, we could use the rhyme test devised by Fairbanks (1958); in this procedure, the client reads 50 phonetically balanced words and a panel of judges scores the recording for intelligibility.

4. Powers (1971b) presents a number of factors to consider when making judgments of severity. How many sounds are defective? Which sounds are they (some sounds have a greater frequency of occurrence)? How consistent are the errors? How important is good speech for the person? What are the attitudes of persons who are important to the client? Some types of articulation defects, a lateral lisp for instance (Silverman, 1976), are rated more negatively by others and thus could be inferred to be more handicapping.

5. Finally, when evaluating a younger client, you will want to compare the child's performance to norms for consonant sound maturation. Consult the work of Smith (1973) and others (Prather, Hedrick, and Kern, 1975; Weybright, 1976). The chart prepared by Sander (1972: 62) is particularly useful [See Figure 6.3].

A PHONEMIC ANALYSIS. The first analytical task is to delineate which sounds the client is having difficulty with; this includes several facets and is termed a phonemic analysis (Van Riper, 1963: 221–223). A phonemic analysis identifies: (1) *which* sound is in error; (2) *what* type of defect it is—omission, substitution, or distortion; and (3) *where* the error occurs—the initial, medial, or final positions.[4]

---

[4]Is it possible to consider all articulation errors as substitutions? See Van Riper and Irwin (1958: 77–78). Is there a medial position? Consult Keenan (1961).

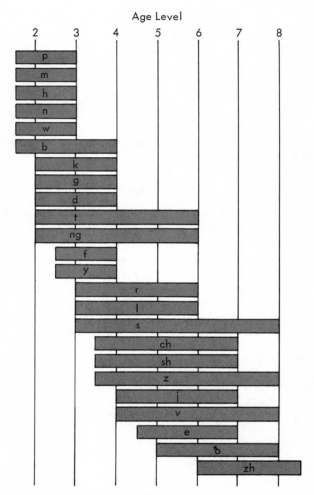

Figure 6.3 Average age estimates and upper age limits of customary consonant production. The solid bar corresponding to each sound starts at the median age of customary articulation; it stops at the age level at which 90 percent of all children are customarily producing the sound (Sander, 1972: 62).

Figure 6.4 presents an articulation inventory worksheet summarizing the results of an evaluation done with an eight-year-old second grader. The child's production of each phoneme was evaluated by having him name a series of pictures; each sound was tested in the initial, medial, and final positions (the column on the far left represents the ages which the majority of children acquire the phoneme). Note the method of recording results:

√ = the sound was produced satisfactorily.
− = the sound was omitted.

Name Ricky S. Age 8 (6/1/56) Sex M Folder # 63-139
Clinician Helgeson Date 4/7/63

DEV AGE		I	M	F	Stimulable
4 1/2	k	✓	✓	✓	
4 1/2	g	✓	✓	✓	
4 1/2	l	✓	✓	✓	
4 1/2	d	✓	✓	✓	
4 1/2	t	✓	✓	✓	
4 1/2	j	✓	✓	✓	
5 1/2	f	✓	✓	✓	
6 1/2	v	✓	✓	✓	
6 1/2	ʃ	S	S	S	Yes
6 1/2	ð	d	d	d	Yes
7 1/2	θ	t	t	t	Yes
7 1/2	tʃ	✓	✓	✓	
7 1/2	dʒ	✓	✓	✓	
7 1/2	s	t	θ	-	Yes
7 1/2	z	d	ð	ð	Yes
7 1/2	r	w	w		Slight
7 1/2	ʒ	x	x	x	No

Key words:

Sounds most noticeably defective:

Sound discrimination:

Vocal phonics:

Oral examination:

Diadochokinetic rate:

Auditory memory:

Hearing:

Other observations:

Figure 6.4 Articulation Inventory Worksheet.

> *s/sh* = substitutions are recorded phonetically.
>
> *x* = the sound was distorted; some clinicians recommend delineating the severity of a distortion as D_1 = mild, D_2 = moderate, D_3 = severe.

In the clinician's notes we discovered this cryptic message: *t/s* (I); *th/s* (M); −*s* (F). Can you put into words what the clinician wrote?[5] In order to show how the raw information is translated into workable messages, we now present a portion of the report we sent to the child's second-grade teacher:

> As you noted in your referral, Ricky has difficulty with several speech sounds. We asked him to name a set of pictures; the pictures were of common objects and contained each sound being tested at the beginning, middle, and end of the words. We found seven sound errors:
>
> *s/sh* He substitutes the /s/for the /sh/—for example, "sip" for "ship."
> *d/th* He substitutes /d/ for the voiced /th/—for example, "dem" for "them."
> *t/th* He also substitutes the /t/ for the voiceless /th/, as "toot" for tooth.
> *s*   Ricky is inconsistent on the /s/. At the beginning of words such as "soup," he substitutes a /t/ and says "toup." In the middle of words he substitutes a /th/ ("bathkit" for "basket"). And he omits the sound when it is at the end of a word.
> *z*   He is also inconsistent on the /z/. At the beginning of words, he substitutes a /d/ for /z/ ("debra" for "zebra") and substitutes the voiced /th/ for /z/ in the middle and at the ends of words ("buth" for "buzz").
> *w/r*   Ricky substitutes the /w/ sound for /r/—for example, "wabbit" for "rabbit."
> *3*   The vowel /r/ sound, as in "bird" and "word" is distorted. This is why, no doubt, you observed that he sounded "eastern."

Although at first inspection, substitution errors may seem random, further experience will reveal a definite regularity. Which phoneme is substituted depends, in part, on how alike the two sounds are—how much they *sound* alike and how much the *movements* that produce that phonemes are similar. Rarely will the /p/ sound be substituted for /r/; however, the /w/ sound is frequently used. You will want to study the work of Van Riper and Irwin (1958: 68–96) and Winitz (1969: 85) and review physiological and acoustic phonetics. In the next unit we will discuss this area of kinetic analysis—how the client produces the error.

A KINETIC ANALYSIS. In the last section we identified *what* sounds the client misarticulated. Now we must discuss *how* he is making the errors; what specifically is the individual doing to produce the phonemes in a defective manner? This is termed a kinetic analysis (Van Riper, 1963: 224–226). Let us provide an example:

> We saw Robin, a university sophomore, for only a cursory appraisal before a weekend vacation. She distorted severely the /l/ and /r/ sounds, but there was something else about the way she produced the tongue-tip phonemes /ch/, /dz/, /t/,

---

[5]/t/ substituted for /s/ in initial position; /θ/ substituted for /s/ in medial position; /s/ omitted in final position.

/d/, and even /n/ that had seemed strange. During the long drive, we remembered Powers' (1971a, p. 845) lucid description of the necessary motor requirements for accurate sound production and tried to relate it to Robin's misarticulation:

1. First, there must be *precision* of movement, precision in terms of *placement* of structures [that's part of Robin's problem, certainly]; movements must be in the right *direction* [she seems okay on that score]; there has to be the right *amount of contact surface* [now, there is a major factor in Robin's /l/ and /r/ distortion]; and the contacts between the articulators must be of the right shape [don't know about this, will have to see what she does when I get back].

2. Articulatory movements must also be made at the right speed. [Robin's rate is slow—yes, her specific articulatory movements are rather slow.]

3. The movements must be made with enough *energy* or *pressure*. [Maybe she has a health problem we don't know about, but her articulation certainly is not very crisp.]

4. [Lastly] there must be *synergy* of the sequential movements of speech, an optimum temporal-spatial integration of movements. [Does she put it all together? Have to scrutinize her more carefully but did notice rather flaccid gross motor behavior—and didn't she say something about having trouble in typing class and being generally clumsy?]

It finally dawned on us that Robin was trying to make the /l/ and /r/ sounds with her tongue tip down; and, since her tongue is so low in her mouth and the tip is forward, she dentalizes the other tongue-tip sounds.

In order to help him change, we need to always start where the client is. We have to identify what he is doing so that we can alter it. This is particularly relevant to disorders of articulation, since the perception and monitoring of speech signals seems to be mediated by motor decoding (Lieberman, 1972). After studying articulatory inconsistencies in the speech of normal children, Gallagher and Shriner (1975a: 174) conclude:

The children's deviations from adult phonological performance was found to be related to motoric difficulties rather than idiosyncratic lexical representation.

Using minature transducers, McGlone and Proffit (1973) found that lateral lispers have bizarre swallowing patterns and poor tongue control. It is important to know how the client is misarticulating.

How does one go about making a kinetic analysis? We use three methods: (1) We ask the client to tell us what he is doing. This is the least productive approach. Although some children seem to be aware (Schuckers et al., 1974), most misarticulators simply cannot tell you what they are doing to produce certain sounds. As they progress in treatment, however, clients should become better informed about what is going on when they talk. (2) Watch what the client is doing. Does his mandible shift to one side when he utters sibilants? Does his tongue tip protrude between his teeth when he says the /s/ sound? Does he appear to substitute sounds requiring fewer motor adjustments for more difficult sounds (Locke, 1972)? What can we see? (3) With our trained ear and knowledge of motor phonetics, we try to duplicate with our own mouth what the client is doing. This is usually the best method of all. Often the client "teaches" us how to make his error, creating an objectivity and sharing that augers well for the outcome of treatment. An example of a clinician's search with a young child:

> How do you do that? Let's see. I put my tongue tip out front, through the teeth "gate," right? Then what? Oh, I see, you squirt the air right through that tiny space around your tongue. Now, let me see if I can do it the way you do. How's that? Not quite the same, huh? Well, I have to learn how to do it the way you do so we can fix that sound up. Let's try again.

We often use a common drinking straw to help identify abnormal air flow on certain consonant sounds. In the future, the diagnostician will have the assistance of highly refined techniques for assessing articulatory kinesiology: although not currently available for clinical use, researchers (Hixon, 1972; Fletcher, McCutheon, and Wolf, 1975) are studying motor speech behavior employing electromagnetic measurements, strain gain measurements, and ultrasonic scanning; a new computer-based instrumental system known as *PAGIS* is being used to diagnose and treat speech defects as well as study normal speech patterns. With this system, researchers detect and measure the pattern of tongue contact against the roof of the mouth and the motions of the lips and jaws during the actual processes of speaking. A National Institute of Health news bulletin (August 10, 1975: 11) described the research:

> Tiny electrodes or "beads" embedded in a thin plate are placed against the roof of the mouth to detect tongue contacts while a video-based system determines lip and jaw activities by scanning and measuring the "beads" attached to the face and one tooth. A computer takes in all the information, processes it and displays it back to a clinician or, in many instances, to the speaker himself.

The kinetic analysis may also reveal obvious motor dysfunctions such as flaccidity or spasticity of the oral musculature, and tremors. Indeed, we often perform a kinetic analysis during an oral peripheral examination (see Chapter 3).

The diagnostician must know all he can about motor phonetics, and it would be wise to review several books concerned with this topic. The publication by Carrell and Tiffany (1960) is an excellent point of departure. For additional information regarding the kinesiology of articulation, consult Van Riper (1963: 224–226) and others (Van Riper and Irwin, 1958: 72; Morley, 1965: 210–225; West, Ansberry, and Carr, 1957: 675–676; and Irwin and Duffy, 1955: 31).

IDENTIFYING SOURCES OF VARIABILITY. *Finding* a client's articulation errors and identifying *how* he produces them is only half the diagnostic task. We must also discover what circumstances improve his speech performance. Does he ever utter his defective sounds correctly? Inconsistency is an important clinical sign; if the client can make his error sound correctly on occasion—or significantly shift his production toward normalcy—the diagnostician considers this a favorable indicator for treatment. There are three reasons why clinicians are anxious to identify sources of variability in their clients' articulatory performances:

1. If the individual can make his error sound correctly under certain conditions, then we can assume he possesses normal capability to improve his articulation during treatment.

2. Inconsistency, especially if the client improves his performance when provided a good model, is a good prognostic sign. In our clinical experience, when we can identify sources of variability in a client's speech performance, we generally find that therapy progresses more rapidly.

3. If the client can modify his articulation performance under certain circumstances, we have a place to commence treatment. These correct productions provide a nucleus for therapeutic attention that may then be extended. The morale of both client and clinician is enhanced if some improvement can be made early in therapy.

We shall discuss four aspects of client variability: connected speech, response to stimulation, key words, and deep testing.

CONNECTED SPEECH. Most articulation inventories are designed to evoke naming responses, but not even the most taciturn of persons speaks only in single words. Speech flows—it is a dynamic, overlapping, incredibly swift activity; although careful listening may distinguish separate speech sounds, in spontaneous utterance each phoneme (phone) is influenced by the others that precede and follow it. This is called coarticulation and may extend across as many as four or five speech sounds (Noll, 1970: 289). Therefore, a complete picture of a client's articulation must include a sample of his spontaneous speech. (Goda, 1970; McLean, 1976; Weston and Leonard, 1976). A recent study supports this notion:

> The results of this study strongly suggest that analysis of connected speech describes a person's habitual articulation behavior more appropriately than does single-word testing. A connected-speech analysis enables one to determine the physiological movement patterns which control both the syllabic and phonetic integrity of the individual's language system (Faircloth and Faircloth, 1970:61).

We have already suggested several ways in which the clinician can obtain a sample of the client's connected speech; let us simply list some of the most common: (1) oral reading; (2) paraphrasing written material; (3) asking questions and holding a conversation; (4) extemporaneous, or impromptu, speaking; and (5) informal, off-guard spontaneous speech.[6]

RESPONSE TO STIMULATION. What impact does the examiner's speech have upon the client, can he then imitate the clinician's standard articulation product? Is there some modification in the direction of normalcy, or doesn't his articulation change at all? Consider again Figure 6.4, which depicts the results of an articula-

---

[6]Is it possible for the clinician to obtain a really spontaneous speech sample free of examiner contamination or irrelevant stimuli? (See Laffel, 1965: 79.)

tion inventory conducted with Ricky, an eight-year-old second grader. Note the column headed *Stimulable*. To illustrate this important diagnostic concept, we include a portion of the student examiner's protocol:

> After I finished the articulation inventory and identified his sound errors, I went back and tested for stimulability. By that time Ricky was getting restless, so I made a game of it. I told him we were going to play follow-the-leader and began by having him model some of my gross motor movements. Then, I started to make some noises, an airplane, a siren, and so forth, and he continued to follow me. Finally, I moved to speech sounds—I started with sounds he could make, the /k/ and /g/—and told him to watch me closely and listen carefully. As you told me, I made the sounds in isolation three times and then nodded for him to imitate my production immediately. He seemed to like this. If he improved with the sounds in isolation, I moved to nonsense syllables and then to words. Anyway, here are the results:

Error Sound	Stimulable
sh	He produced a good /sh/ in isolation, in several syllables ("sha," "shi," "shu," "sho") but reverted to the /s/ when I moved to short words like "ship," "shoot," and "fish."
th	He copied my standard production of isolated syllables and even put them into words. I don't think this is a "defect" as such but rather a cultural thing.
th	Same thing.
s	He can make the /s/ easily, even in complex words like "first." I think we should start therapy with this sound.
z	Ditto. I believe we can correct both of these at the same time.
r	His error changed slightly, from a /w/ to a more lingual sound but only in isolation, not in syllables (I didn't try words).
ω	No response here at all, he didn't budget from his distortion. Guess we will need to search for key words and do a deep test.

> After we finished with the stimulability test, he still seemed interested in following the-leader. So, I brought out the stethoscope and put it on him; he can make an almost acceptable /r/ with very intense and prolonged stimulation but the /ω/ didn't change at all. Guess I should have had him explore different tongue positions but we ran out of time.

Testing for stimulability (Milisen, 1954: 6–7) is an extremely useful diagnostic procedure. If a client can produce his error correctly by imitating a standard model—either in isolation, in nonsense syllables, or in words—then there are generally no serious organic obstacles that would prevent his eventual acquisition of the sound (Darley, 1964: 65).[7] Stimulability is also a useful prognostic sign; clients who can modify their articulation errors by imitating the examiner's standard production improve more swiftly in treatment than those who cannot. Finally, as illustrated in the case of Ricky, when the client has several defective sounds, the stimulability test provides the clinician with a place to begin treatment; it also suggests the *type* of therapy procedures to be used (Winitz, 1969).

---

[7]A similar proposition has been made about stuttering: stutterers are fluent in some circumstances, and therefore they must not have organic impairment. Is this truer of stuttering than of articulation disorders?

KEY WORDS. The clinician should carefully note whether the client occasionally uses the correct sound in certain words. These "key words," as they are called, are valuable in therapy because

> . . . they provide for the person a model in his own mouth for the sound we seek to teach him. We can use these key words to help us perceive the characteristics of the standard sound, both acoustic cues and the postures and movements required for their production. They can be used in discriminating error words from normally spoken words (Van Riper, 1963: 231).

Key words give us a starting point:

> Steve produced a defective /r/ on all the items in the phonemic inventory—single words, blends, and sentences. Near the end of the session, however, he began to talk about space travel (a Gemini space shot had gone off that morning) and out popped "rocket" uttered with a normal /r/ sound. We talked further and noted several other /r/ words, all related to space travel, that Steve said normally. Apparently, the experience of hearing these terms repeated again and again in the context of an exciting vicarious adventure, prompted him to utter them correctly. We started therapy with a unit about space travel; we uttered, and had Steve utter, the key words over and over as we pretended to be astronauts. We used an auditory training unit to heighten his self-hearing; we had him prolong the /r/ sound as he monitored himself with earphones. Gradually, we shifted to more prosaic modes of travel, railroads, cars, and trucks. We strengthened the /r/ and expanded the list of key words. By then Steve had an internal model with which he could scan his speech. His recovery was incredibly swift.

DEEP TESTING. We pointed out previously that in spontaneous, ongoing speech, each sound is influenced and altered by the phonetic context in which it occurs. Phonemes are uttered differently in the company of other phonemes, even as people behave differently depending upon their circumstances and companions. Most articulation tests permit only a superficial assessment of a client's articulation of a given sound; they provide a small sampling of the many possible phonetic environments in which the case's misarticulated sound can occur (Subtelny, Oya, and Subtelny, 1972; Kresheck, Fisher, and Rutherford, 1972). The evidence is clear that misarticulators are inconsistent (Spriestersbach and Curtis, 1951; Curtis and Hardy, 1959) and that these inconsistencies are of great importance for treatment. As speech clinicians we are not just interested in identifying what the client *cannot* do, we must also search diligently for what he *can* do. It is often necessary, then, to delve beneath the surface with a more comprehensive deep-testing device.

Several writers (Powers, 1971b; Van Riper, 1972; Gallagher and Shriner, 1975b) have stressed the importance of more thorough articulation testing. McDonald (1964) devised a sensitive testing instrument, the Deep Test of Articulation, which allows the examiner to evaluate a client's misarticulation of any defective sound in a systematic way and in all possible phonetic contexts. McDonald describes the Deep Test in these words:

> In a "Deep Test of Articulation" the phonetic environment of a sound is manipulated to cause the sound to be articulated as it is preceded by each of the consonants and

vowels and followed by a vowel, and as it is preceded by a vowel and followed by each of the consonants and vowels (1964: 129).

Each phoneme can thus be observed forty or more times as the initiating or terminating sound in a syllable. Since it is the basic unit of speech, it seems appropriate that the focus of testing should be the syllable (Priestly, 1977). Here is a portion of a transcribed session in which the examiner is administering the /s/ portion of the McDonald instrument to a second-grade boy with a lateral lisp:

Clinician: Okay, Tony, we are ready to start with the numbered pages. You understand now that you are to make a funny big word from the names of the objects on the two pictures, like we did in the example "tub-vase," without stopping between the word? Fine! Here is the first one:

1.	housepipe	no change
2.	housebell	no change
3.	housetie	improvement—moderate
4.	housedog	improvement—moderate
5.	housecow	no change
6.	housegun	no change

Note that the word *house*, with a final /s/, is tested as it precedes all other phonemes; the examiner listens carefully to identify any changes in the client's misarticulation. Then, the examiner reverses the procedure so that /s/ follows all other phonemes, thus:

1. cupsun
2. tubsun
3. kitesun

For older clients, McDonald has prepared a series of sentences to be read aloud. The diagnostician will want to be familiar with this test.

We do not routinely administer the *Deep Test of Articulation* during a diagnostic evaluation of a child. We have found that it is too lengthy for initial assessment purposes and that some children experience considerable difficulty blending the two test items into one large word (Goda, 1970). We prefer to use the test during the initial stages of treatment, exploring with the client for loci of improved, or at least altered, sound production. Additionally, we find the *Deep Test* invaluable for charting a client's improvement during the course of therapy.

A LINGUISTIC ANALYSIS. Linguists and speech pathologists interested in language have provided the diagnostician with a new way of looking at articulation disorders (Grunwell, 1975; Ingram, 1976; Parker, 1976; Singh, 1976). Instead of viewing sound production and sound errors as isolated phenomena, articulation is considered "a subsystem of oral language, and that as a subsystem its existence and deficits are inter-related to rather than separate from other aspects of oral language'' (Irwin, 1972: 4). Since phonology is clearly one facet of oral language, children presenting defects of articulation may be considered to have a language problem.

For some time clinicians had observed that children with functional sound errors seemed to be deficient in other language skills. Research (Menyuk, 1964; Vandemark and Mann 1965; Shriner et al., 1969; Marquardt and Saxman, 1972; Panagos, 1974; Kuchon, 1976; Weger, Shattuck and Erickson, 1976) tended to support this notion, particularly with respect to children with more severe or multiple-articulation defects. Moreover, careful phonological analysis showed that the supposed inconsistency of children's misarticulations could be explained in terms of an underlying or subsegmental system.

When experts in linguistics (Haas, 1963; Crocker, 1969; Compton, 1970) examined a misarticulator's errors by the use of feature analysis, it became apparent that the individual did not have a random collection of unrelated sound substitutions. Children with articulation defects did not simply have a ''broken-down'' sound production facility; it was possible, in fact, to identify definite patterns underlying their use of speech sounds. Leonard (1973a) described two basic patterns of misarticulation: a *delayed* or *immature sound system* whereby certain common features expected to be present are absent; and an *idiosyncratic system* in which certain features are misused relative to the standard adult system.

Investigations (Menyuk, 1968; Prather, Hedrick, and Kern, 1975) show that the mastery of the distinctive features which comprise speech sounds follows a definite, systematic progression. Some children take longer to acquire certain features and display, as it were, an immature phonological system.

Another larger group (as high as 70 percent, according to Leonard) acquire articulation in a manner which is at variance with appropriate usage. In this case, the client follows idiosyncratic rules of distinctive feature usage; however, *his* phonological system has logical and coherent principles (Priestly, 1977). According to McReynolds and Huston:

> When articulation errors occur, they may consist of a phoneme system organized differently from the adult phoneme system. The more the systems differ, the more severe the child's articulation problem. The child's system may be complete for the child and as lawful as the adult's, but it is his own system, and his rules are at variance with the adult or the standard system (1971: 155–156).

In terms of diagnosis, then, we shift our focus from the child's sound errors per se to the underlying patterns his errors follow. What are the elements comprising his sound system? What are the phonological rules he employs in using the speech sounds in his particular repertoire?

> A phonologic pattern is defined as occurring when one or more relationships are discovered between phonemes that have at least one major articulation feature in common (Weber, 1970: 137).

In order to discern if a child's misarticulations have an underlying pattern, it is necessary to undertake a distinctive feature analysis: we must see what subsegmental features are present and how he uses them.

What are distinctive features? In this concept, speech sounds are not indivisible entities, but rather are considered to be composed of intersecting subcomponents or attributes (voicing, nasality, etc.) which are termed "features" (Comptom, 1970). Distinctive feature theory attempts to specify the characteristics of phonemes—according to the presence (+) or absence (−) of each feature—that distinguish or contrast one speech sound from another. Let us illustrate with a distinctive feature analysis of /s/ and /θ/, two speech sounds which are often confused by children:

/θ/	features	/s/
(−)	vocalic	(−)
(+)	consonantal	(+)
(−)	high	(−)
(−)	back	(−)
(−)	low	(−)
(+)	anterior	(+)
(+)	coronal	(+)
(−)	voice	(−)
(+)	continuant	(+)
(−)	nasal	(−)
(−)	strident	(+)

To repeat, an anaylsis of phonemes (in this case the /s/ and /θ/) yields a description of each speech sound with respect to the presence or absence of each feature (McReynolds and Engmann, 1975; definitions of the features can be found in Chomsky and Halle, 1968). When particular features (in the example above the feature of "stridency") serve to differentiate one phoneme from another, they are said to be distinct (Weston and Leonard, 1976).

A distinctive-feature analysis reduces all a client's articulation errors (its usefulness is limited primarily to children presenting four or more errors) to a few underlying phonological principles by which he regulates his sound production. Kamara, Kamara and Singh describe the diagnostic procedure:

> By tallying the subject's feature confusions in sound substitutions, as revealed in articulation testing, a pattern will emerge which identifies relative strengths and weaknesses within the subject's phonological system. In addition, a composite phonemic score reveals the overall stability of the subject's phonological system in comparison to a system which is intact. Generally, the smaller the number of distinctive feature differences, the closer or less deviant the error sound is felt to be with the target (1975: 1).

McReynolds and Engmann (1975) have prepared a manual featuring detailed clinical worksheets to guide the diagnostician in performing a distinctive feature analysis. The clinician first obtains a sample of the client's articulation—at least ten productions of each phoneme is recommended; the responses are transcribed carefully according to number of correct productions, errors of omission, substitutions (the actual sound substituted). Finally, using a table of distinctive features, the clinician notes the number of times a particular feature was used by the client, and compares his performance to standard adult usage.

What are the advantages of a linguistic analysis? We see four: (1) it provides a model for understanding articulation disorders in many children; an error on a given feature (for example, voicing) which is shared by more than one phoneme accounts for the misarticulation of many phonemes by reducing the seemingly random errors to a simpler pattern; (2) it provides a gauge of severity; (3) it provides a basis for the selection of a target sound for therapy; the clinician can select the phoneme which shares features with many other misarticulated sounds; and (4) it provides a basis for more efficient therapy (Ritterman and Freeman, 1974; Costello and Onstine, 1976) by facilitating generalization to sound errors not being treated:

> We recently examined a child who substituted plosives for all the fricative consonants. The misarticulation of the fricative sounds was viewed as a surface reflection of an underlying phonological principle—the child's system did not include friction as a "manner of articulation." Instead of teaching one sound at a time, we sought to include the principle of friction within his system of phonology.

Therapy directed toward one sound often improves others that are phonetically similar. Considered within the framework of underlying phonological principles, it makes sense that training in features common to many sounds would result in greater improvement in misarticulation than specific training for each sound error. The basic assumption of a linguistic-analysis approach to the assessment and treatment of articulation disorders is that the elimination of a particular sound error produces a change in the principle underlying the defect, and thus all other errors which arise from that principle will also be eliminated (Compton, 1975).

Despite the many advantages, however, there are a number of factors which limit the application of distinctive-feature theory to clinical problems. First of all, the procedures for assessment as described by McReynolds and Engmann (1975) are quite time consuming; the clinician has to weigh this factor against the purported increase in efficiency. The second limiting factor is the obvious complexity of the system of analysis. But the main drawback is that, on a phonetic level, the distinctive features advocated by Chomsky and Halle have no conceptual reality (LaRiviere, 1974). By that we mean that there is no one-to-one relationship between distinctive features—an acoustic classification—and articulatory production—physiological level (Parker, 1976); the physical act of articulation clearly is not a binary function that is either present ($+$) or absent ($-$), but is multivaried, is a matter of varying degrees. According to Walsh (1974), the categories employed in distinctive-feature analysis are overgeneralized and may encompass too great a phonetic space to be of clinical value. Leonard (1973b: 141–2) points out that "articulation therapy involves giving phonetic instructions. Therefore, the features we deal with must have a specific physical interpretation." Where it is necessary to use a sub-phonemic system of analysis, we advocate with others (Fisher and Logemann, 1971; Leonard, 1973; Walsh, 1974; McLean, 1976; Sommers and Kane, 1974; Eisenson and Ogilvie, 1977; Nation and Aram, 1977) the selection of one based upon a model of *speech production* rather than on a system limited to an abstract classificatory function.

We employ a simple procedure for making a limited linguistic analysis. Let us illustrate with a case example:

Audrey, age four years, seven months, was referred to us by a local school clinician. Her speech was unintelligible. Her developmental and medical history was unremarkable. Her oral peripheral organs were judged to be structurally and functionally normal. Her hearing was within the normal limits for pure tone and speech reception. Her verbal intelligence (Peabody Picture Vocabulary Test) was low normal. Her receptive language seemed normal—she was able to follow rather complex directions. There was some history of familial discord and perhaps reduced environmental stimulation; her parents were estranged and the father left the home for several months, necessitating the mother's employment outside the home.

We administered parts of the Templin-Darley Tests of Articulation (1970) and the McDonald Deep Test of Articulation (1964). We found that the child possessed only six phonemes, /m/, /p/, /b/, /t/, /d/, and /h/. Here is a delineation of her errors:

Standard Sound	Substitution
k	t, h
g	d, h
θ	t
ð	d
n	d

All the rest were substituted by a voiceless, glottal fricative, /h/.

Following the suggestion of Weber (1970) and Beresford and Grady (1968), we examined the child's phoneme system by employing three major articulation features—*place* of articulation, *manner* of articulation, and *voicing*, as shown in the following diagram:

	Labial	Labio-dental	Dental	Alveolar	Palatal	Velar	Glottal
Glide							
Semivowel							
Nasal	m						
Stop	p,b			t,d			
Fricative							h

Audrey had not acquired several aspects of the features that distinguish sounds such as place and manner of articulation. She recognized voicing-unvoicing in the plosives /pb/ and /td/, but yet she substituted the voiceless fricative /h/ for all the glides and other fricatives. Her particular phonological system did not include friction, glides, semivowels, and so on.

Several clinicians (Fisher and Logemann, 1971; Sommers and Kane, 1974; Eisenson and Ogilvie, 1977) advocate similar models for phoneme feature targeting. The language-specific system devised by Walsh (1974: 40) is particularly effective for completing a comprehensive linguistic analysis. An example will illustrate:

> Return to the distinctive feature analysis of /θ/ and /s/. According to this analysis, the common substitution of θ/s would be described as + strident → − strident. Note that this "describes not a change in articulation, but rather the consequence of a change in articulation" Walsh, 1974: 42). The substitution is more efficiently explained as a forward shift of the tongue tip which blocks the production of sibilance. Note also that this description leads directly to a treatment goal.

DYSLALIA, DYSARTHRIA, and DYSPRAXIA. Some children who have been diagnosed as having functional articulation disorders—no readily discernible organic basis for their sound errors—may, on close examination, possess subtle neurological impairments. (Frisch and Handler, 1974; Yoss and Darley, 1974a). Quite often these same children fail to improve despite year after year of treatment; a local survey revealed that as high as 12 percent of clients comprising the caseloads of school clinicians were youngsters with persistent articulation problems.

At the urging of colleagues working in school settings, we searched the literature for information on the persistence of articulatory disorders. The topic had received only limited attention (Dickson, 1962; Wilbeck, 1963; Eberline, 1963; Foster, 1963; Palmer, Wurth, and Kinchloe, 1964; Renfrew, 1966) so we decided to explore the issue as a clinical research project.

Our research is still incomplete (Trevarton, 1975), but preliminary results on sixty subjects do identify clusters of variables. Although each child had been diagnosed as having a "functional" disorder of articulation, the cases comprising the "persistent" group (those students who did not alter their defective sound production in one year of treatment) showed more indications of abnormality, including signs of possible organic impairment. Here is a list of cues, or indicators, frequently found among the children who did not make progress in therapy (italicized items were found in all persisters):

1. *Motor behavior (fine and gross) on the slow and incoordinated end of the normal range*
2. *Dysrythmia of tongue movements, slow oral diadochokinesis, protruding and retracting of the tongue not accomplished swiftly*
3. Drooling
4. Abnormal chewing and swallowing
5. Abnormal dental bites
6. Reading problems
7. Difficulty in attending (frequently says "huh?" but no measured hearing loss; listening in noise is often even more difficult)
8. Reverses sounds, leaves out phonemes in longer words; low on slurvian skills

9. Tends to reverse letters when writing; spelling problem
10. Cannot sound out words (vocal phonics); difficulty sequencing
11. Siblings had speech or language problems
12. Tends to be a follower; initiates conversation less frequently
13. Lower educational achievement of parents
14. Errors of omission

We are also impressed with the great overlap between groups on many of the dimensions studied. Differential diagnosis is not an easy task. By and large, however, the children with persistent disorders of articulation were similar in many respects to subjects described by Chappell (1973) and others (Yost and Darley, 1974a; Yost and Darley, 1974b; Dabul and Bollier, 1976). To assist you in distinguishing between three major categories of articulatory disorders— dysarthria, dyspraxia, and dyslalia—we included Table 6.1, prepared on the basis of our experience and a survey of the literature (see also Project 3). We urge you to carefully study the work of Darley, Aronson and Brown (1975) as well as other sources (Morely, 1965; Milisen, 1966; Carrell, 1968; Luchsinger and Arnold, 1965; West and Ansberry, 1968; Peacher, 1962; Deal and Darley, 1972; Moore, Rosenbeck, and LaPointe, 1976).

ADDITIONAL EVALUATIONAL ACTIVITIES

Diagnosticians often give additional tests to a client who presents an articulation disorder. We shall consider briefly only five aspects which clinicians frequently assess: sound discrimination, auditory memory span, vocal phonics, oral sensory discrimination, and parental attitudes and adjustments. The reader will want to review Chapter 3 regarding examination procedures commonly undertaken with clients.

Sound-Discrimination Testing

Some children with articulatory disorders have difficulty distinguishing sounds from one another. Although the research is far from unequivocal (see reviews by Van Riper and Irwin, 1958; and Winitz, 1969; Powers, 1971a; Sommers and Kane, 1974) there is sufficient evidence to warrant sound discrimination testing for each case, especially children with multiple sound errors (Sherman and Geith, 1967).

> We recently evaluated a second-grade boy who, in addition to having several defective sounds (/s/, /z/, /ch/, /dʒ/, and /ω/) was a poor reader. The child had repeated first grade and the teacher told us, "Bernie doesn't know 'Dick' from 'down'." After scrutinizing Bernie's audiogram—his hearing for pure tone was within normal limits—we decided to administer a rather comprehensive battery of sound-discrimination tests.
>
> We wanted to see how the child would do on an *interpersonal* measure of

Table 6.1 Differential Diagnosis of Dysarthria, Dyspraxia and Dyslalia

	Dysarthria	Dyspraxia	Dyslalia
Definition	Distinct patterns of speech disturbance due to weakness and slowness. Incoordination of speech muscles. Oral movements are disrupted and reflect different types of neuropathology. Articulation, phonation, resonation and prosody may be impaired	Articulation errors, in the absence of muscle slowness, weakness, incoordination, due to disruption of cortical programming for the *voluntary* production of speech sounds	Articulation errors without apparent organic disability
Medical history	Often diagnosed neuropathology	May be apparent or diagnosed neuropathology	Generally unremarkable
Development of speech	Generally delayed	May be delayed	May be slower than normal
Oral peripheral examination	Obvious defectiveness: slow, weak and incoordinated. *Vegetative* functions (sucking, chewing) disturbed as well as speech movements	No obvious dysfunction except when requested to execute *voluntary* movement. Vegetative functions performed adequately	Generally unremarkable. May be slower than normal

Table 6.1 Cont'd.

	Dysarthria	Dyspraxia	Dyslalia
Articulation	Simplification a. distortions b. substitutions Errors consistent More complex units (clusters of consonants) are more difficult More errors in final position Errors consistent with neurological record Severity related to extent of neuro-muscular involvement	Complication a. transpositions, reversals b. perseverative and anticipatory errors c. fewer distortions, more substitutions, intrusive additions Errors increase proportionate to word weight (grammatical class, difficulty of initial consonant, position in sentence and word length) Fewer errors in spontaneous performance Inconsistency is key sign	
Repeated utterance	Same performance	Make repeated attempt and may achieve correct performance. Appears to grope or struggle for correct production	May improve depending on amount of auditory-visual stimulation

190

Table 6.1 Cont'd.

	Dysarthria	*Dyspraxia*	*Dyslalia*
Rate	Deterioration of performance with increased rate Slow rate of speech	Performance improves at faster rate Disturbances of prosody: stuttering-like struggle reactions; slow, labored speech during voluntary attempts	Generally does poorer at increased rate Normal rate of speech
Response to stimulation	May alter performance slightly to match auditory-visual model. Best response to demonstration of specific articulatory gestures	Best performance if sees and hears model. Does better if provided one stimulation and given several chances to match the model	Variable, may demonstrate normal capacity
Associated disabilities	Reading, spelling, writing problems	Reading, spelling, writing problems Some have difficulty with auditory discrimination Some have difficulty with oral stereognosis	More difficulties with language arts than in normals; may be secondary to speech disorder
Treatment	Assistance in making compensatory adjustments	Direct training in listening and repeating	

discrimination; we selected the *Templin Short Test* (1943) and the *Wepman Auditory Discrimination Test* (Wepman, 1958). The Templin instrument features paired nonsense syllables that the examiner utters, and the child indicates if the pair are "same" or "different." Bernie seemed bored with this task but he made only seven errors—which exceeds the norms for his grade level. The Wepman test consists of word pairs (for example, pat/pack, coast/toast, badge/badge) which are read to the client, who judges whether they are the same or different. Again, Bernie performed well, missing only two items (thimble/symbol and clothe/clove). The diagnostician should keep in mind that, (1) children under the age of eight may have difficulty understanding the task of judging "same" and "different" (Beving and Eblen, 1973); (2) in some cases, errors on a sound discrimination task may, in fact, be linguistic errors steming from the limited grammatical and phonetic clues (Schwartz and Goldman, 1974); and, (3) the Wepman test may introduce bias by not using the two response categories equally (Vellutino, DeSetto and Steger, 1972).

Recalling the conclusion which Aungst and Frick (1964: 83) reached in their research in sound discrimination, "The ability to discriminate between paired auditory stimuli presented by another speaker is unrelated to the ability to judge one's own speech production as correct or incorrect," and the advice that the clinician should tailor his discrimination assessment procedures to his particular client (Spriestersbach and Curtis, 1951), we moved to more sensitive tasks.

We devised an *intropersonal* test of discrimination: we uttered short words (for example, "sail," "ship," "earth," "chop") twice, once using Bernie's errors and once correctly. His job was to "catch" the mistakes. We mixed the order of errors and correct sounds and used five word pairs for each defective phoneme. At first he didn't understand the task, so we gave him several examples. He liked "catching" us and did very well except for the /ω/ list, where his missed three of the five items.

Finally, we concluded the examination with three *intrapersonal* tests of auditory discrimination (Aungst and Frick, 1964): Bernie and the examiner made a short tape recording wherein they both named a set of stimulus pictures. The clinician simulated the child's error on some items and uttered others correctly. When the tape was played back, the child was asked to compare his production to that of the clinician. He missed seven of fifteen items and requested several playbacks of the recording.

We then had the child name another set of pictures (some containing his error sounds, others without any error sounds) and asked him to tell us immediately if he had said it "right" or "wrong." He was unable to do this task, shrugged, and played with the electrical cord on the machine after naming each picture.

After a short break, we listened to the tape made during the test of instantaneous judgment just described. We asked Bernie to tell us which words were said correctly and incorrectly. Even on the test of delayed judgment, he experienced considerable difficulty, missing thirteen of twenty items. Our clinicial findings were similar in many respects to research showing that breakdowns in discrimination tend to be specific to articulation errors (Monnin and Huntington, 1974; McReynolds, Kohn and Williams, 1975; Williams and McReynolds, 1975; Locke and Kutz, 1975).

In addition to the instruments already mentioned, there are several other tests of sound discrimination (Goldman, Fristoe and Woodcock, 1970; Aten, 1973; Prather, Miner and Addicott, 1971). The *Ohio Test of Articulation and Perception of Sounds* (Irwin, 1973; 1974) is particularly useful since it is well standardized and incorporates many of the assessment procedures described in the case example. It features tasks that measure both inter- and intra-personal discrimination.

In some cases, the diagnostician will want to administer additional tests to evaluate auditory perceptual skills. The instruments devised by Kimmel and Wahl

(1970), Lindamood (1969) and Goldman, Fristoe, and Woodcock (1975) are useful in this regard.

Auditory Memory Span

A few of our clients with articulation disorders have considerable difficulty retaining information in "immediate memory." In some instances, a child simply cannot seem to attend to a series of items presented auditorily—an ability necessary for the acquisition of speech—and repeat them back. As with sound discrimination, the research on the relationship between articulatory defectiveness and auditory memory span is not conclusive (Wintz, 1969: 178–180; see also the work of Locke, 1969; Locke and Kutz, 1975). Saxman and Miller (1973) found that children with articulatory deficiencies were inferior to normal-speaking children on a sentence-recall task and inferred that it was due to diminished linguistic capacity rather than short-term memory disturbance. However, we commonly include an assessment of retention span in an evaluation of clients presenting error sounds.

To test for auditory memory span, the examiner may use digits, speech sounds, nonsense syllables, and sentences of progressively longer length. Items such as digits are presented one per second; the client either repeats the items or writes them down. Norms may be found in various source books (Berry and Eisenson, 1959: 503; Van Riper, 1963: 477–478; Irwin, 1965: 396–397). Baker and Leland (1959) have published a test of auditory memory span that employs words and syllables. The clinician should be aware that anxiety tends to reduce retention span.

Clients with limited auditory-memory span experience considerable difficulty in therapy. Happily, however, in our experience specific training in the retention of longer and longer units often meliorates the condition.

Vocal Phonics

Van Riper (1963: 479–480) has devised a simple test for determining a client's ability to *analyze* (break a word down into its sound elements) and *synthesize* (assemble a word from its component sounds) language units. We find vocal phonics to be an extremely useful concept not only for diagnostic purposes, but also for therapy. Children who do poorly in vocal phonics, especially synthesis tasks, need considerable training in this aspect, along with conventional articulation therapy.

Most children are delighted with games involving mystery or guessing and find tests of phonetic analysis and synthesis particularly intriguing. Here is how one clinician introduced a test of vocal phonics (synthesis) to a young child:

> Do you know that I can stretch words out like rubber bands? Watch me say the name for this thing (points to nose) and s-t-r-e-t-c-h it way out: n . . . .o . . . .z. What did I say? That's right, nose . . . .n . . . .o . . . .z. Now, you did very well and let's see if you can put back together some words that I am going to stretch way apart. P . . . . at, J . . . . u.

A more formal measure of auditory synthesizing ability may be obtained by using the instrument devised by Oliphant (1971). In this test (standardized on first-grade children) a child listens to phonemes, holds them in memory, blends them into a correct sequence and then assigns meaning to the sequence. The test features three units, each with ten test words; words comprised of two, three, and four phonemes are used. If the child.does not respond correctly to an initial presentation, he is offered a multiple-choice format.

Oral Sensory Discrimination

The relationship between oral sensation and perception and speech proficiency has received considerable research attention (Bosma, 1967; 1970; Dellow et al., 1970; Putnam and Ringel, 1972; Moreau and Lass, 1974; Marshall, Sharrow, Yairi, 1977). While not all misarticulators have difficulty with oral sensory discrimination, clients with multiple sound errors and those in certain diagnostic subgroups—for example, tongue-thrusters—may manifest disturbances (Schlanger, 1976). At present, clinical application is somewhat limited and we are sometimes called upon to improvise an oral sensory test battery for particular children:

> We encountered Julie while certifying caseloads in a rural area of Upper Michigan. The public-school clinician had been working with the child for three years—Julie was now in the fourth grade—but with only minimal results. Although she exhibited no gross abnormality of the oral area, her lalling persisted; the clinician reported that Julie seemed uncertain of movements and positioning of her tongue when asked to assume various articulatory postures. Remembering the work of McCall (1969), we decided to do some gross clinical testing of the child's lingual-tactile sensation and perception.
>
> First, we assessed tactile *sensitivity*—could she detect the presence of a stimulus? Using a cotton wisp, we lightly brushed Julie's tongue at various locations; interestingly, she made more errors on the right than on the left side, and her responses became progressively more certain and swift as we moved away from the tip toward the dorsum. Next, we tested for tactile *localization*—could Julie identify the precise spot we touched with a surgical stick? Using a schematic drawing of the tongue, the child attempted to locate the exact point of stimulation. Again, we noted that Julie was more accurate away from the tongue tip and on the left side.
>
> We also wanted to evaluate *tactile acuity*—could she detect minimal changes in stimuli? The only materials we could find to assess this dimension of lingual sensitivity were an old set of stainless steel weights borrowed from the chemistry teacher. Sterilizing them carefully in alcohol, we placed them gently on Julie's tongue (at the midline) and asked her to judge their relative weight. She had no difficulty with this admittedly gross task, nor did she experience any difficulty identifying various *textures* (emery board, eraser, cotton, polished block of marble). Recalling some research (Ringel, Burke, and Scott, 1968) which showed that speakers with articulation defects experience more difficulty identifying shapes orally (*oral form recognition*), we searched about the school for suitable stimulus objects to use with Julie. The only items we could find were some small plastic letters and a number of small bracelet charms. Julie may simply have been fatigued at this

point, but she did miss over half the items presented. We had borrowed a pair of calipers from the metal shop to test for *two-point discrimination,* but Julie was tired and we abandoned the evaluation.

We saw the child later at the Speech and Hearing Clinic for a more thorough evaluation. At that time we administered the *Florida Oral Form Recognition Measure* (Williams and LaPoint, 1971). The stimulus materials for this test consist of small plastic forms attached to stainless steel orthodontic wire. Julie was blindfolded. The forms were placed in her mouth one at a time and she was asked to select the appropriate one from a score sheet. She identified the star form correctly but missed all the others.

Julie was referred to a neurologist, who confirmed our impression of lingual-sensory deficit. The speech clinician altered his therapy with the child to include tongue exercises, point-to-point matching in the oral area, oral object identification, and compensatory articulatory positioning. The child is still in therapy, but at our last visit showed significant improvement.

In our clinicial experience, difficulty with tactile localization and oral form recognition are more closely related to misarticulation than are other measures. Children with multiple sound errors (four or more sounds), lallers, and omitters often exhibit problems of oral sensory discrimination. The reader will want to consult the work of Silverman (1972) for another method of assessing intra-oral form identification (Lass et al., 1972). The use of vibratory stimulation may prove useful in evaluating other aspects of oral sensory discrimination (Fucci, 1972; Telage and Fucci, 1973).

Parental Attitudes and Adjustments

We must have some information about the parents of our clients. What role, if any, have they played in the child's articulation disorders? Although we quite agree with McDonald (1962) that disturbed families often tend to develop handicapped children, we are not particularly impressed by research efforts comparing parents of articulatory-defective children with parents of normal-speaking children (Bloch and Goodstein, 1971). Only a few parents of cases with whom we have worked actually neglected or psychologically abused their children. There were some evil parents who seemed not to care about their offspring, a few who tormented their children with their own private demons, and some who propelled and pushed them like pawns in the status game. But most parents are simply people with their own distinct needs and interests. We must come to realize that parents are not just vehicles to further our therapeutic goals. When we find those who do have problems that impinge upon our client's treatment program, it is our responsibility to see that they get the help they need; we should not just criticize them and thus explain away our own failure.

The best way to find out about our client's parents is to talk with them (Emerick, 1969). On occasion, we have administered one of the published attitude and adjustment inventories (Schaefer and Bell, n.d.; Wiley, 1955; Roth, 1961; Wyatt, 1964), but we have never felt comfortable using them. We prefer interviewing. The specific areas of exploration will depend, of course, upon the particular case being evaluated. There are, however, several general areas of inquiry: the amount and type of stimulation the parents provided during the child's speech development; the parent's expectations regarding the child's development, particularly his acquisition of speech; the child's communication patterns at home; the child's need for speech; how the family deals with the child's speech difference at home; how the parents have tried to help the child's defective articulation. In addition, the clinician is interested in evaluating the speech models the parents provide for their child.

PROGNOSIS

In Chapter 3 we discussed prognosis in a general way, defining the concept as professional premonitions regarding a client's potential for treatment. Now we will consider two aspects of clinical forecasting in articulation disorders: (1) determining the most effective place to begin therapy; and (2) delineating factors involved in predicting the outcome of therapy.

Where should we begin therapy? If a client has several sound errors, which one (or more than one) should we treat first? In a real sense, we have already answered the query; the data we obtain by performing the various diagnostic procedures outlined above will no doubt lead the clinician to an auspicious starting point. Let us review the factors we consider in deciding where to begin. On the basis of our experience, we have ranked the factors listed below according to their clinical importance; however, each client must be examined carefully to determine the relative impact each of these aspects will have on his particular problem:

1. We prefer to select the most stimulable sound error.
2. We consider the client's preference: Which sound error does he most wish to eliminate?
3. We determine which sound error, if improved, would make the client's speech pattern less conspicuous. Three major considerations are: the relative *frequency* in the spoken language of the various sounds in error (the /s/ sound occurs more frequently than /ch/); the *nature* of the error (lateral distortions are more conspicuous than t/th substitutions); and the *type* of error (omissions are the most conspicuous, then substitutions and distortions).
4. We like to select a sound that is phonetically easier. The /th/ is easier to produce than the /r/ because it involves fewer oral adjustments.
5. We prefer to start with the most visible sound. If a client has errors on both /f/ and /r/, for example, we would usually begin with the /f/ sound.
6. We consider the norms for consonant sound maturation when working with children. If a six-year-old misarticulates /k/, /g/, and /s/, therapy would generally begin with the plosives since a child of that age should have acquired /k/ and /g/ but not necessarily /s/.

It is easy to present such a list, but it is quite another thing to weigh the various factors and reach a decision for a real client. Turn back to the case of Ricky (pp. 146–148 and Figure 5). Considering the aspects we have listed, determine if you agree with the student clinician's selection of the sound error with which to begin therapy. Many clinicians prefer to conduct trial therapy and select a particular sound—or underlying pattern of sound errors—only after extensive clinical scrutiny of the case. How might a clinician employ the concept of distinctive features (including "markedness") to select a target sound?

Prognosis also means predicting the outcome of therapy. What are the prospects for success? We do not have any final answers, but treatment does seem more effective if the following factors obtain:

1. If the client can correctly produce his error sounds when provided a standard model (Moore, Burke, Adams, 1976)
2. If the client has few errors—the more sounds misarticulated, the poorer the prognosis
3. If the client is inconsistent in his sound error
4. If the client can synthesize sounds into words (vocal phonics)
5. If the client is motivated to improve his speech
6. If the client's mental age is within normal limits
7. If the client's auditory memory span is within normal limits
8. If the client can locate his own errors
9. If the client does not have other speech or language abnormalities
10. If the client's parents, teacher, and peers are willing to cooperate
11. If the client is relatively free of negative personality traits
12. If the client is not receiving powerful reinforcement for abnormal speech
13. If the client can come frequently to therapy
14. If the client shows swift improvement during trial therapy
15. If the client has personal assets from which he derives satisfaction
16. If the client is relatively free from health problems

Again, it is rather easy to prepare lists; it is a far more difficult task to *apply* these variables, weigh them carefully, and then make a prediction for a given client. We have long hungered for a better way to identify patterns in the hundreds of variables involved in clinical success and failure with our clients. Perhaps the reader will discover one.

PROJECTS AND QUESTIONS

1. Can persons not trained in speech pathology identify speech defects as accurately as experienced clinicians? If they cannot, how does this influence our definition of a speech defect? How reliable are various incidence survey methods? How do parental

assessments compare with those of teachers and clinicians? Review the following articles before responding to the questions:

DIEHL, C., and C. STINNETT (1959). "Efficiency of Teacher Referrals in a School Speech Testing Program." *Journal of Speech and Hearing Disorders*, 24: 34–36.

CALNAN, M., and K. RICHARDSON (1976). "Speech Problems in a National Survey: Assessments and Prevalences." *Child Care, Health and Development*, 2: 181–202.

CLAUSON, G., and N. KOPATIC (1975). "Teacher Attitudes and Knowledge of Remedial Speech Programs." *Language Speech and Hearing Services in Schools*, 6: 206–210.

OYER, H. (1959). "Speech Error Recognition Ability." *Journal of Speech and Hearing Disorders*, 24: 391–394.

SIEGEL, G. (1962). "Experienced and Inexperienced Articulation Examiners." *Journal of Speech and Hearing Disorders*, 27: 28–35.

WERTZ, R., and M. MEAD (1975). "Classroom Teacher and Speech Clinician Severity Ratings of Different Speech Disorders." *Language, Speech and Hearing Services in Schools*, 6: 119–124.

ZEHRBACH, R., (1975). "Determining a Preschool Handicapped Population." *Exceptional Children*, 42: 76–83.

2. What does Renfrew (1966) mean by the persistence of the open syllable? Of what relevance is this to predicting articulatory maturation? Review the follow-up study (Renfrew and Gleary, 1973): of the ten subtests used, which were of the greatest predictive value?

3. See if you can expand Table 6.1 to include *dysglossia, dysaudia,* and *psycholalia.* In order to provide you a start, here are some articles regarding *dysaudia:*

DODD, B. (1976). "The Phonological Systems of Deaf Children." *Journal of Speech and Hearing Disorders*, 41: 185–198.

OLLER, D., and C. KELLY (1975). "Phonological Substitution Processes of a Hard-of-Hearing Child." *Journal of Speech and Hearing Disorders*, 39: 65–74.

SHER, A., and E. OWENS (1974). "Consonant Confusions Associated with Hearing Loss above 2000 Hz." *Journal of Speech and Hearing Research*, 17: 669–681.

WILCOX, J., and H. TOBIN (1974). "Linguistic Performance of Hard-of-Hearing and Normal Children." *Journal of Speech and Hearing Research*, 17: 286–293.

4. Why does Locke (1968) question the use of the number of sounds in error as a measure of severity?

5. Consider how you might use the concept of "markedness" in making a linguistic analysis. Consult the following article:

McREYNOLDS, L., D. ENGMANN, and K. DIMMIT (1974). "Markedness Theory and Articulation Errors." *Journal of Speech and Hearing Disorders*, 39: 93–103.

6. What diagnostic implications can you identify in the following research:

MOORE, W., J. BURKE, and C. ADAMS (1976). "The Effects of Stimulability on Articulation of /s/ Relative to Cluster and Word Frequency of Occurrence." *Journal of Speech and Hearing Research*, 19: 458–466.

MANNING, W., N. KEAPPOCK, and S. STICK (1976). "The Use of Auditory Masking to Estimate Automatization of Correct Articulatory Production." *Journal of Speech and Hearing Disorders*, 41: 143–149.

7. Design a test of auditory discrimination that fulfills the following criteria: (a) demands an immediate response from the child; (b) includes self-listening tasks; and (c) interrupts the child's oral motor responses (rehearsal of faulty articulation patterns) with which he listens.

8. Which of the following variables are related to intra-oral recognition of geometric forms: age, sex, educational level, length of time taken per form. To find the answers, consult this study:

WILLIAMS, W., and L. LAPOINTE (1971). "Intra-Oral Recognition of Geometric Forms by Normal Subjects." *Perceptual and Motor Skills,* 32: 419–426

9. What ideas can you glean from the following articles:

ARNDT, W., et al (1977). "Identification and Description of Homogeneous Subgroups within a Sample of Misarticulating Children." *Journal of Speech and Hearing Research,* 20: 269–292.
HEDRICK, D., M. CHRISTMAN and L. AUGUSTINE, L. (1973). "Programming for the Antecedent Event in Therapy." *Journal of Speech and Hearing Disorders,* 38: 339–344.

10. What is included on the Reitan-Indiana Neuro-Psychological Test Battery? See the following investigation:

FRISCH, G., and L. HANDLER (1974). "A Neuropsychological Investigation of 'Functional Disorders of Speech Articulation'." *Journal of Speech and Hearing Research,* 17: 432–445.

11. A treatment plan follows logically from the nature and scope of a worker's clinical assessment. Can you discern what form the following clinicians would employ in diagnosing clients with misarticulations?

FORMAAD, W. (1974). *Articulation Therapy Through Play.* Glen Ridge, N.J.: Exceptional Press.
MYSAK, E. (1976). *Pathologies of Speech Systems.* Baltimore, Md.: William & Wilkins Co.

BIBLIOGRAPHY

ANDERSON, V., and H. NEWBY (1973). *Improving the Child's Speech,* 2nd Ed. New York: Oxford University Press.
ATEN, J. (1973). *Denver Auditory Phonemic Sequencing Test.* Denver: University of Denver.
AUNGST, L., and J. FRICK (1964). "Auditory Discrimination Ability and Consistency of Articulation of /r/." *Journal of Speech and Hearing Disorders,* 29: 76–85.
AVANT, V., and C. HUTTON (1962). "Passage for Speech Screening in Upper Elementary Grades." *Journal of Speech and Hearing Disorders,* 27: 40–46.
BAKER, H., and B. LELAND (1959). *Detroit Tests of Learning Aptitude.* Indianapolis: Bobbs-Merrill.
BARRETT, M., and J. WELSH (1975). "Predictive Articulation Screening." *Language, Speech and Hearing Services in Schools,* 6: 91–95.
BERRY, M., and J. EISENSON (1956). *Speech Disorders.* New York: Appleton-Century-Crofts.
BEVING, B., and R. EBLEN (1973). "Same and Different Concepts and Children's Performance on Speech Sound Discrimination." *Journal of Speech and Hearing Research,* 16: 513–517.
BLACK, M. (1964). *Speech Correction in the Schools.* Englewood Cliffs, N.J.: Prentice-Hall, Inc.

BLOCH, E., and L. GOODSTEIN (1971). "Functional Speech Disorders and Personality: A Decade of Research." *Journal of Speech and Hearing Disorders*, 36: 295–314.

BOSMA, J., ed. (1967). *Symposium on Oral Sensation and Perception*. Springfield, Illinois: C.C. Thomas.

BOSMA, J., ed. (1970). *Second Symposium on Oral Sensation and Perception*. Springfield, Illinos: C.C. Thomas.

BRYEN, D. (1976). "Speech-Sound Discrimination Ability on Linguistically Unbiased Tests." *Exceptional Children*, 42: 195–202.

BRYNGELSON, B., and E. GLASPEY (1962). *Speech in the Classroom* (with speech improvement cards), 3rd ed. Chicago: Scott, Foresman & Company.

BURKLAND, M. (1967). "Use of Television to Study Articulation Problems." *Journal of Speech and Hearing Disorders*, 32: 80–81.

BZOCH, K. (1974). *Bzoch Error Pattern Diagnostic Test*. Gainesville, Florida: University of Florida.

CARRELL, J. (1968). *Disorders of Articulation*. Englewood Cliffs, N.J.: Prentice-Hall, Inc.

CARRELL, J., and W. TIFFANY (1960). *Phonetics: Theory and Application to Speech Improvement*. New York: McGraw-Hill Book Company.

CARTER, E., and M. BUCK (1958). "Prognostic Testing for Functional Articulation Disorders Among Children in the First Grade." *Journal of Speech and Hearing Disorders*, 23: 124–133.

CHAPPELL, G. (1973). "Childhood Verbal Apraxia and its Treatment." *Journal of Speech and Hearing Disorders*, 38: 362–368.

CHOMSKY, N, and M. HALLE (1968). *The Sound Pattern of English*. New York: Harper & Row.

COMPTON, A. (1970). "Generative Studies of Children's Phonological Disorders." *Journal of Speech and Hearing Disorders*, 35: 315–339.

———, (1975). "Generative Studies of Children's Phonological Disorders: a Strategy of Therapy." in S. Singh, ed. *Measurement Procedures in Speech Hearing and Language*. Baltimore: University Park Press.

COOPER, E.; R. PARRIS; and M. WELLS (1974). "Prevalence of and Recovery from Speech Disorders in a Group of Freshmen at the University of Alabama." *Journal of the American Speech and Hearing Association*, 16: 359–361.

COSTELLO, J., and J. ONSTINE (1976). "The Modification of Multiple Articulation Errors based on Distinctive Feature Theory." *Journal of Speech and Hearing Disorders*, 41: 199–215.

CROCKER, J. (1969). "A Phonological Model of Children's Articulation Competencies." *Journal of Speech and Hearing Disorders*. 34: 203–213.

CURTIS, J., and J. HARDY (1959). "A Phonetic Study of Misarticulation of /r/." *Journal of Speech and Hearing Research*, 2: 244–257.

CYPREANSEN, L.; J. WILEY; and L. LAASE (1959). *Speech Development, Improvement, and Correction*. New York: Ronald Press.

DABUL, B., and B. BOLLIER (1976). "Therapeutic Approaches to Apraxia." *Journal of Speech and Hearing Disorders*, 41: 268–276.

DANILOFF, R. (1973). "Normal Articulation Processes," in *Normal Aspects of Speech, Hearing and Language*, ed. F. Minifie, T. Hixon and F. Williams. Englewood Cliffs, N.J.: Prentice-Hall, Inc.

DARLEY, F. (1964). *Diagnosis and Appraisal of Communication Disorders*. Englewood Cliffs, N.J.: Prentice-Hall, Inc.

———, A. ARONSON, and J. BROWN (1969a). "Differential Diagnostic Patterns of Dysarthria." *Journal of Speech and Hearing Research*, 12: 246–269.

——— (1969b). "Clusters of Deviant Speech Dimensions in the Dysarthrias." *Journal of Speech and Hearing Research*, 12: 462–496.

DARLEY, F.; A. ARONSON; and J. BROWN (1975). *Motor Speech Disorders*. Philadelphia: W. B. Saunders.

DEAL, J., and F. DARLEY (1972). "The Influence of Linguistic and Situational Variables on Phonemic Accuracy in Apraxia of Speech." *Journal of Speech and Hearing Research*, 15: 639–653.

DELLOW, P. et al. (1970). "Oral Assessment of Object Size." *Journal of Speech and Hearing Research*, 13: 526–536.

DICKSON, S. (1972). "Difference between Children Who Spontaneously Outgrow and Children who Retain Functional Articulation Errors." *Journal of Speech and Hearing Research*, 5: 263–271.

DIEDRICH, W. (1971). "Procedures for Counting and Charting a Target Phoneme." *Language, Speech and Hearing Services in Schools*, 5: 18–32.

DRUMWRIGHT, A. (1971). *The Denver Articulation Screening Exam*. Denver: University of Colorado Medical Center.

————, et al. (1973). "The Denver Articulation Screening Exam." *Journal of Speech and Hearing Disorders*, 38: 3–14.

EBERLINE, L. (1963). "Persistence of Articulatory Disorders." Master's thesis, Texas Women's University.

EDMONSON, W. (1960). *The Laradon Articulation Scale*. Denver, Colo.: Laradon Hall.

EWARDS, K., and J. ANDERSON (1972). "A factor-analytic Study of the Articulation of Selected English Consonants." *Journal of Speech and Hearing Research*, 15: 720–728.

EGLAND, G. (1970). *Speech and Language Problems*. Englewood Cliffs, N.J.: Prentice-Hall, Inc.

EISENSON, J., and M. OGILVIE (1963). *Speech Correction in the Schools*, 2nd ed. New York: Macmillan.

EISENSON, J., and M. OGILVIE (1977). *Speech Correction in the Schools*, 4th ed. New York: Macmillan.

ELBERT, M.; R. SHELTON; and W. ARNDT (1967). "A Task for Evaluation of Articulation Change: 1. Development of Methodology." *Journal of Speech and Hearing Research*, 10: 281–288.

FAIRBANKS, G. (1958). "Test of Phonemic Differentiation: The Rhyme Test." *Journal of the Acoustical Society of America*, 30: 596–600.

———— (1960). *Voice and Articulation Drillbook*, 2nd ed. New York: Harper & Row.

FAIRCLOTH, M., and S. FAIRCLOTH (1970). "An Analysis of the Articulatory Behavior of a Speech-defective Child in Connected Speech and Isolated-word Responses." *Journal of Speech and Hearing Disorders*, 35: 51–61.

FISHER, H., and J. LOGEMANN (1971). *The Fisher-Logemann Test of Articulation Competence*. Boston: Houghton-Mifflin.

FLETCHER, S.; M. MCCUTCHEON; and M. WOLF (1975). "Dynamic Palatometry." *Journal of Speech and Hearing Research*, 18: 812–819.

FLUHARTY, N. (1974). "The Design and Standardization of a Speech and Language Screening Test for Use with Preschool Children." *Journal of Speech and Hearing Disorders*, 39: 75–88.

FOSTER, S. (1963). "Language Skills for Children with Persistent Articulatory Disorders." Master's thesis, Texas Women's University.

FRISCH, G., and L. HANDLER (1974). "A Neuropsychological Investigation of 'Functional' Disorders of Speech Articulation." *Journal of Speech and Hearing Research*, 17: 432–445.

FRISTOE, M., and R. GOLDMAN (1968). "Comparisons of Traditional and Condensed Articulation Tests Examining the Same Number of Sounds." *Journal of Speech and Hearing Research*, 11: 583–589.

FUCCI, D. (1972). "Oral vibro-tactile sensation: An Evaluation of Normal and Defective Speakers." *Journal of Speech and Hearing Research*, 15: 179–184.

FUDALA, J. (1970). *The Arizona Articulation Proficiency Scale*, rev. ed. Beverly Hills, Calif.: Western Psychological Services.

GALLAGHER, T., and T. SHRINER (1975a). "Articulatory Inconsistencies in the Speech of Normal Children." *Journal of Speech and Hearing Research*, 18: 168–175.

———— (1975b). "Contextual Variables Related to Inconsistent /s/ and /z/ Production in the Spontaneous Speech of Children." *Journal of Speech and Hearing Research*, 18: 623–632.

GARRETT, E. (1973). "Programmed Articulation Therapy," in *Articulation and Learning*. ed. W. Wolfe and D. Goulding. Springfield, Illinois: C.C. Thomas.

GILLESPIE, S., and E. COOPER (1973). "Prevalence of Speech Problems in Junior and Senior High Schools." *Journal of Speech and Hearing Research*, 16: 739–743.

GODA, S. (1970). *Articulation Therapy and Consonant Drill Book*. New York: Grune & Stratton.

GOLDMAN, R., and M. FRISTOE (1967). "The Development of a Film-strip Articulation Test." *Journal of Speech and Hearing Disorders*, 32: 256–262.

———— (1969). *Goldman-Fristoe Test of Articulation*. Circle Pines, Minn.: American Guidance Service.

————, and R. WOODCOCK (1969). *Goldman-Fristoe-Woodcock Test of Auditory Discrimination*. Circle Pines, Minn.: American Guidance Service.

GOLDMAN, R.; M. FRISTOE; and R. WOODCOCK (1976). *Goldman-Fristoe-Woodcock Auditory Skills Battery*. Circle Pines, Minn.: American Guidance Service.

GRUNWELL, P. (1975). "The Phonological Analysis of Articulation Disorders." *British Journal of Communication Disorders*, 10: 31–42.

HAAS, W. (1963). "Phonological Analysis of a Case of Dyslalia." *Journal of Speech and Hearing Disorders*, 28: 239–246.

HAM, D. (1971). *The Evaluation of Sounds: An Articulation Index for the Young Public School Child*. Springfield, Ill.: C.C. Thomas.

HAWS, E. (1975). *The Haws Screening Test for Functional Articulation Disorders*. Salt Lake City: Educational Support Systems.

HEJNA, R. (1963). *Developmental Articulation Test*. Ann Arbor, Mich.: Speech Materials.

HIXON, T. (1972). "Some techniques for Measuring the Biomechanical Events of Speech Production: One Laboratory's experiences," in *Orofacial Function: Clinical Research in Dentistry and Speech Pathology*. ed. R. Wertz. ASHA Report 7 Washington, D.C.: American Speech and Hearing Association.

HULL, F. et al. (1969). *National Speech and Hearing Survey*. Washington, D.C.: Department of Health, Education and Welfare.

INGRAM, D. (1971). *Edinburgh Articulation Test*. London: Edward Arnold Company.

———— (1976). *Phonological Disability in Children*. London: Edward Arnold Company.

IRWIN, J., and J. DUFFY (1955). *Speech and Hearing Hurdles*. Columbus, Ohio: School and College Service.

———— (1972). "The Triota: A Computerized Screening Battery." *Acta Symbolica*, 3: 26–38.

———— (1972). *Disorders of Articulation*. Indianapolis: Bobbs-Merrill.

IRWIN, R. (1965). *Speech and Hearing Therapy*. Pittsburgh: Stanwix House.

———— (1973). *The Ohio Tests of Articulation and Perception of Sounds*. Pittsburgh: Stanwix House.

———— (1974). "Evaluating the Perception and Articulation of Phonemes of Children, ages 5 to 8." *Journal of Communication Disorders*, 7: 45–63.

JOHNS, D., and F. DARLEY (1970). "Phonemic Variability in Apraxia of Speech." *Journal of Speech and Hearing Research*, 13: 556–583.

JOHNSON, W.; F. DARLEY; and D. SPRIESTERSBACH (1963). *Diagnostic Methods in Speech Pathology*. New York: Harper & Row.

JORDON, E. (1960). "Articulation Test Measures and Listener Ratings of Articulation Defectiveness." *Journal of Speech and Hearing Research,* 3: 304–319.

KAMARA, C.; A. KAMARA; and S. SINGH (1975). *The Distinctive Feature Wheel*. Athens, Ohio: Speech and Hearing Systems, Inc.

KEENAN, J. (1961). "What Is Medial Position?" *Journal of Speech and Hearing Disorders,* 26: 171–174.

KIMMEL, G., and J. WAHL (1970). *Screening Test for Auditory Perception*. Johnstown, Pa.: Mafex Associates.

KRESHECK, J.; H. FISHER; and D. RUTHERFORD (1972). "A Study of /r/ Phones in the Speech of Three-Year-Old Children." *Folia Phoniatrica,* 24: 301–312.

———, and E. SOCOLOFSKY (1972). "Imitative and Spontaneous Articulation Assessment of Four-Year-Old Children." *Journal of Speech and Hearing Research,* 15: 729–733.

KUCHON, P. (1976). "Relations Among Defective Articulatory Patterns and Selected Morphologic and Syntactic Patterns in 1st Grade Children." Doctoral dissertation, City University of New York.

LAFFEL, J. (1965). *Pathological and Normal Language*. New York: Atherton Press.

LARIVIERE, C., et al. (1974). "The Conceptual Reality of Selected Distinctive Features." *Journal of Speech and Hearing Research,* 17: 122–133.

LASS, N., et al. (1972). "Assessment of Oral Tactile Perception: Some Methodological Considerations." *Central States Speech Journal,* 23: 166–173.

LIEBERMAN, P. (1972). *Speech Acoustics and Perception*. Indianapolis: Bobbs-Merrill.

LINDAMOOD, C., and P. LINDAMOOD (1969). *Lindamood Auditory Conceptualization Test*. Boston: Teaching Resources Corporation.

LOCKE, J. (1968). "Questionable Assumptions Underlying Articulation Research." *Journal of Speech and Hearing Disorders,* 33: 112–116.

——— (1969). "Short-term Auditory Memory, Oral Perception and Experimental Sound Learning." *Journal of Speech and Hearing Research,* 12: 185–192.

——— (1972). "Ease of Articulation." *Journal of Speech and Hearing Research,* 15: 194–200.

LOCKE, J., and K. KUTZ (1975). "Memory for Speech and Speech for Memory." *Journal of Speech and Hearing Research,* 18: 176–191.

LEONARD, L. (1973a). "The Nature of Deviant Articulation." *Journal of Speech and Hearing Disorders,* 38: 156–161.

——— (1973b). "Some Limitations in the Clinical Application of Distinctive Features." *Journal of Speech and Hearing Disorders,* 38: 141–143.

LUCHSINGER, R., and G. ARNOLD (1965). *Voice-Speech-Language*. Belmont, Calif.: Wadsworth.

MARQUARDT, T., and J. SAXMAN (1972). "Language Comprehension and Auditory Discrimination in Articulation Deficient Kindergarten Children." *Journal of Speech and Hearing Research,* 15: 382–389.

MARSHALL, P.; M. SHARROW; and E. YAIRI (1977). "Short-term Memory Factors in Oral Retention." *Journal of Speech and Hearing Research,* 20: 344–349.

MCCALL, G. (1969). "The Assessment of Lingual Tactile Sensation and Perception." *Journal of Speech and Hearing Disorders,* 34: 151–156.

MCDONALD, E. (1964). *Articulation Testing and Treatment*. Pittsburgh: Stanwix House.

——— (1968). *A Screening Deep Test of Articulation*. Pittsburgh: Stanwix House.

——— (1962). *Understand Those Feelings*. Pittsburgh: Stanwix House.

MCGLONE, R., and W. PROFFIT (1973). "Patterns of Tongue Contact in Normal and Lisping Speakers." *Journal of Speech and Hearing Research,* 16: 456–473.

McLEAN, J. (1976). "Articulation," in *Communication Assessment and Intervention Strategies*. ed. L. Lloyd. Baltimore: University Park Press.

McREYNOLDS, L., and K. HUSTON (1971). "A Distinctive Feature Analysis of Children's Misarticulations." *Journal of Speech and Hearing Disorders*, 36: 155–166.

———; D. ENGMANN; and K. DIMMITT (1974). "Markedness Theory and Articulation Errors." *Journal of Speech and Hearing Disorders*, 39: 93–103.

———, J. KOHN; and G. WILLIAMS (1975). "Articulatory-defective Children's Discrimination of Their Production Errors." *Journal of Speech and Hearing Disorders*, 40: 327–338.

———, and D. ENGMANN (1975). *Distinctive Feature Analysis of Misarticulations*. Baltimore: University Park Press.

MECHAM, M.; J. JEX; and J. JONES (1970). *Screening Speech Articulation Test*. Salt Lake City: Communication Research Associates, Inc.

MENYUK, P. (1964). "Comparison of Grammar of Children with Functionally Deviant and Normal Speech." *Journal of Speech and Hearing Research*, 7: 109–122.

——— (1968). "The Role of Distinctive Features in Children's Acquisition of Phonology." *Journal of Speech and Hearing Research*, 11: 138–146.

———, and S. ANDERSON (1969). "Children's Identification and Reproduction of /w/ and /r/." *Journal of Speech and Hearing Research*, 12: 39–52.

MILISEN, R. (1966). "Articulatory Problems," in *Speech Pathology*, ed. R. Rieber and R. Brubaker. Philadelphia: J.B. Lippincott, Co.

———, et al. (1954). "The Disorder of Articulation: A Systematic Clinical and Experimental Approach." *Journal of Speech and Hearing Disorders*, Monograph Supplement 4.

MONNIN, L., and D. HUNTINGTON (1974). "The Relationship of Articulatory Defects to Speech-Sound Identification." *Journal of Speech and Hearing Research*, 17: 352–366.

MONSEES, E., and C. BERMAN (1968). "Speech and Language Screening in a Summer Head Start Program." *Journal of Speech and Hearing Disorders*, 33: 121–126.

MOORE, W.; J. BURKE; and C. ADAMS (1976). "The Effects of Stimulability on Articulation of /s/ Relative to Cluster and Word Frequency of Occurrence." *Journal of Speech and Hearing Research*, 19: 458–466.

———; J. ROSENBECK; and L. LaPOINTE (1976). "Assessment of Oral Apraxia in Brain-Injured Adults." in *Clinical Aphasiology*, ed. R. Brookshire. Minneapolis: BRK Publishers.

MOREAU, V., and N. LASS (1974). "A Correlational Study of Stimulability, Oral Form Discrimination and Auditory Discrimination in Children." *Journal of Communication Disorders*, 7: 269–277.

MORLEY, M. (1965).. *The Development and Disorders of Speech in Childhood*, 2nd ed. Baltimore: William and Wilkins.

MOWRER, D.; R. BAKER; and R. SCHUTZ (1968). "Operant Procedures in the Control of Speech Articulation." *Operant Procedures in Remedial Speech and Language Training*. ed. H. Sloane and B. Macaulay. Boston: Houghton Mifflin.

MULLEN, P., and R. WHITEHEAD (1977). "Stimulus Picture Identification in Articulation Testing." *Journal of Speech and Hearing Disorders*, 42: 113–118.

NATION, J., and D. ARAM (1977). *Diagnosis of Speech and Language Disorders*. St. Louis: Mosby.

NEAL, W. (1976). "Speech Pathology Services in the Secondary Schools." *Language, Speech and Hearing Services in Schools*, 7: 6–16.

NIH News Feature (1975). August 10: 11–12. Washington, D.C.: National Institute of Health.

NOLL, J. (1970). "Articulatory Assessment." In *Speech and the Dentofacial Complex: The State of the Art.* American Speech and Hearing Association, Report No. 5.

OLIPHANT, G. (1971). *Oliphant Auditory Synthesizing Test.* Cambridge, Mass.: Educators Publishing Service.

PALMER, M.; C. WURTH; and J. KINCHLOE (1964). "The Influence of Lingual Apraxia and Agnosia in 'Functional' Disorders of Articulation." *Cerebral Palsy Review,* 25: 7–9.

PANAGOS, J. (1974). "Persistence of the Open Syllable Reinterpreted as a Symptom of Language Disturbance." *Journal of Speech and Hearing Disorders,* 39: 23–31.

PARKER, F. (1976). "Distinctive Features in Speech Pathology: Phonology or Phonemics." *Journal of Speech and Hearing Disorders,* 41: 23–39.

PAYNTER, E., and T. BUMPAS (1977). "Imitative and Spontaneous Articulation Assessment of Three-Year Old Children." *Journal of Speech and Hearing Disorders,* 42: 119–125.

PEACHER, W. (1962). "Dysarthria-Lesions of the Nervous System Causing Articulatory Disorders," in *Voice and Speech Disorders: Medical Aspects,* ed. N. Levin. Springfield, Ill.: C.C. Thomas.

PECKHAM, C. (1973). "Speech Defects in a National Sample of Children Aged Seven Years." *British Journal of Communication Disorders,* 8: 2–8.

PEINS, M., and M. PETTAS (1963). "A College Speech Improvement Course." *Speech Teacher,* 12: 37–40.

PENDERGAST, K., et al. (1966). "An Articulation Study of 15,255 Seattle 1st Grade Children with and without Kindergarten." *Exceptional Children,* 33: 541–547.

———, et al. (1969). *Photo Articulation Test.* Danville, Ill.: Interstate Printers and Publishers.

POWERS, M. (1971a). "Functional Disorders of Articulation: Symptomatology and Etiology," in *Handbook of Speech Pathology and Audiology,* ed. L. Travis. New York: Appleton-Century-Crofts.

——— (1971b). "Clinical and Educational Procedures in Functional Disorders of Articulation," in *Handbook of Speech Pathology and Audiology,* ed. L. Travis. New York: Appleton-Century-Crofts.

PRATHER, E. (1960). "Scaling Defectiveness of Articulation by Direct Magnitude-Estimation." *Journal of Speech and Hearing Research,* 3: 380–392.

———; D. HEDRICK and C. KERN (1975). "Articulation Development in Children Aged 2 to 4 Years." *Journal of Speech and Hearing Disorders,* 40: 179–191.

———; A. MINER; and M. ADDICOTT (1971). *Washington Speech Sound Discrimination Test.* Danville, Illinois: Interstate Printers and Publishers.

PRIESTLY, T. (1977). "One Idiosyncratic Strategy in the Acquisition of Phonology." *Journal of Child Language,* 4: 45–65.

PUTNAM, A., and R. RINGEL (1972). "Some Observations of Articulation During Labial Sensory Deprivation." *Journal of Speech and Hearing Research,* 15: 529–542.

RENFREW, C. (1966). "Persistence of the Open Syllable in Defective Articulation." *Journal of Speech and Hearing Disorders,* 31: 370–373.

———, and L. GEARY (1973). "Prediction of Persisting Speech Defects." *British Journal of Disorders of Communication,* 8: 37–41.

RILEY, G. (1971). *Riley Articulation and Language Test.* Los Angeles: Western Psychological Service.

RINGEL, R.; K. BURKE; and C. SCOTT (1958). "Tactile Perception: Form Discrimination in the Mouth." *British Journal of Disorders of Communication,* 3: 150–155.

———, and S. EWANOWSKI. "Oral Perception: I. Two-point Discrimination." *Journal of Speech and Hearing Research,* 8 (1965):389–398.

————, and H. FLETCHER. "Oral Perception: III. Texture Discrimination." *Journal of Speech and Hearing Research,* 10 (1967): 642–649.

RITTERMAN, S., and N. FREEMAN (1974). "Distinctive Phonetic Features as Relevant and Irrelevant Stimulus Dimensions in Speech Sound Discrimination Learning." *Journal of Speech and Hearing Research,* 17: 417–425.

ROBERTS, D. (1967). "The Term Dyslalia: Its Uses and Value." *Journal of the Australian College of Speech Therapists,* 17: 44–52.

ROE, V., and R. MILISEN (1942). "The Effect of Maturation upon Defective Articulation in Elementary Grades." *Journal of Speech Disorders,* 7: 37–50.

ROGERS, W. (1972). *Picture Articulation and Screening Test.* Salt Lake City: Word Making Production.

ROSENBEK, J.; R. WERTZ; F. DARLEY (1973). "Oral Sensation and Perception in Apraxia of Speech and Aphasia." *Journal of Speech and Hearing Research,* 16: 22–36.

ROTH, R. (1961). *The Mother-Child Relationship Evaluation.* Beverly Hills, Calif.: Western Psychological Services.

SANDER, E. (1972). "When are Speech Sounds Learned?" *Journal of Speech and Hearing Disorders,* 37: 55–63.

SAXMAN, J., and J. MILLER (1973). "Short-term Memory and Language Skills in Articulation-Deficient Children." *Journal of Speech and Hearing Research,* 16: 721–730.

SCHAEFER, E., and R. BELL (n.d.). *Parental Attitude Research Instruments and Normative Data.* Bethesda, Md.: National Institute of Mental Health.

SCHLANGER, P. (1976). "Oral Stereognostic Ability Among Tongue Thrusters With Interdental Lisp, Tongue Thrusters Without Interdental Lisp and Normal Children." *Perceptual and Motor Skills,* 42: 259–268.

SCHNEIDERMAN, J. (1955). "A Study of the Relationships between Articulatory Ability and Language Ability." *Journal of Speech and Hearing Disorders,* 20: 359–364.

SCHUCKERS, G., et al. (1974). "Children's Verbal Awareness of Articulation Gestures." *Journal of Communication Disorders,* 7: 239–245.

SCHWARTZ, A., and R. GOLDMAN (1974). "Variables Influencing Performance on Speech Sound Discrimination Tests." *Journal of Speech and Hearing Research,* 17: 25–32.

SHANKS, S.; M. SHARPE; and B. JACKSON (1970). "Spontaneous Responses of First-Grade Children to Diagnostic Picture Articulation Tests." *Journal of Communication Disorders,* 3: 106–117.

SHERMAN, D., and W. CULLINAN (1960). "Several Procedures for Scaling Articulation." *Journal of Speech and Hearing Research,* 3: 191–198.

————, and A. GEITH (1967). "Speech Sound Discrimination and Articulation Skill." *Journal of Speech and Hearing Research,* 10: 277–280.

SHRINER, T., et al. (1969). "The Relationship Between Articulation Defects and Syntax in Speech Defective Children." *Journal of Speech and Hearing Research,* 12: 319–325.

SIEGEL, G. (1967). "Interpersonal Approach to the Study of Communication Disorders." *Journal of Speech and Hearing Disorders,* 32: 112–120.

SILVERMAN, S. (1972). "Degeneration of Dental and Orofacial Structures," in *Orofacial Function: Clinical Research in Dentistry and Speech Pathology,* ed. R. Wertz. Report No. 7. American Speech and Hearing Association.

SILVERMAN, E. (1976). "Listener's Impressions of Speakers with Lateral Lisps." *Journal of Speech and Hearing Disorders,* 41: 542–547.

SINGH, S. (1976). *Distinctive Feature Theory: Theory and Validation.* Baltimore: University Park Press.

SMITH, M., and S. AINSWORTH (1967). "The Effect of Three Types of Stimulation of Articulatory Responses of Speech Defective Children." *Journal of Speech and Hearing Research*, 10: 333–338.

SMITH, N. (1973). *The Acquisition of Phonology*. New York: Cambridge University Press.

SOMMERS, R.; S. COX; and C. WEST (1972). "Articulatory Effectiveness, Stimulability and Children's Performance on Perceptual and Memory Tasks." *Journal of Speech and Hearing Research*, 15: 579–589.

————, and A. KANE (1974). "Nature and Remediation of Functional Articulation Disorders," in *Communication Disorders*. ed. S. Dickson. Glenview, Ill.: Scott, Foresman and Company.

SPRIESTERSBACH, D., and J. CURTIS (1951). "Misarticulation and Discrimination of Speech Sounds." *Quarterly Journal of Speech*, 37: 483–491.

SUBTELNY, H.; N. OYA; and J. SUBTELNY (1972). "Cineradiographic Study of Sibilants." *Folia Phoniatrica*, 24: 30–50.

SWIRL SPEECH ARTICULATION KITS (1973). Cincinnati: American Book Company.

TELAGE, K., and D. FUCCI (1973). "Vibrotactile Stimulation: A Future Clinical Tool for Speech Pathology." *Journal of Speech and Hearing Disorders*, 38: 442–447.

TEMPLIN, M. (1943). "A Study of Sound Discrimination Ability of Elementary School Pupils." *Journal of Speech and Hearing Disorders*, 8: 132.

————, and F. DARLEY (1970). *The Templin-Darley Tests of Articulation* 2nd ed. Iowa City: University of Iowa Bureau of Educational Research and Service.

TREVARTON, L., ed. (1975). *An Exploratory Investigation of School Age Children Manifesting Persistent Disorders of ARTICULATION*. Marquette, Mich.: Northern Michigan University.

TURTON, L. (1973). "Diagnostic Implications of Articulation Testing." In *Articulation and Learning*, ed. W. Wolfe and D. Goulding. Springfield, Ill.: C.C. Thomas.

VANDEMARK, A., and M. MANN (1965). "Oral Language Skills of Children with Defective Articulation." *Journal of Speech and Hearing Research*, 8: 409–414.

VAN HATTUM, R., ed. (1969). *Clinical Speech in the Schools: Organization and Management*. Springfield, Ill.: Charles C Thomas.

VAN RIPER, C. (1963). *Speech Correction: Principles and Methods*, 4th ed. Englewood Cliffs, N.J.: Prentice-Hall, Inc.

———— (1972). *Speech Correction: Principles and Methods*, 5th ed. Englewood Cliffs, N.J.: Prentice-Hall, Inc.

————, and R. ERICKSON (1968). *Predictive Screening Test of Articulation*. Kalamazoo, Mich.: Western Michigan University Press.

————, and J. IRWIN (1958). *Voice and Articulation*. Englewood Cliffs, N.J.: Prentice-Hall, Inc.

VELLUTINO, E.; L. DESETTO; and J. STEGER (1972). "Categorical Judgment and the Wepman Test of Auditory Discrimination." *Journal of Speech and Hearing Disorders*, 37: 252–257.

WALSH, H. (1974). "On certain Practical Inadequacies of Distinctive-Feature Systems." *Journal of Speech and Hearing Disorders*, 39: 32–43.

WEBER, J. (1970). "Patterning of Deviant Articulation Behavior." *Journal of Speech and Hearing Disorders*, 35: 135–141.

WEGER, R.; SHATTUCK, J.; and R. ERICKSON (1976). *Language Comprehension and Articulation: A Study of Children Entering Kindergarten in Grand Rapids*. Grand Rapids, Mich.: Center for Educational Studies.

WEPMAN, J. (1958). *Auditory Discrimination Test*. Chicago: Language Research Associates.

———— and A. CARR (1957). *The Rehabilitation of Speech*, 3rd ed. New York: Harper & Row.

WEST, R., and M. ANSBERRY (1968). *The Rehabilitation of Speech,* 4th ed. New York: Harper & Row.

WESTON, A., and L. LEONARD (1976). *Articulation Disorders: Methods of Evaluation and Therapy.* Lincoln, Nebraska: Cliff Notes, Inc.

WEYBRIGHT, G. (1976). "The Development of Consonants /t/ and /k/ in the Speech of Preschool Children." *Journal of Speech and Hearing Disorders,* 41: 134–135.

WILBECK, M. (1963). "An Investigation of Certain Factors in Children with Persistent Functional Articulation Disorders." Unpublished Master's thesis, University of Houston.

WILEY, J. H. (1955). "A Scale to Measure Parental Attitudes." *Journal of Speech and Hearing Disorders,* 20: 284–290.

WILLIAMS, G., and McREYNOLDS, L. (1975). "The Relationship Between Discrimination and Articulation Training in Children with Misarticulations." *Journal of Speech and Hearing Research,* 18: 401–412.

WILLIAMS, W., and L. LAPOINT (1971). *Florida Oral Form Recognition Measure.* Gainesville, Florida: University of Florida.

WINITZ, H. (1969). *Articulatory Acquisition and Behavior.* New York: Appleton-Century-Crofts.

WOLFE, W., and D. GOULDING (1973). *Articulation and Learning.* Springfield, Ill.: Charles C. Thomas.

WOOD, K. (1949). "Measurement of Progress in the Correction of Articulatory Speech Defects." *Journal of Speech and Hearing Disorders,* 14: 171–174.

WOOLF, G., and R. PILBERG (1971). "A Comparison of Three Tests of Auditory Discrimination and Their Relationship to Performance on a Deep Test of Articulation." *Journal of Communication Disorders,* 3: 239–249.

WYATT, G. (1964). *Language Learning and Communication Disorders in Children.* New York: The Free Press.

YOSS, K., and F. DARLEY (1974a). "Developmental Apraxia of Speech in Children with Defective Articulation." *Journal of Speech and Hearing Research,* 17: 399–416.

——— (1974b). "Therapy in Development and Apraxia of Speech." Language, Speech and Hearing. Services in Schools, 5: 23–31.

7

Stuttering

The prolonged search for understanding of the problem of stuttering (or stammering, which means the same thing) has produced an extensive, confusing, and conflicting literature. Although more has been written about the disorder than any other impairment of communication, its basic nature still eludes researchers and clinicians. In fact, we are moved to paraphrase a famous comment attributed to Winston Churchill: We cannot explain stuttering, it is a riddle wrapped in a mystery inside an enigma.

If experts who have investigated the disorder (Adams, 1976; Wingate, 1976; Webster, 1977; Bloodstein, 1977; Cooper, 1977) acknowledge that they are plagued by unanswerable questions about stuttering, consider the dilemma of the student. Confronted with the vast body of information, a plethora of etiological possibilities, and an array of treatment paradigms, each with its advocates, it is easy to despair:

> After a semester of very intense study, abstracting scores of articles, poring over microfilmed dissertations, and participating in lengthy seminar discussions, one of our more literate students appended this parody of a popular folk song to her comprehensive final examination—
>
> "I've looked at stuttering from both sides now,
> From research and clinical and still somehow
> It's stutterings illusions I recall,
> I really don't know stuttering at all!"

Yet, for some beginning clinicians, the dramatic nature of the disorder and even the confusion among experts have a fascinating appeal; they present a challenge. Perhaps this is a good place to review the fund of reliable truth we possess on stuttering, as filtered through our perceptual biases.

Sifting through the mounds of written material to find facts about stuttering is like sluicing poor placer dirt: the reader has to do an incredible amount of winnowing before even small specks of truth emerge (Hoffer, 1969). Perhaps revealing more temerity than good sense, we present below a list of "facts" about stuttering gleaned from the literature and an extensive clinical practice. For purposes of exposition we have eschewed lengthy lists of references. Each item can be documented, however, even though some might disagree with our particular selection or interpretation:

1. Stuttering as a disorder has existed throughout recorded history (and probably before).

2. Stuttering is found among all peoples of the world; its relative incidence and its forms vary across cultures (the most commonly reported incidence in the United States is slightly less than 1 percent).

3. Stuttering is a disorder of childhood, generally having its onset before the age of six; rarely does it begin in older persons, and when it does it may be a distinct subtype of the disorder (for example, neurotic stuttering).

4. Stuttering is found more frequently among males.

5. The overt characteristics of stuttering tend to be more severe among males.

6. Stuttering exhibits a familial incidence pattern.

7. Stuttering may be precipitated (and perpetuated) by certain environmental events, particularly the impact (in a critical, demanding way) of significant others—usually the parents.

8. Stuttering tends to appear more frequently in children described as "sensitive," who may be more vulnerable or susceptible to stress. Stutterers may have a lower threshold for autonomic arousal.

9. Stuttering tends to appear more frequently in children who were slow in acquiring speech or who manifest certain inadequacies of oral communication (articulation errors, language disturbances) other than fluency breakdowns.

10. Stuttering, in its developed state, has both overt and covert dimensions.

11. Stuttering is intermittent in occurrence. Many stutterers exhibit a decrease in blocking with repeated oral readings of the same material; moments of stuttering also tend to occur consistently on particular words.

12. The basic speech characteristics of stuttering consist of relatively brief part-word repetitions (phonemic, syllabic) and prolongations. These oscillations and fixations may be audible or silent, and tend to occur more frequently at the beginning of an utterance and on words and phrases motorically more complex—longer words, less frequently used words.

13. Stuttering tends to change in form and severity as the individual matures.

14. Stuttering tends to exhibit cycles of frequency and severity in a given individual.

15. Stuttering is apparently "outgrown" by a significant number of individuals.

16. Stuttering, in its developed form, consists largely of escape and avoidance behavior; that is, much of the overt abnormality results from the individual's attempt to cope with the emission of the basic speech characteristics described in Number 12.

17. Stuttering is also characterized by speech and voice abnormalities other than disfluency—narrow pitch range, vocal tension, lack of vocal expression—which can be detected in nonstuttered speech. These anomalies *may* reflect a basic impairment of phonation (difficulty initiating phonation, making consonant-vowel transitions), respiration (abnormal reflex activity), or cortical integration; they *may,* however, simply be effects of stuttering.

18. Stuttering, in its developed form, is often associated with an expectancy or anticipation of its occurrence.

19. Stuttering is a personal problem; individuals who stutter report fear, frustration, social penalties, dissatisfaction with themselves, lower level of aspiration, felt loss of social esteem. There is a tendency for problems common to all human beings to become associated with the speech disturbance.

20. Stuttering is a social-psychological event. The acoustic and visual phenomena that occur during the motor act of stuttering are noxious stimuli in a communicative context, and listeners tend to react in various explicit or implicit ways. The stutterer tends in turn to react to these listener responses.

For more detailed discussions of stuttering, the reader should consult the work of Van Riper (1971) and others (Sheehan, 1970; Emerick and Hamre, 1972; Fransella, 1972; Gregory, 1973; LeBrun and Hoops, 1973; Bloodstein, 1975; Eisenson, 1975; Rieber, Brubaker and Gelder, 1977; Wingate, 1976). We trust that we have not discouraged the reader unduly by our somewhat somber presentation; for, even though the fluency disorder of stuttering remains a tantalizing mystery, there is much that we can do to help persons who seek our services. We hope to show by our case presentations and discussion that if we focus on the *client,* rather than the disorder, our mission becomes clearer.

DIFFERENTIAL DIAGNOSIS

There are two important dimensions of differential diagnosis in regard to fluency disorders: identifying subtypes within the stuttering population; and distinguishing the problem of stuttering from other conditions in which speech fluency is also disrupted.

Are there different kinds of stuttering? Does the label *stuttering* impart a linguistic unity to a generic disorder that may encompass several disparate types of fluency disturbances? We are not able to answer those questions, but we do know that, clinically, stuttering wears a variety of sad and confining disguises. Although the research is negligible in this area, we have seen several distinct subtypes—for example, interiorized and exteriorized stutterers (Douglass and Quarrington, 1952), predominantly clonic and predominantly tonic stutterers, clients who feature escape techniques, those who are addicted to avoidance, those who can predict an occurrence of stuttering, and those who cannot (Silverman and Williams, 1972). Perhaps there are even variations in stuttering which stem from cultural influence (Leith and Mims, 1975). We find these distinctions useful in planning therapy; persons with different behavioral histories require different management. Several observers have noted and attempted to classify subgroups of stutterers, but as yet no one system has been accorded widespread acceptance (see Project 1).

We are concerned not only with types of stutterers but also with varieties of fluency disturbance. There are several kinds of fluency breakdowns that can be confused with stuttering. In our clinical experience we have seen individuals with five rather distinct forms of abnormal disfluency:

1. Episodic stress reaction. It is well known that most speakers exhibit some degree of disfluency—revisions, interjections, word and phrase repetitions, and the like. Furthermore, everyone occasionally stutters (part-word repetitions and prolongations) at some point. In fact, speech fluency is a sensitive barometer of a person's psychological and physical integrity. Stress, particularly communicative stress, tends to increse a speaker's disfluency; Van Riper (1963) speculates that there is a positive relationship between communicative stress and progressive deterioration of speech:

> With minor stress, repetitions of sentences or phrases occur; with more stress, words are repeated, with even more pressure, the oscillating occurs on syllables. When complete disruption occurs but the urge to speak still remains, first prolongations of an audible sound (''mmmmmmmother'') are shown and finally even this breaks down to a silent posture (Van Riper, 1963: 320).

Other situations of stress, such as battle conditions (Gavis, 1964; Grinker and Spiegal, 1945), intense excitement, emotional upheaval, and stage fright can also precipitate a fluency breakdown.

Fluency breakdowns due to episodic stress show a number of consistent identifying features: an acknowledged source of intense or prolonged stimulation; tension overflow throughout the body (including the oral area), which may also produce a tremulous voice; an exacerbation of ''normal'' disfluency—broken words, incomplete phrases, interjections, repetitions of whole words; some part-word repetitions, usually syllabic but always with the correct vowel, never with the $\partial/$ vowel replacement; no avoidance, fear, rarely any penalty—perhaps some embarrassment after the incident is over. Finally, the most crucial characteristic is that the disfluency decreases markedly or stops when (or shortly after) the stress terminates. It is likely that all but the most stoic of persons have experienced an episodic fluency breakdown. It is interesting to note that laymen often react to stutterers with the same advice often tendered to persons under stress: ''calm down,'' ''take it easy,'' ''slow down,'' and so on. The unfortunate consequence of such recommendations, for some stutterers, is an elaborate charade they play, attempting to simulate speakers under stress, often feigning confusion or bewilderment.

2. Neurotic or hysterical stuttering. Most stutterers, particularly confirmed adult cases, acquire a negative feeling tone about their problem. One of our clients summarized it succinctly when he said, "Stutterers are bugged because they are plugged." A few stutterers, however, show symptoms of a primary neurosis—they are "plugged because they are bugged." For these individuals, stuttering is a maladaptive solution to an acute psychological problem:

> Colleen, an eighth-grade parochial-school pupil, began to stutter suddenly following the death of her parents in an automobile accident. She collapsed upon hearing the tragic news and remained mute, almost transfixed and catatonic, for several hours. During the planning for the funeral and the extended period of the wake, she started to stutter—a monotonous repetition of the initial syllable of words. She showed no struggle, no avoidance behavior. She looked directly at the auditor when she spoke and smiled bravely. We followed this case closely until the remission of stuttering two months later, and her disfluency was always the same—it never varied in form or severity from situation to situation. When she read a passage several times, she did not show the typical reduction (adaptation) in stuttering. School documents, as well as interviews with several relatives, indicated that Colleen had had no prior speech difficulty. One maternal aunt whom we interviewed did recall, however, that the girl had several "spells" of uncontrolled weeping and laughing during her first menses a year before. The child had received an incredible amount of attention and solace after her parents' death—perhaps even more so because of her "stuttering" —from sympathetic adults.

Neurotic stuttering is characterized by a sudden onset (often in an older child), a monosymptomatic speech pattern, little situational variation, and seeming unconcern or indifference; the individual may be experiencing chronic stress or a sudden acute emotional upheaval; there may be a history of neurotic symptoms (Van Riper and Gruber, 1957: 16; Freund, 1966: 139–140).

3. Fluency breakdowns following brain injury. We have observed disfluency in clients suffering from Parkinson's disease, some types of cerebral palsy, and other neurological impairments. There are also reports of fluency disruptions in alcoholism, drug addiction, and in patients afflicted with dialysis dementia (Madison et al., 1977). Several aphasics with whom we have worked, particularly those clients who show good progress in word-finding but have residual syntactic difficulty, exhibited fluency breakdowns superficially similar to stuttering:

> Miss Horn had suffered an aneurysm in the Circle of Willis leaving her hemiplegic, apraxic, and with mild expressive aphasia. When we examined her, almost a year after the cerebral vascular episode, her speech pattern resembled clonic stuttering. She would begin a word, repeat a phoneme or syllable several times, back up and try again; if blocked once more, a repetition might reverberate almost endlessly. She frequently pounded on the table as if to time her utterances. We could discern no

evidence of fear or avoidance, just severe frustration. Interestingly, when she spoke or read swiftly her fluency increased dramatically; she also talked quite freely when distracted from closely monitoring the act of speaking. Here is a sample of her speech taken from a tape recording during a group therapy session: "I can't—I can't (sigh) . . . I-I-I-I have tr-trouble with my, ah, with my speech . . . and, ah, my leg is, is, you know, stiff. . . ."

The disfluencies noted are rather typical—whole-word repetitions, revisions, interjections, broken words, gaps in the flow of speech. This client had difficulty formulating messages and then programming the proper motor sequences to utter the thought; unlike stutterers who have difficulty getting started, Miss Horn's fluency breakdowns occurred at any point in a sentence (see Luchsinger and Arnold, 1965; Farmer, 1975; Boller, Albert and Denes, 1975).

4. Stuttering among the retarded. Some observers have reported a rather high prevalence of stuttering among mentally retarded, especially mongoloid, children (Van Riper, 1971: 42–45). We are frankly puzzled by these reports since our experience agrees quite closely with the findings of Sheehan, Martyn, and Kilburn (1968) and Martyn, Sheehan, and Slutz (1969). We found only one stutterer in a population of 217 severely retarded children (ages four to twelve) in a residential hospital. It was our impression that the group of children evaluated, which included a large number with Down's syndrome, simply did not have a sufficient flow of speech on which to stutter; the majority were limited to one- or two-word utterances or an assortment of unintelligible grunts. Interestingly, we did observe stuttering emerge in two mongoloid children during a language-building program.

We have seen several stutterers among public-school special education ("educable") pupils; it is our impression that the relative incidence of stuttering in this group is similar to that in most published surveys for normal school-age populations. Their stuttering behavior exhibited the following characteristics: (1) an uncomplicated, typically clonic or repetitive, pattern; (2) little word or sound fear; (3) no anticipation of difficulty—most of these clients showed little awareness of their disfluency; and (4) almost no avoidance behavior (except sullen withdrawal). Frustration and struggle were the predominant features. These children responded best to a treatment program that stressed a direct attack on the motor act of stuttering, employing mirror work and imitation of the clinician.

5. Cluttering. Cluttering is sometimes confused with stuttering:

Ralph was referred to us as a stutterer by his critic teacher during his semester of student teaching. When we examined him, he revealed no fears or avoidances, exhibited only a few part-word repetitions, and had no fixations; he said that he enjoyed talking, did a lot of it, and that he was asked frequently to repeat himself, "especially when I talk fast." His speech was swift and jumbled; it emerged in rapid torrents until he jammed up, and then he surged on again in another staccato outburst. In spontaneous talking, his message was characterized by disorganized sentences and poor phrasing; he would start to tell us something, lose the train of thought, and then change the content in midsentence. He slurred sounds and omitted and transposed words and phrases; he said "plobably," "posed," and "pacific" for "probably," "supposed," and "specific." Ralph's speech was sprinkled with spoonerisms ("darn bore" for "barn door") and malapropisms (he talked of smoke "bellowing" out a chimney, and was indignant about Wilbur Mills and Fanny Fox jumping in the "Tidy" Basin). He gave the overall impression of being in great haste. When we asked him to slow down and speak carefully, there was a dramatic improvement, but he soon forgot our admonishment and reverted to his hurried, disorganized style. By and large, Ralph was unaware and indifferent to his fluency problem. He was an impatient, impulsive young man, always on the go. His course work was characteristically done in a great, almost compulsive, rush; he had difficulty reading, and his handwriting was a scrawl.

The distinguishing features of cluttering and stuttering have been succinctly summarized by Weiss (1964; see particularly p. 69) and Freund 1966: 140–144). Consult also the work of Novak (1975) and others (Rieber, Breskin and Jaffe, 1972; Hutchinson and Burke, 1973). The diagnostician should be aware, however, that some stutterers may also exhibit features associated with cluttering; and it may be necessary to determine which fluency problem is primary (generally cluttering) or the most problematical.

Each of the fluency disorders described above requires distinctly different clinical management, even though the objective distortion of the speech signal may be somewhat similar. The diagnostician must keep in mind that a speech disorder involves more than a disturbance in the acoustic characteristics of an individual's oral output.

In order to better reveal the diagnostician in action, the remainder of the present chapter will be devoted to case presentations. We shall describe the assessment of a young child reportedly beginning to stutter, the evaluation of school-age children, and conclude with a lengthy review of appraisal for adult clients.

EVALUATION AT THE ONSET OF STUTTERING

Experienced clinicians agree that the problem of stuttering is much easier to prevent in children than to treat in chronic adult clients. Indeed, the early detection and management of children beginning to stutter is one of the most significant contributions a speech clinician can make. The diagnostician must seek answers for a great many questions: Is the child stuttering? If he is stuttering, how far has the disorder progressed? When did it begin? What factors were associated with the onset of the problem? How aware is the child that his speech is blocked? How do listeners attempt to help him, and how does he respond to their efforts? How can we alter the child's environment to prevent the problem from getting worse?

Throughout this volume we have repeatedly suggested that diagnosis and therapy are not separate undertakings. The careful assessment of a client's problem is often therapeutic; only by working with an individual for a period of time do we truly come to know the dimensions of his problem. This is particularly true in the management of children beginning to stutter. In order to illustrate the activities of the diagnostician-clinician, we present below a case study of a 3½-year-old child brought to the clinic as an "incipient" stutterer. Our account is chronological and reports what was done from the initial contact to the termination of treatment. The family was seen for a total of six counseling sessions (not including brief follow-up contacts) over a period of two months.

The Case of Stephen Wood

In many cases, a physician is the first professional to be consulted by parents, and the clinician is wise to enlist the support of local pediatricians in the early identification of children beginning to stutter (Emerick and Teigland, 1965). Stephen Wood, however, was referred to the clinic by his maternal uncle, who had received therapy for stuttering in a different community and knew of the senior author through his publications. Mr. Wood called us at home one weekend in midsummer and asked if we would see his son as soon as possible. He told us that Stephen had begun to stutter several months before—around the Christmas holiday, he thought. He added:

> At first he did it only occasionally. Even now it comes and goes in waves. Some days he will be talking along just fine and then, bang!—he stutters badly. We ignored it for a while, but when it persisted we told him to "take his time" and "think what he wanted to say." He doesn't like it when we give him advice; I noticed the other day he put his hand over his mouth and walked away when he got stuck. We are really worried that we may have waited too long.

We agree with Wyatt (1969) that the onset of stuttering is a crisis situation in which swift intervention is absolutely essential. It was arranged to see Stephen and his parents on Monday. We praised Mr. Wood for calling and suggested that Stephen did not need to know the real purpose of the visit to the speech clinic; we advised him to simply tell the child that his parents had to see some people at the university and he could come along and play a few of the interesting games they had for children.

In planning for the evaluation, we delineated several objectives that would guide our efforts:

1. determine if the child is stuttering;
2. if he is, identify at what stage or level of development the disorder has progressed;
3. obtain the parent's perception of the onset and current status of the problem;
4. sample the child's general level of functioning in regard to auditory, motor, and language abilities; and,
5. perhaps most important, commence the development of a counseling relationship with the parents.

We assigned an undergraduate student clinician to observe Stephen and his parents in the clinic waiting room. She was to unobtrusively watch the parent-child interaction and submit a descriptive report to us before we interviewed Mr. and Mrs. Wood. Here is what she wrote:

> The child is well-dressed and well-groomed. At first he sat on his father's lap, but when he saw the toy box he climbed down and played with the farm animals. He talked constantly, asking questions, commenting on what was taking place outside, and describing his animal parade. I heard some repetitions in his speech, especially when he was trying to get his parents to attend to him. I noticed that Mrs. Wood always called him "Stephen," not "Steve" or "Stevie." Does that mean anything?

Before examining a child individually, we like to chat informally with both the youngster and the parents. We do this primarily to observe if the parents are reacting in an overt way to the child's speech. When the child is asked a question, do the parents attempt to answer for him? Do they point out instances of stuttering to the examiner? Do they signal their presence by non-verbal behavior—gestures, postures, and the like? How does the child respond to this?

We took the family on a brief tour of the speech clinic, ignoring Stephen and chatting with Mr. and Mrs. Wood. Ushering them into a playroom, we invited the child to sample the toys while we talked with his mother and father. Gradually, we edged closer to the boy and casually began to join his play, commenting on what his cars were doing, and asking him some questions. Soon he was chattering to the clinician. We noted several repetitions—all on small words, pronouns like "he," "I," "you"—but they were easy and rhythmical. When he attempted to utter the word "blue", however, he use the schwa vowel on the first two repetitions (b—b—blue-blue). Only one prolongation was heard, and occurred when he asked a question beginning with the word "how." Mrs. Wood tensed noticeably and looked at the examiner questioningly when Stephen repeated and hesitated. Once, she finished a word for the child when he had repeated it five times. We could discern little overt reaction on the part of Mr. Wood except he did slump in his chair and look out the window when his wife completed Stephen's utterance. We now needed a larger sample. Would his speech change if his parents left the room? How would he respond to stress?

On a prearranged signal, a graduate student came in and asked Mr. and Mr. Wood if they would like to see the rest of the "school." Stephen glanced up briefly as his parents left, but continued playing and talking with the examiner. No increase in disfluency was noted.

Diagnosticians observe two clinical rules when examining young children thought to be starting to stutter: they use indirect means of obtaining a speech sample, and they never do anything that might bring the child's disfluency to his attention. Employing play as a vehicle, it was very easy to engage Stephen in conversation. With some more reluctant children we have used puppets, extended periods of self-talk, or projective drawings (Bar, 1973). But we also must have some idea of the impact of stress upon the child's fluency. Slowly and subtly at first, we began to hurry the play and to interrupt Stephen in midsentence with our own message. We asked him a question, and before he could finish his answer, we asked another. Then, when he tried to respond or direct the examiner's attention to some facet of our joint play, we looked away from him and purposely dropped toys on the floor and noisily scurried to pick them up. We gauged the communicative stress carefully, watching for changes in the child's speech. Following this, we once again resumed an easy, relaxed style of interaction with the youngster. We abandoned the play for a moment, feasted on a salted peanut, and went to get a drink of water. Returning to the room with Stephen, the examiner pointed to a log building set and said, "We really should build a barn for the animals . . . but, golly, I have to do some school things first. Say, if you helped me, maybe we could get done faster, okay?" Stephen eagerly volunteered to "help" administer a hearing screening test, a measure of receptive vocabulary, and several tasks to assess motor skills. We thanked the child for coming in to see us, and started him on the barn-building project with a student clinician while we prepared for the interview with Mr. and Mrs. Wood. But first, while our impressions of Stephen were clear and fresh, we recorded these observations:

> The child is not a stutterer in the sense of a fully developed symptom pattern, but he did exhibit several forms of abnormal disfluency: multiple repetitions, an occasional intrusive schwa vowel, and a few prolongations. The repetitions occurred most often on the initial word of an utterance. During a free-play situation, he repeated on approximately 9 to 11 words per hundred; the number of repetitions per unit ranged from three to as many as nine. The repetitions were easy and rhythmical—in the same tempo and speed as the rest of his speech. The intrusive schwa vowel occurred when he repeated words beginning with blends—*bl*ue, *str*aw, and *tr*actor. Stephen prolonged only four times and always on vowels, always in the initial position. There is little tension, forcing or gaps in his speech; nor is there obvious evidence of "awareness"—he speaks constantly with an excellent vocabulary and good grammar. When communicative stress was introduced, the disfluency was exacerbated: the number of repetitions increased. My impression is that "listener loss" produced the most stress, then "interruption," "hurrying," and finally "questioning." Stephen's hearing is normal, and he scored in the ninety-ninth percentile on a measure of receptive vocabulary. Motor behavior seems adequate: gait, stance, throwing, block-building, and skipping all appeared normal. At this point in time (note: the diagnostician must be aware that at the onset of the disorder stuttering is characteristically intermittent and he may see the child on a "good" day), although Stephen shows several danger signs (see Figure 7.1) of developing stuttering, the problem can probably be dealt with by environmental intervention.

The clinician needs experience distinguishing normal from abnormal disfluency in the speech of young children. An excellent color film developed and narrated by Eugene Walle (1974) depicts each of the eight danger signs of developing stuttering through the use of freeze-frames and slow-motion views; only children presenting actual fluency disorders were filmed. An unusually effective feature of the film is a gauge (see Figure 7.1) by which the diagnostician can judge the severity of the problem.

Prior to meeting with Mr. and Mrs. Wood, we checked our observations

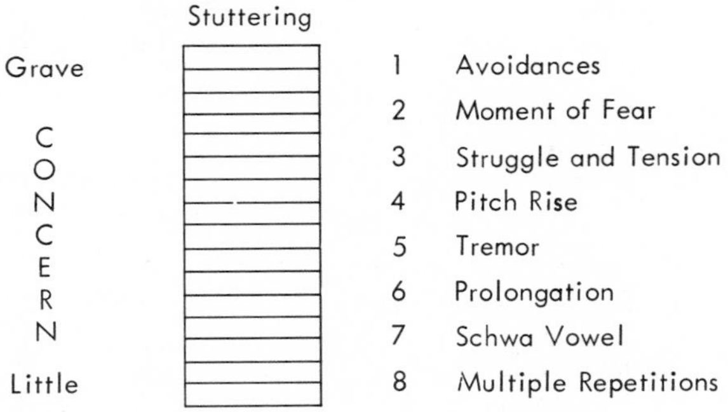

Stuttering

Grave

C
O
N
C
E
R
N

Little

1 Avoidances
2 Moment of Fear
3 Struggle and Tension
4 Pitch Rise
5 Tremor
6 Prolongation
7 Schwa Vowel
8 Multiple Repetitions

Figure 7.1 The Danger Signs of Developing Stuttering (adapted from Walle, 1974).

with those of a graduate student who had monitored the entire diagnostic session behind a one-way mirror. Her findings are summarized on a clinical worksheet (Figure 7.2) designed to facilitate identification of children beginning to stutter. (See Van Riper, 1971: 28, for a clinical schema to differentiate stuttering and normal disfluency; consult also the checklist devised by Cooper, 1973 and the work of Adams, 1977).

Initial interview with Mr. and Mrs. Wood. The initial interview with a parent of a child beginning to stutter is of critical importance. We must establish our professional competence, demonstrate our genuine interest, and convince the parents that we can be trusted. In short, our primary task in this initial contact is to build a relationship for subsequent counseling sessions. We also listen carefully to the parents presenting story: How do they see the child and his problem? In their view, what might have caused it? What do they identify as their role in the onset of the child's stuttering? What expectations and apprehensions do they have regarding the nature and outcome of treatment?

Let us emphasize here that this is *their* story: hear them out. It is not the proper time to take a lengthy case history; there will be plenty of time for a careful review of the background of the problem in subsequent interviews when the parents can then profit from an objective review of the situation. Guilt, which is almost always present in these sessions, must not be engendered by the interviewer's questions or commentary.

We prefer to record these initial interviews; this frees us from the onus of note taking, and we can devote our entire attention to the respondent. It also permits repeated review of the session. Here is a resumé of our initial interview with Mr. and Mrs. Wood:

At the outset of the interview, both parents pressed the examiner for his impressions of Stephen's speech problem. We told them that we were pleased with our findings and would explain in detail after we had a chance to hear from them. Mrs. Wood was the main informant; her husband corroborated dates and added minor details. Both

Name: Stephen Wood   Birthdate: 1/4/73   Date: 7/12/76   File: #76-271
Observer: M. Ruffatto   Situation: "joint play"

1. Repetitions: whole word x syllabic x phonemic _____

   a. Frequency of repetitions: No. per word   3-10 _____
                                  No. per hundred words   11 _____
   b. Speed of repetitions: same rate as fluent speech _____
   c. Tempo: even, regular _____
   d. Co-articulation
        (is appropriate vowel used in repetition?): _schwa noted on_
        blends--5 times _____
   e. Evidence of tension-struggle: _____ none _____
   f. How are the repetitions terminated: _no surge or stoppage_

2. Prolongations: syllabic x vocalic   x   consonant _____
                   articulatory posture _____
   a. Frequency: ___ four _____
   b. Duration: _less than one second_ _____
   c. Change in pitch: ___ no _____
   d. Stoppage of air-flow/phonation: ___ no _____
   e. Repetitions end in prolongations or silent postures: __ no _
   f. Evidence of tension-struggle: ___ none _____
   g. Inappropriate articulatory postures: _____ no _____

3. Response to Communicative Stress:

   a. Type of stress: b. Response:
      loss of listener   repetitions increased,
      hurrying him   noted on pronouns
      interruptions
      overlapping questions

4. Awareness

   a. Eye contact: ___ seemed normal ___ b. Facial flushing no signs __
   c. Eyeblink rate: ___ 19 ___   26
                     (base rate)   (disfluency)
   d. Motor behavior: ___ no signs ___
   e. Verbalizes about speech problem: _not observed_
   f. Behavior following disfluency: _continued talking and playing_

5. Advanced features:

   a. Evidence of frustration: _____ none _____
   b. Evidence of avoidance: _____ none _____
   c. Breathing disturbance: _____ none _____
   d. Facial contortion, extraneous body movements: ___ none __
   e. Tremor: ___ none _____

6. Other observations: _He appears somewhat small for his_
   age but his movements are quick and well-coordinated.
   His articulation skills are excellent and he generates
   long, complex sentences.

Figure 7.2 Clinical Worksheet: Onset of Stuttering

parents appeared tense and uncertain—Mrs. Wood seemed especially anxious. Throughout the interview her vocal quality was querulous, and her eyes filled with tears several times as she related the onset of Stephen's speech problem.

The youngster began to stutter seven months ago, during the Christmas Holidays. At this time both sets of grandparents were visiting and the home was filled with a great deal of excitement and confusion. Mrs. Wood even remembered the very first instance when she noted that Stephen was having trouble—when he attempted to name items in a picture dictionary book he had received as a gift. When we asked her to describe the child's speech at that time, she said he repeated letters—k, m, n. Mr. Wood added that Stephen also seemed to draw out some letters, but his wife insisted that this came later. After the holidays the problem seemed to go away, only to reappear a few weeks later; now, they agreed, there are fewer days when the child is free of speech interruptions. It was also during the holidays that Mrs. Wood discovered that she was pregnant with their second child (Philip, Jr. was born in early June, 1976), and she wondered what impact this had on Stephen. She admitted that she has had very little time to spend with him since the baby was born.

The parents described Stephen as an active, inquisitive child. He began to talk early and enjoys describing events; he provides a running commentary when the family goes for a ride or on some other outing. Mr. Wood added that his son is very adult oriented and, in fact, interacts with neighborhood children as if he were a parent instead of a playmate.

Mrs. Wood confided that she is very concerned about Stephen because her younger brother stuttered severely and she had observed how the disorder hampered his education and social life. She does not want the same thing to happen to Stephen. "Although I have tried to be permissive," she confessed, "I find myself adopting the same rigid perfectionism that characterized my own parents."

The parents have attempted to manage the fluency problem by asking Stephen to "slow down," "take his time," and "think what he intends to say." They have also suggested that he whisper the word first before trying to say it out loud. These home remedies do not seem to help.

It is important that parents obtain some closure during these initial interviews, so we related our findings briefly:

Stephen does indeed have some breaks in his speech, more than normal for a child of his age. He is doing some stuttering but it is still the 'good kind': he is not struggling or avoiding and, most important, he doesn't seem to be very aware that talking is tough (We drew a rough sketch of the stuttering gauge depicted in Figure 7.1 and showed them that Stephen exhibited only the three early danger signs of stuttering). We want to prevent the disorder from developing further and cannot do anything without your help. We need to find out why he is having speech breaks; we need to know when he does it, under what circumstances. In short, we have to start looking at behaviors, at what he *does*, not a condition he *has*. In many cases like this, if we identify and alter certain environmental situations, the child stops stuttering. Stephen's speech will likely get worse if we ask him to stop or change the way he is talking. Talking is automatic, and the more he tries to think and plan how he is speaking, the more tangled up he will get. You were very wise to bring him in now, before the fear and frustration had a chance to develop. Let's plan on meeting again tomorrow, and together we can begin to review Stephen's background and then decide how to gather information on what is happening now.

Plan of treatment. The therapeutic management of children beginning to stutter is largely indirect: we work for changes in the environment through parental counseling and education.[1] In the case of Stephen Wood, our treatment plan included four basic goals:

1. to deal with parental emotions and resistance;
2. to obtain a careful case history;
3. to review the nature and onset of stuttering; and
4. to provide general and specific suggestions for altering the home situation and parent-child interaction.

For purposes of discussion, we will consider each goal separately, although it is rarely possible to do this in clinical practice. Note the interplay of diagnosis and therapy as we review our activities relative to the four goals.

HANDLING EMOTION AND RESISTANCE. The first (and continual) task in a counseling relationship is to deal openly with the client's emotions. A person's feelings are primary. Consequently, at the outset of the second session with Mr. and Mrs. Wood we encouraged them to relate what impact our initial interview had had. Again, Mrs. Wood was the main respondent and here, in part, is what she said:

> We were really dumbfounded—but relieved in a way too—when you said that Stephen does not need active therapy . . . but you would be seeing us today. Last night after the children were in bed, we sat down and reviewed what has happened the past seven months. There is a great deal of hurry and tension in our home, especially when we have to go somewhere; it seems like we are always trying to hasten Stephen along so we can make some deadline. We tend to talk too much, too swiftly and in a complicated fashion to him—maybe we are expecting too much, too early because he is so bright and verbal. Anyway, we feel just sick that we may be responsible for his problem.

We let Mrs. Wood talk it out, nodding occasionally and expressing our interest and understanding. When she had finished, we searched for the right words:

> Most parents feel a bit guilty when their children begin to stutter. They sense that they may have caused the problem—a notion which unfortunately is reinforced by many laymen. Parents, especially the mother, are blamed for everything negative about their youngsters. And stuttering is such a highly visible problem; the neighbor kid might wet the bed every night, but no one else need know. No doubt you were a bit

---

[1]Most parents with whom we have worked responded well to the program of counseling and education *(Phase One)* illustrated by the case of Craig Ryan (Schuell, 1949). In a few instances, however, it has been necessary to become more directive *(Phase Two),* spelling out exactly how the household must be reorganized (Johnson, 1961; see also Van Riper, 1961: 110–111). In only a small number of cases have we had to move to *Phase Three:* some adamant parents became amenable to counseling and recommendations only after stormy sessions with several adult stutterers. Although we do not like to, it is also possible (and occasionally necessary) to work directly with the child (Van Riper, 1963: 371–373).

surprised when I indicated that I would be seeing you and not Stephen. I'm very glad that you told me how you feel and that you are open and honest, because it's difficult to deal objectively with a problem when feelings get in the way. An undercurrent of guilt or resentment makes the problem very difficult to clear up. As I pointed out yesterday, you were most wise to bring Stephen in now when we—you and I as a team—can sort out and eliminate those things that produce speech breaks. We can't change what happened, but that's not nearly so important as what's going on right now. We can alter the present. Here is the phone number of the Munsons; last year they were in the same situation you are, and they volunteered to talk with other parents. A problem shared is a problem lessened. Now, why don't we get started by reviewing all the aspects that we can think of?

THE CASE HISTORY. We seek more than information when we compile a case history. A parent's careful review of the many factors involved in his child's problem tends to foster objectivity. It also shifts the focus away from a general impression of "trouble" to observation of specific behavior. We include a portion of our case history of Stephen Wood:

History of the speech problem. Stephen began to "stutter" approximately seven months ago. Onset occurred, according to the parents, when he faltered at naming pictures in the presence of a group of relatives. No prior history of speech, language or hearing difficulty. Both parents have offered various forms of advice with no lasting effect. Disfluency consists of syllabic repetitions and a few prolongations. No negative reactions from playmates or adult visitors. Disfluency has been cyclic but became more persistent in the last month.

Developmental history. Normal (first) pregnancy. No untoward conditions associated with delivery. Described as an "active" baby. Sat up at three months, walked at eleven months, and spoke first word at twelve months. Usual childhood colds and flu, but no high fevers. Father describes the child as "adult-oriented" and officious in his relationship with other youngsters.

Family. Glenda Wood, age twenty-eight. Married six years. Homemaker. Earned a two-year certificate in business management after completing high school, and worked several years in a bank. Describes herself as perfectionistic and compulsive about order and cleanliness.

Philip Wood, age thirty-one. Federal health inspector. College degree, currently taking graduate work in health planning.

Additional items to assess in obtaining a case history include: 1) a specific review of any familial incidence of stuttering; 2) the impact, if any, of relatives or babysitters upon the child; 3) a description of how the child spends a typical day; and, 4) a description of any prior professional treatment. Case-history forms may be found in Wingate (1976) and other sources (Johnson, Darley and Spriestersbach, 1963; Nation and Aram, 1977).

THE NATURE AND ONSET OF STUTTERING. The second interview with Mr. and Mrs. Wood was devoted mainly to obtaining a case history. By this time they were insistently curious: What is stuttering? What causes it? What did we mean when we said that Stephen still had the "good kind" of stuttering? We gave them a copy of a short pamphlet (Emerick, 1970) written for parents whose children are beginning to stutter and asked that they read it carefully and discuss its contents. (There are several excellent publications concerning the onset of stuttering: Lassers, 1945; Pennington, 1955; Johnson, 1959; Robinson, 1960; Murphy, 1962; Mulder, 1960; Sander, 1959) Perhaps, we warned, portions of the booklet might make them feel a bit guilty; we reminded the parents that our purpose was to convey information, not to point an accusing finger. Finally, we asked Mr. and Mrs. Wood to record their observations regarding Stephen's speech breaks.

> It is often helpful if we put down on paper some of the things we see and hear about the way our child is talking. It will help obtain a clearer picture of the child's situation. Try to be as objective and honest as you can in making your observations. Use the chart (Figure 7.3) at the end of the pamphlet. In the four squares you record what you observed (and the date) with respect to the questions listed along the border. For example: Mrs. E. made an effort on January 19, to study Mary's nonfluency. She found that the child was mainly repeating first sounds of words (muh-muh-Mommy). Mrs. E. put this information, with the date, in one of the four blocks opposite the first question. She then followed down the page and put her other observations about Mary's reactions in the rest of the blocks opposite the questions.
>
> It will be helpful to you to see under what circumstances the child is experiencing the most speech interruptions. To whom was he talking? What was he talking about? What happened immediately before he began to talk? What happened when he was trying to talk? If, for example, you note that the child's speech interruptions occur most frequently when he is competing with his brothers and sisters for speaking time, then you will readily see what needs to be corrected in order to help him. Using this chart, we will be able to find the reasons for an increase in the child's speech interruptions. Once we know *how* and *why* the child is hesitating, we are less apt to label his behavior as stuttering; we concentrate less on the speech and more on the circumstances. Also, we can then take steps to smooth out the circumstances that seem to increase the child's speech interruptions.

We find often that simply asking parents to monitor the antecedents and consequences of their child's speech disfluencies is sufficiently motivating to engender change. Environmental events which disrupt a child's flow of speech become obvious when parents begin to chart.

At the end of the second counseling session Mr. and Mrs. Wood were visibly relieved. Before they left, they asked what they could do to help besides observing. It is important that parents be provided with suggestions when they ask for them:

> Once we identify the factors associated with Stephen's fluency disruptions, we can act to eliminate or reduce them. In the meantime, however, there are several things you can do: 1) be the best listener you can be—not all the time obviously, but arrange it so when you *can* listen to him, do it *totally;* 2) talk simply with him, using short sentences and a slow, relaxed tempo; throw in an easy repetition now and then—and if he asks about it, tell him even big people make mistakes when they talk; 3) arrange to have some quiet times alone with him where he has you one-on-one with no distractions; 4) try to relax the standards or expectations you have for his behavior, at least for now; he is still a small boy even though he seems so adult-like; and, finally, 5) whenever he does have difficulty talking, make sure you complete the communication—let him know that the message, not the struggle, was paramount.

SPEECH CHART		
What type of speech inter- ruptions did the child have (repeating sounds or words; hesitations, changing his sentences)?	date: .... date:	date: .... date:
Did he appear to be tense or struggle with the speech interruptions?	date: .... date:	date: .... date:
Did he seem to be aware that he was having the interrup- tions; did he react to them? If so, how did he react?	date: .... date:	date: .... date:
To whom was he talking when the speech interruptions were noted?	date: .... date:	date: .... date:
What was he talking about?	date: .... date:	date: .... date:
What had happened immediately prior to his speaking (was he interrupted, ignored, ex- cited, frustrated, tired)?	date: .... date:	date: .... date:
What was happening--what was the listener doing--when the child was talking? (Did they offer advice, look away, become tense, etc.?)	date: .... date:	date: .... date:

Record number of times:						
1. Demand for speech						
2. Child told "no" or "don't"						
3. Child was interrupted while talking						
4. Parental conflict or tension						

5. Gave child speech advice,
   such as "stop and start
   over," "take a deep
   breath," "slow down."						

Figure 7.3 Form for Recording Parental Observations of Speech Interruptions.

ALTERING HOME AND PARENT-CHILD INTERACTION. We held four additional counseling interviews with Mr. and Mrs. Wood during the remainder of the summer school session. These meetings were devoted to analyzing the parent's observations of Stephen's speech behavior; we also made a number of suggestions designed to reduce fluency disruptors. The best suggestions came from the parents themselves. The primary focus of this book does not permit a complete account of this phase of counseling with the family. We have included only fragments to illustrate the clinician's role in modifying the home and parent-child relationship:

> Mr. and Mrs. Wood held a conference each evening to review their observations of Stephen's speech disfluency. They slowed the pace of activity in the home and reduced the demands upon the child. Mrs. Wood enrolled in a program of Parent Effectiveness Training offered through the local school system. They both agreed that the most effective modification they made was improving their listening habits; once the child realized that his parents were actively attending, his incessant chatter declined dramatically. Almost immediately the repetitions and prolongations disappeared.

It has been our experience that most parents are amenable to making changes that will benefit their child, if the rationale is explained to them and if it is obvious that the clinician is totally commited to the prevention of stuttering. In order to assist mothers and fathers in altering their interaction with youngsters beginning to stutter, we have offered a wide variety of suggestions. Here are just a few: allow the child to express his fears and anger; count the number of times you say no each day, and reduce these by half; devise stable and consistent rules for behavior; balance the ratio between demand and support so the balance shifts to the latter. We often make a home visit, not only to observe the child in a naturalistic setting, but also to demonstrate that our concern is far more than casual.

There are two additional tools that we have found helpful in parent counseling. Some parents are unaware of the impact of negative comments on their children, and we have had to show them how to analyze their verbal interaction. We loan them a portable tape recorder and ask them to collect samples of conversations with their child. Then, using the research of Egolf et al. (1972) and Kasprisin-Burrelli, Egolf and Shames (1972), we show them how to categorize positive and negative statements. This graphic procedure helps them to become more creative, more supportive in their interaction with the child.

The other tool we use in helping parents are two excellent films: *Family Counseling* (Walle, 1975) and *Is it Me Is it You?* (Walle, 1977). Both films are invaluable in helping parents understand how they can help children overcome the broken and hesitant speech they often display between two and six years of age.

Outcome of Treatment

By the end of August Stephen was exhibiting no signs of stuttering except occasionally when he was very excited. Once, when a large dog knocked him off his tricycle, he was disfluent for several hours; but Mrs. Wood managed the traumatic event in a calm, supportive manner. Mr. and Mrs. Wood met with the Munsons (parents who had undergone counseling when their child was beginning to stutter), and the women formed a close friendship. Now both mothers make presentations in our university classes. A frequent fringe benefit of counseling parents is the personal gains they derive; Mr. and Mrs. Wood report that they feel better, their home is more relaxed, and they enjoy their children much more.

Prognosis

We are very impressed with the efficacy of treatment for young children beginning to stutter. When the clinician can intervene before the child develops fear and avoidance reactions, and if the parents are amenable to counseling, the prognosis for recovery is excellent. Our own records on 173 cases, admittedly limited and incomplete, reveal an astounding success ratio of 84 percent. There are several factors that the clinician must consider when estimating a client's prospects for recovery:

1. How long has the child been stuttering? The older the child is and the longer his exposure to adverse environmental reactions, the poorer his prognosis.
2. What type and intensity of environmental reactions has the child been exposed to? Our cases who experienced slapping or other forms of physical abuse had the worst prognoses.
3. Is the child aware that he has difficulty speaking? (See Figure 6.1). The more heedful the child is of his speech interruptions, the less positive the prognosis.
4. What type of speech disfluency characteristics are present? The more danger signs present (see Figure 7.1)—in particular, cessation of phonation, stoppage of air-flow, moment of fear—the poorer the prognosis.
5. How amenable are the parents to counseling? The presence of parental psychopathology is an extremely poor sign for prognosis.
6. What is the child's level of intelligence? We have had more limited success with "slow" children.
7. Are there organic or neurotic factors that figure in the onset of stuttering? Chances for recovery are more limited if either is present.

Our clinical success or failure with children beginning to stutter is also related to the characteristic pattern of factors present at the onset of stuttering. Apparently, there are several ways of becoming a stutterer, and a careful scrutiny of 173 cases seen over the past fifteen years revealed four basic patterns (see Van Riper, 1971: 104–117):

Pattern one. The most typical form (92 cases) of onset in our clinical experience is that of the bright, alert, and sensitive child (Robinson, 1964: 59) who may have low frustration tolerance. This child began to talk early and was considered normal in all respects. The parents are not unusually demanding or rejecting but often are very busy and involved people; most often they are simply not properly informed about speech development in young children. The child cannot seem to keep up with the pace of the house or may be overwhelmed trying to match the fluency of others; there are many fluency disruptors present. Our records show complete recovery in all cases we treated.

Pattern two. This pattern was the next most frequent (41 cases) in our clinical sample. The child is average or above in intelligence but may have an articulation problem. The parents are typically ambivalent and inconsisent in their child-rearing; they may have implicit or explicit standards that are unusually high. The mother tends to be malcontent. Some critical episode such as changing schools or the birth of a sibling may precipitate the stuttering:

> Bobby, age three, was an only child. His mother was seven months pregnant when he suddenly began to stutter following an altercation with his father over finishing all the food on his plate. The father, a navy veteran, was an exceptionally perfectionistic and demanding individual. He insisted that the home be vacuumed and scrubbed daily and flew into a rage if items were not in their proper place. He actually conducted a daily inspection of Bobby's room and chalked up demerits (no dessert) if his shoes and toys were not lined up in a military manner. Mrs. Baker was completely overwhelmed and dominated by her husband; she even talked about him to Bobby in hushed and reverent tones as "our father." We must confess that we failed miserably to alter the home situation, and our latest check revealed that Bobby is now stuttering quite severely.

Despite our failure in the case described briefly above, the prognosis in Pattern Two is quite good. The significant variable is parental cooperation. In some cases, the parents have been seen jointly by a family service agency.

Pattern three. A significant number (29 cases) of children exhibited a third type of onset. The child is almost always "slow" or below average not only in intelligence but in many other respects. He is usually delayed in speech and language development. Often there is a history of disease or injury; the child may show signs of neurological impairment such as motor clumsiness, mixed cerebral dominance, and slow diadochokinetic rate. The general impression is that of inadequacy—a lack of capacity to think and talk—not only in the child but also in the parents (Andrews and Harris, 1964). The parents—almost one-third of our Pattern Three cases were being raised by only the mother—seem to be marginal persons who have produced marginal children. They have low socioeconomic status. Almost in every case, the child was said to have stuttered since he began to speak. Prognosis is only fair or guarded in these cases. Therapy is generally more prolonged than in Pattern One and Two, and our success ratio is less than 50 percent.

Pattern four. This final mode of onset is relatively rare (11 cases). The child is usually normal or above in intelligence. The onset of stuttering is sudden and severe and always seems to follow some traumatic episode.

Theophilis, age six, began to stutter severely when the tip of his right index finger was nipped off in an automatic barn cleaner. His father, a successful dairy farmer and part-time Pentecostal preacher, had warned the boy not to play in the barn. Indeed, he had filled the boy with fears of sin and hellfire; he prayed over and protected the child from evil in a thousand intricate ways. Easily excited and disorganized by emotional stimuli, the boy feared the dark, wet his bed almost nightly, and altogether was a miserable, cowed little boy.

Prognosis in these Pattern Four cases is poor. We can only report one unequivocal success among the nine cases we have seen. These children and their families needed so much more than we could offer; we now refer them to a skilled child psychologist.

We have often wondered how much we actually did for some of these cases. Would they have gotten better without our help, due simply to the passage of time and some internal recovery potential in the child? Did we do any good? In most instances, however, the recovery from stuttering occurred too swiftly after the initiation of therapeutic practices (two weeks to several months) to be attributed to spontaneous recovery (Wingate, 1964; Shearer and Williams, 1965; Sheehan and Martyn, 1970). Consult the work of Wyatt (1969: 310–312) for a list of variables contributing to and inhibiting progress.

EVALUATION OF THE SCHOOL AGE CHILD

Appraising and treating elementary-school stutterers is particularly challenging. This group of children, approximately seven to twelve years old, is no longer beginning to stutter; they are not simply repeating and hesitating. They struggle noticeably when speaking and attempt to avoid or disguise their difficulty; they are frustrated and bewildered by their behavior. The self-perpetuating cycle has started, and it is now necessary to deal directly with the stuttering.

The clinician is faced with several thorny problems when planning an examination of a young stutterer: (1) Young children frequently lack the insight and cooperation necessary to analyze their problem objectively and rationally. (2) Children are reluctant or unable to freely verbalize their internal feelings. (3) Children can face unpleasant and feared experiences only with great difficulty; they don't understand enduring temporary discomfort for a future payoff. (4) The speech clinician is associated in the child's mind with the teaching personnel, who may in some cases be penalizing or disturbing listeners. In addition, the clinician may find himself identified with authority figures; this tends to undermine a trusting relationship. (5) Lastly, and perhaps most significantly, the child usually has no choice about entering therapy; most likely he is brought for evaluation by his parents, referred by a teacher, or identified by a speech clinician.

As Van Riper (1973: 427) points out, however, there are several advantageous factors in working with youngsters who stutter:

The disorder is still not fully developed in the child. Its component behaviors have not had as long a history of reinforcement. They are not fixed. The avoidance and struggle reactions are less complex. Morbidity is lower. Living primarily in the present, past trauma are less important in the design of therapy. The child stutterer forgets his unpleasant experiences more swiftly than the adult who often nurtures them. The child's fears also seem more transitory and his malattitudes less severe. The clinician finds that the child's resistances are more open and direct; we do not find the ingenious sabotage which often characterizes the adult stutterer. And perhaps most important of all, the child has not interiorized the stuttering role to the degree manifested by the adult.

Some clinicians continue to deal with young stutterers as if their problem were incipient or onset in nature. They talk in hushed voices about rhythm problem and report that they are "watching" a child who stutters. Parents and teachers are advised to refrain from using the word "stuttering." Literature concerning the onset of stuttering is sent home which, in the absence of counseling and follow-up, merely increases the parents' guilt. This leads to an elaborate conspiracy of silence that only makes matters worse:

> To pretend that there is no speech defect when it is obvious to the child and everyone else is folly, since this pretense will only make him feel he is doing something unclean, as well as unspeakable (Van Riper, 1961: 114).

In their uncertainty lest they do something harmful and create "stuttering," such clinicians do nothing at all. The emperor has no stuttering problem. Perhaps this is one reason why the children, taking their cue from their elders, so frequently *act* as if they were not greatly concerned about their speech (Silverman, 1970).

The diagnostician will find that these youngsters respond to an honest, straightforward clinical approach. With preschoolers and early elementary children, we use descriptive language—"tensing," "getting stuck,"—to inquire about their speaking difficulty, not out of any fear of the word stuttering, but simply because the term either doesn't mean much to the child or, in some cases, is too negatively charged. It is better to refer to different ways of *talking* when assessing younger children (Williams, 1971). Here is a fragment taken from a recording of a recent diagnostic session with a seven-year-old child. The examiner is trying to elicit the little girl's own description of her fluency problem:

> These are your eyes. You use them for seeing. Do you have any trouble seeing? These are your ears. You use them for hearing. Do you have any trouble hearing? This is your mouth. You use it for talking. Do you ever have any trouble talking?

With later elementary children, we use a frank, direct style. The clinician must establish trust and confidence by showing the client that he is competent, that he *knows* about the problem of stuttering. He does this by demonstrating that he understands what it feels like to stutter, by revealing a bit about himself, and by his willingness to touch stuttering without fear or distress. Notice how swiftly the clinician accomplishes those objectives in the following example:

> "Hello. I suppose you're wondering what's going to happen today. You know that I am a speech-correction teacher and that my job is to help you get rid of your stuttering. But you don't know what kind of person I am except that I'm a stranger

and you often have more trouble talking to a stranger. And you don't know how much I'll make you talk or how much stuttering you'll have. So you're probably a bit scared. You don't have to be, because today I'm going to do most of the talking.

"You noticed that I didn't ask your name. That's because I know that saying your name is often one of the hardest things there is to do. How did I know that? It's because I have worked with other kids who've stuttered—a lot of them. And it's because I had to do a lot of stuttering myself when I was learning to be a speech-correction teacher. I had to go into stores and stutter like this [Demonstrates] and like this . . . and like this . . . and many other ways, too. I had to know how it looked and how it felt. And at first, I was sure scared and embarrassed—especially when I had to do it on the phone or to one of my classmates. Once, it almost seemed to run away with me and I couldn't stop. So I think you'll find that I can understand how you feel when you stutter. I also learned how to help the stutterer and I want to help you. So let's get started.

"The first thing I've got to do is to know *how* you stutter. Let me give you some samples and ask you if you've ever had that kind of stuttering. How about this kind? [Therapist illustrates a very severe and unusual form of stuttering.] You don't have that kind? Good! One of the kids I worked with had that kind when we first started. How about this kind? . . . Or this? . . . [Therapist gradually shows models of decreasing abnormality and unfamiliarity.] But I bet you've often had some like this, haven't you? [Illustrates.] (Van Riper, 1964: 30–31)

An Assessment Plan

The evaluation of a young stutterer does not differ greatly in substance from an assessment of an older individual (with children, environmental, parental, and school factors are more important); therefore, we will defer a detailed description of diagnostic procedures until a later section of this chapter. In order to reveal the range of information generally sought, however, we have included an outlined assessment plan prepared by a diagnostic team comprised of a faculty member and graduate students. The plan was compiled for the evaluation of a ten-year-old child referred to a university speech clinic by a public-school clinician:

Assessment Plan for Alan Schlicher

I. *Identifying Information*

Obtain all the usual information regarding address, grade level, etc. This can be obtained from Ms. Hronkin, the referral source, or in the parent interview. Be sure to inquire about living arrangements: Ms. Hronkin mentioned that a paternal grandfather may reside with the family and apparently he is a dominant force in the family (reportedly, he is against Alan receiving speech therapy and insists he overcame stuttering by eating mashed potatoes!)

II. *Description of Stuttering*

A. Global description: what are the salient descriptive features of Alan's stuttering behavior? Is it basically fixative or oscillative? Are there long silent periods of internal struggle or does he exhibit a more overt pattern?

B. Core behaviors: make an analysis of the repetitions and prolongations observed—the number of oscillations per unit, tempo, duration, and so forth.

C. Tension-struggle features: using the items on the Summary Sheet (Figure 7.4), note the occurrence and location of any ancillary behaviors.

D. Frequency: this analysis will serve as our baseline for re-evaluation of Alan so we need to be especially precise. Collect data (count repetitions, prolongations, other salient features of his moments of stuttering) on at least three types of speech samples—reading, paraphrasing, and spontaneous speech. We can compute the relative frequency of stutterings per minute, or per total words uttered, by analyzing the videotape later. One word of caution: stuttering is notoriously ephemeral and it is very difficult to obtain reliable baselines. Ryan (1969) recommends recording data in three different sessions in order to count reliably and define specific behaviors. (He also includes more speaking tasks—echoic, naming pictures, speaking with puppets, etc.)

E. Severity: We will use the *Riley Stuttering Severity Instrument* (Riley, 1972); this instrument employs the three dimensions of frequency, duration, and physical concomitants and yields a score which can be converted to a percentile. A severity measure like this (particularly when it allows the examiner to score a client on a common scale of 0 to 100) is useful when communicating the results of the evaluation to the parents, teacher, even the child himself. The severity scales devised by Johnson, Darley, and Sprietersbach (1963: 281) and others (Andrews and Harris, 1964: 5; Wingate, 1976: 319) are also useful.

F. Variations in frequency/severity: Explore with the child and his parents whether his stuttering comes and goes in cycles, which situations or listeners provoke variations in his problem, and whether there are any words or sounds that are particularly difficult. Determine what impact delayed auditory feedback and masking noise have upon his speech.

G. How does the child try to control his stuttering? What techniques has he devised for coping with speech interruptions? How effective are they?

H. Can the child predict when he is about to stutter? Ask him if he can; but also have him underline words he thinks he might stutter on as he reads silently a simple passage. Have him read it aloud and determine the degree to which he can accurately predict his stuttering.

I. What is the client's post-stuttering behavior? Does he continue talking, give up, become angry, or cry? Does he appear indifferent?

III. *Attitude Dimension*

This is the most difficult and least reliable aspect of the evaluation. Some information can be obtained through observation of Alan and his parents and by what they say about the problem. We can also administer several self-inventory scales (see particularly Chapman, 1969) or have him do some projective drawings (Bar, 1973). What is the child's attitude toward treatment? How much does he know about stuttering? Has he been teased at school or home because of his problem?

IV. *Case History*

We will want to obtain background information with respect to four basic areas: history of general development (motor, language, social), onset and development of stuttering, medical history, and family history. These areas can be explored in the parent interview.

V. *Present Functioning*

A. Personality: describe the child's personality in general terms (shy, aggressive, etc.) and identify any special features (fears, tics, nail biting, etc.) which may apply to him. Ascertain his special interests or hobbies.

B. School: obtain information relevant to his academic and social adjustment in school.

C. Related testing: is a psychological or medical referral indicated? Perform screening evaluations on the child's motor behavior, hearing, and language ability. The latter is particularly important since there is some evidence that children who stutter may have a language disability (Wyatt, 1969; Andrews and Harris, 1964) although the research is equivocal (Perozzi and Kunze, 1969; Perozzi, 1970; Williams and Marks, 1972; Manning and Riensche, 1976).

D. Diagnostic session: how did the child behave during the diagnostic session? What could be discerned about his level of motivation? How did he respond when put under communicative stress? How did he respond to trial therapy?

Prognosis

Since 1962 when we set out to devise a therapy program for young stutterers (Emerick, 1970), we have seen a total of ninety-one children and have consulted with public-school clinicians about many others. According to our records, and they are frankly incomplete in follow-up, sixty-two children made a total recovery and are no longer considered stutterers by parents, peers, or teachers; an additional sixteen children made considerable improvement or are still undergoing treatment; the thirteen remaining youngsters made little or no improvement. What factors are crucial for improvement? What variables should the diagnostician consider when making a prognosis?

According to our records, the most significant improvement in therapy was noted in those cases where the following factors obtained:

1. No prior record of unsuccessful treatment (children identified and treated unsuccessfully as "primary" stutterers did poorly in our program; an absence of treatment seems more conducive to success than a history of therapeutic failure)

1. Identifying Information

    Name:_____ Birthdate:_____ Sex:_____ School:_____
    Address:_____ Teacher:_____ Grade:_____
                       Phone:_____ File Number:_____
    Family Structure:_____
                 (Father)   (age) (education)   (occupation)

                 (Mother)   (age) (education)   (occupation)

                 (sibling)   (age) (sibling)   (age)
                 Living arrangements:_____

II. Description of stuttering
    A. Global description:_____
    B. Core behaviors:

       repetitions   prolongations   C. Tension - Struggle
                                                       features:

    No./unit_____   duration_____   tremor_____
    Tempo_____   pitch change_____   avoidances_____
    Co-articulation_____ how terminate_____   retrials_____
    How terminate_____ _____   starters_____
    _____   _____   breathing_____
                                                 head_____
                                                extremities_____

                                                  eyes_____

    D. Frequency: E. Severity:
        reps. prolong. — — #words time Riley scale_____
                                           other_____
    read
    para-
    phrase
    sponta-
    neous

    _____
    _____

    F. Variations in frequency/severity: G. How does client contorl?_____

         cycles_____
         situations/listens   H. Can client predict?_____
           when worst_____
           when best_____
           ever absent_____   I. Post-stuttering behavior:____
           (e.g. alone,_____
           singing,_____
           with pets)_____

           words/sounds_____
           DAF/masking_____

Figure 7.4   Evaluation of Young Stutterers: Summary Sheet

III. Attitude dimension

    A. Client's attitude   C. Others:
       To stuttering:_____

                                     Siblings:_____
       To treatment:_____
                                     Other children:_____

    B. Parental attitude: Other adults:_____

IV. Case History

    A. General development (motor, language, social):
    B. Onset and development of stuttering:
       Parental explanation_____client's_____
       How has it changed?_____
       Treatment_____

    C. Medical History
    D. Family History

                    Paternal   Maternal

      stuttering   _____   _____
      speech defects_____   _____
      twinning   _____   _____
      diabetes   _____   _____
      others   _____   _____

V. Present functioning

    A. Personality: C. Related testing:

      description_____ psychological referral_____
      special features:
        sensitive_____   medical referral_____
        tics_____
        fears_____   motor_____
        others_____   hearing_____
                          language_____
      interests/hobbies:_____ other_____

                         D. Diagnostic session:

    B. School: response to examiner_____
                         estimate of motivation_____
      academic_____   response to stress_____
      social_____
                         trial therapy_____

       E. Prognosis and recommendations:_____
        _____
        _____
        _____

Figure 7.4 Cont'd.

2. *Cooperative parents, willing to participate meaningfully in a program of counseling*

3. More severe stuttering pattern; mild stutterers showed little improvement

4. *A predominantly clonic stuttering pattern featuring struggle and escape* (children who had become adept at avoidance generally had more difficulty)

5. Cooperative teachers and other school personnel

6. *No other significant problems* (reading difficulty, a scholastic problem independent of stuttering, etc.)

7. When *the child has other resources* (expertise in scouting, athletics, music)

8. When group therapy can be utilized

9. *When it is possible to schedule intensive therapy* (at least three, preferably four, contacts a week)

10. When the child can tolerate imitating various stuttering patterns (not necessarily his own) demonstrated by the examiner

All of the factors listed are significant prognostically; however, Items 2, 4, 6, 7, and 9 loom as the most critical to recovery. According to research already cited, a large number of individuals apparently outgrow stuttering between its onset and young adulthood. Certain variables, severity and family history among others, are related to spontaneous recovery and we suggest that the reader review these investigations carefully (see Emerick and Hamre, 1972). For a convenient checklist of variables that are related to prediction of chronic stuttering, see the work of Cooper (1972; 1973).

For an account of therapy for young stutterers, including case studies of clinical successes and failures, see the publication by Emerick (1970). You will find much that is helpful in the contributions of Chapman (1959) and others (Willis, 1965; Van Riper, 1964; Goven and Vette, 1966; Simpson, 1966; Stennett, 1967; Anderson, 1970; Fox and Connelly, 1970; Savage, 1970; Williams, 1971; Violon, 1973; Silverman, 1974; Polow, 1975; Heistad, 1977).

ASSESSMENT OF THE ADULT STUTTERER

The disorder is fully developed in the adult (adolescent and older) client: speech interruptions are more complex and characteristically compulsive; fears and apprehensions become chronic; avoidance, disguise, and negative attitudes hamper and distort the individual's relationships with others. At this stage a speech breakdown is not simply a response, it is also a stimulus—the problem has become cyclic and self-reinforcing. Clinicians agree that the treatment of stuttering at this advanced stage is complicated and exceedingly difficult.

There is a bewildering array of treatment approaches, each with a diagnostic strategy for the problem of stuttering. It is our position that no legitimate form of therapy should be denigrated, because all types of remediation have been effective with certain clients. On the other hand, no form of therapy is successful with *all* clients. On balance, then, it is reasonable to conclude that a multidimensional approach, a form of assessment and treatment which includes as many features of the disorder as possible, will yield the most lasting results.

In fact, there is overwhelming advocacy in the literature for a broad-based program of treatment for persons who stutter; clinician-investigators from all theoretical persuasions support a form of therapy which attends to the needs of the total person (Prins, 1970; Cooper, 1971; Egolf, Shames and Blind, 1971; Perkins, 1973; Perkins et al., 1974; Andrews and Cutler, 1974; Ingham, Martin and Kuhl, 1974; Ingham, 1975; Guitar, 1976; Klevans and Lynch, 1977). Typically, the authors cited conclude that no single conceptual framework can cope adequately with all aspects of a stutterer's problem. Perkin's comments are representative:

> The ideal program for adult stutterers is not likely to fit exclusively within operant concepts, motor-linguistic concepts, or psychotherapeutic concepts (1973: 283).

Williams's conclusions are more specific:

> Keep in mind that all a clinician can do is to help a stutterer learn to change his way of *speaking*, to change his *emotional reactions* toward himself and his listeners, and, most important, to *adjust* to those changes (1974: 9). (Italics ours)

There appears to be a great deal of agreement, then, that the best, the most successful treatment for stuttering includes activities that help the individual alter his habitual ways of *behaving, feeling*, and *thinking*—as those three elements relate to communication in general and fluency breakdowns in particular.

We believe that the same triad—speech disfluencies, emotional reactions, and mental constructs—also offers the best focus for assessment of the adult stutterer (Table 7-1). Quite obviously, our classification is arbitrary, and there is

Table 7-1 Overview of Assessment of Adult Stutterers

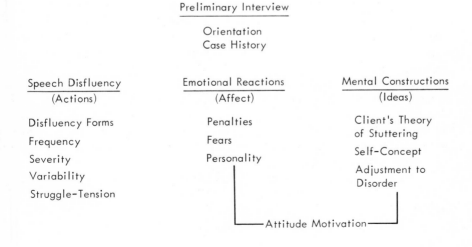

Preliminary Interview

Orientation
Case History

Speech Disfluency	Emotional Reactions	Mental Constructions
(Actions)	(Affect)	(Ideas)
Disfluency Forms	Penalties	Client's Theory of Stuttering
Frequency	Fears	Self-Concept
Severity	Personality	Adjustment to Disorder
Variability		
Struggle-Tension		

Attitude Motivation

considerable overlapping among the three dimensions. For example, a tremor can be *described* as an aspect of speech disfluency; the number of times it occurs can be counted; the anatomical locus, its duration, and release characteristics can be documented. A tremor "happens" to a person, and we also need to obtain a subjective report of what he *experiences* (panic, frustration, anger) before, during, and after its occurrence. Finally, it is important to ascertain what meaning the struggle pattern has for him—what is his *intent* or purpose in attempting to speak the way he did? Does he believe that talking requires a ritualistic pattern of tensing and forcing?

The evaluation process described below may seem unnecessarily lengthy and complicated. We believe that the more information we have about a client, the more complete our picture of how he acts, feels and believes, the better will be our prospects for therapeutic success. Remember too that we are presenting an ideal, comprehensive assessment procedure, and the clinician may, in many situations, adumbrate the outline to fit the needs of a particular individual. By all means, the evaluation delineated here can, and no doubt should, be conducted over several clinical sessions.

Preliminary Interview

Prior to undertaking formal observation and testing, we like to perform an intake interview. This preliminary clinical session is designed to accomplish five objectives: (1) to inform the client what to expect in the diagnostic session; (2) to obtain routine information; (3) to determine why he is coming to treatment at this particular time; (4) to assemble historical information; and, (5) to establish a working relationship.

Since we want the client to be a partner in the exploration of his problem, we feel it is important for him to know *what* we intend to do and *why* we propose to do it. By structuring the clinical transaction so the stutterer knows what role he is to play in his own recovery, we are establishing a therapeutic contract. Eliminating the mystery also reduces anxiety. The clinician will find it helpful to verbalize the apprehensions, embarrassment, and reservations which clients often bring to a diagnostic session.

Routine information includes the client's name, address, phone number—all the relevant identifying information (see Figure 7.4). Although generally we obtain this information by direct inquiry, in some instances when interviewing very severe stutterers, we have them fill out a standard questionnaire form. There will be sufficient opportunity later, when the client feels more comfortable with the examiner, to elicit speech samples.

The third objective of the intake interview is to determine why the client is coming (or being sent) to a speech clinician at this particular point in time. Has the individual undergone a "bottoming-out" experience, a severe crisis in his social, occupational, or educational life? What does he expect from treatment? What do others expect of him? Answers to these questions are useful in determining the client's motivation and in making a prognosis.

We feel that it is important to assemble historical information in the following areas: onset and development of stuttering; education; social adjustment; vocation; and avocation. In order to implement changes in a client, we need to know as much as possible about who he is and how he came to be the person he is now. If we ignore the salient features of the client's case history, we are likely to repeat old mistakes without knowing it.

Finally, the initial contact with a client is of inestimable importance in establishing a working relationship. We tried to discern the critical factors involved in an unusually swift rapport established with a client we worked with in a treatment demonstration project (Starkweather, 1972). The preliminary interview had been held in the stutterer's home town:

> (1)The clinician demonstrated his interest by coming to the stutterer's home base. (2) The clinician is also a stutterer—we did mention this source of identification but we did not dwell on it. (3) We talked straight and tough to Joe, told him exactly what the institute entailed. Some clinicians think that a velvet-glove, Pollyanna approach is effective, but stutterers suspect this tactic, for they know deep inside that solving their problem will not be easy. (4) We invited him to take a chance, we extended a challenge which implied faith in his capabilities; everyone needs an open horizon to aim for in life's journey, and maybe we simply showed Joe the beckoning mirages ahead. Other features could be listed—we somehow revealed our competence even in that brief exchange, we showed that we could be trusted, and we verbalized for him the lack of hope we saw in his sad features.

Analysis of Disfluency

The clinician's primary mission in evaluation of a stutterer is to perform a careful analysis of the individual's speech disfluency behavior. An analysis should include a thorough description of the stuttering pattern (topography) and measures of the relative frequency with which various features of the pattern occur. The disfluency assessment accomplishes two basic purposes: it delineates the behaviors to be altered and provides a base measure to which the worker can refer when monitoring the impact of treatment.

The first step in the disfluency analysis is to obtain a representative sample of the client's speech. The operative word here is *representative;* stuttering is an intermittent disorder, and the amount of difficulty an individual has is contingent upon the speaking task, the situation, and other variables. If it is possible, there are obvious advantages to collecting samples of the client's "real" communication in naturalistic settings—the playground, informal group situations, the family dinner table. Generally, however, clinicians rely on data obtained from three speaking tasks: oral reading, paraphrasing, and conversation. A standard passage can be used for the reading and paraphrasing tasks. Be sure to tape record, or better videotape, the session and note down the time elapsed for each segment of the total sample; it will then be easier to specify rather precise frequency and severity values. We always ask the stutterer to discuss both neutral topics (hobbies, sports, vacations) and threatening topics (family, school, dating) to insure that we obtain a range of speaking difficulty. It is important also to know what produces stress and how the individual responds to it; we experiment in the session with things like hurrying the client, feigning listener loss, and asking him to repeat.

An overall description. We commence the analysis with a global description of the individual's speech behavior. What is his normal speech like in terms of rate, rhythm, degree of tension, articulation, and voice? What are the salient features of his stuttering pattern? Here is how we described one client's disfluency:

> Predominantly fixative blocks, almost on every word (except a few stereotyped social ritual expressions or trite asides, which are generally uttered fluently) with little variation in frequency or severity in three types of talking—reading aloud, paraphrasing, and spontaneous conversation. Overall impression is of extreme tension as he moves slowly and deliberately from word to word.

Core behaviors. The lowest common denominators of the problem of stuttering are repetitions (oscillative phenomena) and prolongations (fixative phenomena). Although most individuals have either predominantly clonic or predominantly tonic disfluency patterns, all stutterers exhibit both forms of speech interruption. A key feature of the disfluency analysis, therefore, is a precise description of these core behaviors.

With respect to *repetitions,* we want to identify the size of the unit (phrase, whole word, syllable), the number of oscillations per unit, their tempo and degree of tension involved, and how they are terminated. Are there silent oscillations of articulatory postures? Does the client perform an articulatory posture—does he assume, for example, a bilabial valving posture prior to emission of air and sound when attempting to utter the word "Bat"? Does he have difficulty finding the proper vowel during the course of the repetitions? Here is a checklist we use for observing repetitions:

Size of unit (record examples)
1. phrase _____
2. whole word _____
3. syllable _____
4. articulatory posture (silent oscillation)
   a. pre-forming _____
   b. incorrect posture
Co-articulation _____
Tempo _____
Tension _____
How terminated

In terms of *prolongations,* we are interested in the anatomical site of the fixations, whether they are silent or audible, how long they last, degree of tension involved and how they are terminated. Here is a description of the fixations of a client with very severe stuttering; note the delineation of a sequence of behaviors:

> *Fixations* of articulatory postures: silent plosives and affricatives, or audible prolongation on semivowels and fricatives; fixations may last as long as thirty seconds and be as brief as three seconds with an average duration of eight seconds; airflow shut off initially at lip or tongue-tip and gum-ridge valves, and as tension increases the locus of fixation shifts to the larynx; a fixation may be released with a surge of tension or with a deep breath and a retrial. If neither works and the tension increases, a tremor is noted.

Struggle-tension features. Very rarely does a client exhibit *only* repetitions and prolongations. Anyone who has observed stutterers know that they appear tense and often make irrelevant sounds and movements while attempting to speak. Stutterers display a wide variety of these mannerisms, and they may vary in frequency of occurrence and degree of involvement in particular clients; some individuals manifest an astounding array of eye blinking, head jerking, postponement rituals, and other behaviors, while others appear relatively quiescent, at least overtly. Most, if not all, of these mannerisms seem to be artifacts of the individual's efforts to speak smoothly, to disguise or eliminate fluency breakdowns. Some of the behaviors no doubt arise from following bad advice (long delays may follow from continual admonitions to "think what you are going to say and then say it"); others seem to stem from autonomic arousal overflow, from efforts at self-help, or from superstitious conditioning. Regardless of their origin, all the "accessory features" appear to be a variety of coping behavior that is designed to either avoid or escape from the core forms of speech interruption. It is ironic that they make the individual's problem all the more obvious.

Clinical assessment of a client's struggle-tension features has two facets: a catalogue of specific mannerisms and a description of the behaviors in a time sequence. The first task is basically taxonomic—identification of the specific mannerisms displayed by the individual. The diagnostician can either devise her own checklist (see Figure 7.4 for a beginning) or choose from several published inventories. Borrowing from the "physical concomitants" portion of the *Riley Severity Instrument,* a clinician could create a simple form for recording observations of a client's pattern:

Extraneous sounds
  speech related _____
  _____

  not related _____
  _____

Facial expressions
  jaw jerking _____
  tongue protrusion _____
  _____

Head Movements

_____

_____

Extremities movement
    arms and hands _____

_____

The Iowa form (Johnson, Darley, and Spriestersbach, 1963: 279–280) is a good choice, but we prefer the *Southern Illinois Behavior Checklist* (Brutten and Shoemaker, 1974) because it is very comprehensive (it lists ninety-seven different behaviors) and is designed so that both the client and the clinician can record the presence of various mannerisms. The Behavior Checklist is one part of a comprehensive diagnostic procedure, the *Behavior Assessment Battery* prepared by Brutten and his associates.

Regardless of the particular format employed, it is obvious that the diagnostician will not be able to identify all of the stutterer's struggle-tension characteristics in a single session. We recommend that the worker pay particular attention to four common forms of escape behavior, and document as many of the client's avoidance techniques as possible.

The following four tension-struggle features are especially noxious to both the stutterer and his listeners:

1. TENSION. Identify the *site* of excess tension, its *extent* (devise a simple rating scale), and *impact* (distracting, impeding) upon the act of speaking. Does the stutterer have any voluntary control over the tension? Some forms of excess muscular activity will be obvious to the examiner; in some instances, however, the clinician will have to rely upon the client's report.

2. TREMOR. A stuttering tremor—rapid vibratory activity of various muscle groups which often follows a surge of energy to a fixated articulatory posture—is a devastating experience for the stutterer. Real panic is precipitated by a sudden loss of self-control. We must specify the anatomical *site* (the trigger points), measure the *duration,* and specify how the tremors are *released.* We include the following description of one client's tremor (again note the specification of a behavioral time sequence):

> The tremor starts at the right corner of his mouth, spreads rapidly down the right side of his face and neck; if the fixation is long (over five seconds), the tremor may extend into Joe's right arm to his index finger which is extended in a gesture that seems to say, "just a minute."

3. RELEASE BEHAVIORS. What are the stutterer's strategies for terminating strings of repetitions and escaping fixative blocks? Does he time the utterance with a movement of his head, hands, or feet? Does he redouble his efforts and blurt out

the word in a sudden surge of energy? Or, does he wait interminably for the "right" moment to proceed? Here is a description of releasing behaviors observed in a severe stutterer:

> *Release behaviors* included in order of frequency of use: sudden surge of tension, often accompanied by postural shift; a tongue-sucking sound ("tsk"); sucking and lip-licking movements; a spitting motion which may or may not be accompanied by saliva. The latter three release devices are infrequently used to initiate a speech attempt or as transitions between fixations seemingly to keep his oral mechanism moving.

4. STOPPAGES OF AIR-FLOW AND PHONATION. Inspect the client's speech performance for evidence of momentary occlusions of the airway. Where do these take place—the lips, velum, larynx? Are there indications of abnormal breathing—rapid, shallow respirations, flaring of the nostrils, attempts to speak on the last bit of exhaled air?

Some recent research (Gautheron et al., 1973; Webster and Furst, 1975; Schwartz, 1974, 1976) suggests that persons who stutter may have basic physiological difficulties in the coordination of respiration, phonation, and articulation. Hutchinson (1975) found several distinct and unusual aerodynamic patterns associated with stuttered speech; the implication is that stuttering may be an anomalie in the initiation, timing, and maintenance of airflow and phonation. Schwartz (1976) describes the respiratory abnormality observed in stutterers as a primitive airway dilation reflex; a laryngospasm with complete abduction of the vocal folds is triggered by "kinks" or stoppages of the airway by the core repetitions and prolongations. Further research is needed to clarify the possible role of "glottal spasms" and aerodynamic anomalies in the onset and perpetuation of stuttering. At present the instrumentation employed by investigators in this area is impractical for diagnostic purposes; however, biofeedback (EMG) techniques may be one method of detecting the location of airflow and phonation stoppages.

We are also interested in *how much* and *what types* of avoidance behavior the client exhibits. Clinically, avoidance behavior is an important feature to deal with since it tends to reinforce and compound the stutterer's difficulty. Rather than diminishing, fears tend to incubate and grow when a person recoils from them; avoidances keep the apprehension high and the problem expanding.

Avoidance behavior may take several forms. It is useful, we feel, to identify two broad categories which we have termed *primary* and *secondary*. Primary avoidance is characterized by the speaker's attempts to alter the act of speaking per se: although evading, the individual is still utilizing oral communication as his battleground. Several types of primary avoidance may be identified:

> 1. STARTERS. Starters are words, sounds, gestures, or rituals that stutterers use to get the flow of speech initiated. Often a series of starters may become chained together in an elaborate delaying tactic.
> 2. POSTPONEMENT. Some stutterers attempt to delay the act of speaking or of uttering a specific word by utilizing periods of silence (pretending to think what they

intend to say), by ritualistic devices (licking of lips, stereotyped body movements), or with verbal stalling or filibustering.

3. RETRIALS. A retrial is another form of postponement whereby the stutterer lets the needle stick on the part of the sentence that he has uttered fluently. Some stutterers back up and repeat a sentence or phrase over and over again in a vain attempt to hurdle the barrier of a feared word.

4. CIRCUMLOCUTIONS. Some stutterers become very adept at selecting words on which they feel they will not stutter, at rearranging sentences to evade encounter with their anticipation of impending difficulty. Often this makes the individual sound stupid and silly.

5. ANTI-EXPECTANCY. In this type of avoidance, the stutterer attempts to alter the communicative context to reduce or eliminate his anticipation of difficulty. He may do this by talking in an accent, speaking in a rhythmic manner, or with over-precise articulation; he may do it by making a joke of everything, or even by singing. One stutterer told us that he usually pulled into a gas station, rolled down the window, and sang brightly, ''Fill 'er up to the brim.'' Anti-expectancy is the most malignant type of primary avoidance because it (a) produces more fluency than the other types, thus increasing the dread of stuttering, (b) lets the stutterer masquerade as a fluent speaker, and (c) tends to distort the individual's self-concept.

Secondary avoidance is characterized by reduction in or cessation of communication: the stutterer retreats from the act of talking. Although many clients manifest both primary and secondary avoidance behavior, some individuals in the more advanced stages of the disorder employ the latter almost exclusively. There are two basic types of secondary avoidance:

1. *Reducing verbal output or not talking at all*--Silence is viewed as protective, and there are some stutterers who would rather sit silently and be thought a fool than to open their mouth and betray their disorder.

2. *Depending upon others for communication*—Many stutterers have had, at one time or another, a relative or friend who talked for them and protected them from verbal demands. We have even seen a few stutterers who were almost totally dependent upon another person for communication with the outside world.

FREQUENCY OF DISFLUENCY. How often does the client stutter? After making an inventory of the specific behaviors that comprise a client's pattern of stuttering, the diagnostician will want to determine the frequency with which moments of stuttering (a global measure) and components of the block (a molecular analysis) are emitted. More specifically, the clinician seeks answers to the following four questions:

1. We like to obtain a global measure first: *on how many words did the client stutter relative to the total number of words uttered?* This procedure yields a ratio (or percentage) of stuttered words to the total number of possible words. Some workers use the syllable as the unit of measure and record the number of stuttered syllables relative to the total number of syllables uttered. Another way to obtain a frequency measure is to compute the number of moments of stuttering for a given time segment; the worker divides the number of stuttered words by the time spent talking, and obtains a simple ratio of stutterings per minute.

Some stutterers talk very slowly; a range from 130 to 250 words per minute is considered normal; Wingate (1976) suggests that 200 syllables per minute be used as a normative frame of reference if the diagnostician prefers to use syllables as the unit of measure. Although they emit very few moments of stuttering, their speech patterns are clearly abnormal. It is helpful to record the rate of each client's speech, since one index of recovery from stuttering is an increase in the number of words uttered for a given time segment.

Beginning diagnosticians may find it difficult to reliably count moments of stuttering, and we suggest they make several assessments of the same speech sample; it is also helpful to compare results with other clinicians.

2. *What is the relative rate of emission of the various components of the moment of stuttering?* A simple frequency count of moments of stuttering masks differences in the extent to which the elements of a block vary (Brutten, 1975). A moment of stuttering is, after all, a process, not a static entity, and its components—core behaviors and coping mannerisms—are probably different kinds of events. Here is a portion of a molecular analysis:

Tasks

Components	reading	conversation	total
part-word reps	/ / /	L+H / / /	11
fixations		/ / /	3
retrials		/ / /	3
lipsmacking	/ /	L+H / / / /	11
head movement		/	1
eyes closed	/	/ / / /	5

3. *Do the various components which comprise the moments of stuttering vary together in any regular manner?* Do the subelements increase or decrease simultaneously? As one component increases, do others decrease in rate of occurrence? Does there seem to be a sequential pattern of behaviors—first an eye blink, then a head movement, etc. . . . . ?

4. *Does the frequency of moments of stuttering—or its components—vary by time segments?* Does it vary by type of speaking task—reading, paraphrasing, conversation? Is there evidence of adaptation or consistency in successive reduplications of the same material?

It is important to remember that we are counting instances of behavior for specific purposes—as one measure of severity and, more important, to establish a base rate for monitoring the impact of treatment. Some workers we know carry the counting aspect to an absurd level and tend to obscure the client with all their charts.

Severity. There are several extant measures of stuttering severity (already cited), but none has achieved a high degree of precision. Clinically, in our work with adult stutterers, we prefer to use the Van Riper Severity Equation (1971: 224–225) because it includes so many of the pertinent variables:

$$S = aF + bD_1 + cD_2 + dT_1 + eT_2 + fA + gE$$

where—

F = frequency of stuttered words as a percentage of spoken words.

D_1 = average duration of a stuttering moment

D_2 = duration of the longest stuttering moment

T_1 = average tension of a stuttering moment

T_2 = amount of tension in the stuttering moment of greatest tension

A = amount of avoidance

E = amount of emotional involvement.

Van Riper includes a profile of stuttering severity which we find useful in assessment of an adult client:

Scale	Frequency	Tension-Struggle	Duration	Postponement-Avoidance
1	under 1%	none	under ½ sec.	none
2	1- 2%	rare but present	average ½ sec.	less than 5%
3	3- 5%	usual but mild	average 1 sec.	5-10%
4	6- 8%	severe	average 2 sec.	11-12%
5	9-12%	very severe	average 3 sec.	21-31%
6	13-25%	overflow to eyes and limbs	average 4 sec.	31-70%
7	More than 25%	overflow to trunk	average longer than 5 sec.	more than 70%

Any estimate of severity should include also the client's own perceptions of the magnitude of his problem. The clinician can obtain the stutterer's self-rating of severity in the interview or by administering the *Perceptions of Stuttering Inventory* (Woolf, 1967). The *PSI* is an instrument devised to assess three dimensions of stuttering behavior—struggle, avoidance, and expectation—as perceived by the stutterer; it yields a profile while the examiner can then compare to scores obtained by a reference group of stutterers.

Variation in frequency and severity. We have alluded several times to the fact that stuttering is an intermittent disorder. Variations in the frequency and severity of stuttering are of interest to the diagnostician for several reasons. There may be specific cues (sounds, words, speaking situations) associated with exacerbation or remission of stuttering, and the identification of these variables may be useful for treatment. It may be possible to commence arraying the various cues in a hierarchy desensitization; it demonstrates to the client that his disorder is subject to variation and that change is possible. Finally, by knowing what factors reduce stuttering, the clinician will be able to distinguish between temporary fluency and genuine remedial gains.

When evaluating an adult who stutters we search for evidence of several types of variability:

CYCLES OF STUTTERING. Does the individual report daily, weekly, or monthly variations in the frequency and severity of his stuttering? If so, do these swings seem to be related to personal or environmental variables? We asked five stutterers to keep careful records of the frequency and severity of their stuttering for several months, and compared the results to computerized charts of their intellectual, emotional, and physical biorhythms. Although the correlations were low, we did observe a negative relationship between frequency of stuttering and the emotional dimensions for four of the clients. See the work of Quarrington (1956) and Sheehan (1969) for information on cyclic variations in stuttering.

SITUATION-LISTENER VARIABLES. The diagnostician should review the types of speaking situations and listeners that increase or decrease the client's stuttering. This can be accomplished by interviewing the person or by having him fill out a checklist. The clinician can devise a form for recording data (simply list different speaking situations, topics of conversation, etc.) or use a published inventory (Johnson, Darley, and Spriestersbach, 1963: 288–290). The *Speech Situation Checklist* prepared by Brutten and Shoemaker (1974) is particularly useful; the client is asked to rate himself on the degree of emotional response and severity of speech disruption in fifty-one life situations. Shames and Egolf (1976: 40–41) list various circumstances (audience size, specific people, different talking situations) and suggest tactics for sampling actual speech behavior under those conditions.

In addition to listing the conditions under which stuttering is increased or reduced, the diagnostician should ask the client to rank order the items in terms of speech difficulty and emotional impact.

WORD AND SOUND FEARS. Many stutterers report that they have particular difficulty with certain words and speech sounds. We make a list of these items and then determine later, by examining the speech sample, if he does in fact stutter more on some sounds or words. During trial therapy we like to show the client how he can ameliorate his stuttering by picking his most feared word or sound; it can be a very vivid demonstration of the efficacy of treatment.

RESPONSE TO ALTERING LISTENING-SPEAKING SET. The final aspect of an assessment of variability involves a determination of the impact of altering the client's listening-speaking set. There are several ways to do this: delayed auditory feedback, masking noise, biofeedback, choral reading. We even have the client try to voluntarily suppress either moments of stuttering or particular sub-elements (avoidances, grimaces, or other mannerisms). The ease with which a client's pattern of disfluency is altered is related to prognosis: the more resistant the stuttering is to change, the less favorable the predicted outcome of treatment. Some clients are startled, and heartened, to learn that their stuttering pattern is not immutable, that they can change the way they talk.

Expectancy. Most stutterers can tell—on some level of awareness—when they are going to stutter; some can predict quite accurately when they will have difficulty, as this illustration shows:

> Joe read a passage silently, marking words on which he thought he would stutter if he read the same passage aloud; when he did read it aloud, his prediction was 93 percent accurate. He described his anticipation of stuttering in this manner: "I know I am going to have trouble getting the word out, and I feel inside like someone is going to jump on me." His posture is consonant with his report—his shoulders bend forward and sag down in a cowed, shrinking manner.

Anticipation of stuttering is unpleasant, to put it mildly, and acts as a trigger to release a chain of coping behaviors—tension, avoidance, struggle. Thus, it is important to discern a client's level of expectancy.

Efforts at self-therapy. Sometimes it is difficult, if not impossible, to distinguish between the stuttering behavior and the things the person does to help himself talk without stuttering. We have already described how the clinician makes an inventory of the core behaviors and the struggle-tension features. In this section we are concerned with the most salient methods which the client employs to "help himself talk without stuttering." Do they really help, or do they impede the flow of speech? How committed is he to these techniques as a "solution" to his difficulty? Keep in mind that all these behaviors, which we classify as self-defeating, represent his best efforts at solving the dilemma of his disfluency. They have been successful on occasion and he will resist their removal in treatment.

Post-stuttering behavior. How does the client behave after he has stuttered? Does he report feelings of guilt, hostility, embarrassment, or shame? Does he withdraw? Does he experience relief? Here is how a clinician described the post-stuttering behavior manifested by one stutterer:

> He lowers his eyelids, feigns a relaxed or indifferent posture, and may spit silently several times (as if saying, "I just stuttered, but so what, I am still cool and it does not bother me."). Covertly, however, the client reports feeling "stupid" and "inferior" after stuttering.

The facets of a complete disfluency analysis are summarized in Table 7-2.

Table 7-2 Summary of Disfluency Analysis

1. *Global description*	2. *Core behaviors* —repetitions —prolongations
3. *Struggle-tension features* —tension —tremor —release —airflow-phonation —avoidances	4. *Frequency* —molar —molecular
5. *Severity*	6. *Variability* —cycles —situation-listeners —word-sound fears —trial therapy
7. *Expectancy*	8. *Efforts at self-therapy*

9. *Post-stuttering behavior*

Evaluation of Emotional Reactions

According to several authoritative reviews of available research (Sheehan, 1970; Bloodstein, 1975; Wingate, 1976), as well as extensive clinical evidence, stutterers are not psychologically different from non-stutterers; the fluency breakdown is not symptomatic of neurosis or psychosis. Nor do stutterers as a group exhibit a "typical" personality.

We are not insinuating, however, that persons who stutter are undisturbed or emotionally quiescent about their speech problem. In fact, because oral communication is such a significant human attribute, an impairment of speech, particularly one that has no obvious overt basis and is intermittent in nature, affects a person in a very human sort of way. It is a common clinical observation that stuttering does contaminate, to varying degrees, how clients *feel* about themselves and about persons with whom they interact. Would it not be rather unusual for the individual to have no or very little emotional reaction to a disorder that disrupts his personal, occupational, educational, and social functioning? Experienced clinicians report that stutterers exhibit the same range of emotions seen in persons afflicted with other disorders that disrupt significant aspects of human functioning.

Although there is no "typical stuttering personality," there are a number of emotional reactions which are commonly observed during diagnosis and treatment. Stutterers, on the average, are not as well adjusted as non-stutterers; they have lower levels of aspiration and lower self-esteem; they tend to exhibit patterns of social withdrawal, sometimes associated with feelings of anger, resentment, shame, and fearfulness. Feelings of frustration, embarrassment, and hostility are also common. We are not impugning that stuttering is *caused* by emotional factors—except in the sense that they compound the individual's problem—but rather that they are a *consequence* of stuttering. Our position is that the clinician must recognize the importance of the negative feelings associated with stuttering and deal with them openly in diagnosis and treatment.

It is generally wise for the diagnostician to regard his observations and test scores as tentative, working assumptions. This guideline is particularly relevant when evaluating a client's emotional reactions to stuttering. Because of the sensitive and personal nature of the clinical tasks, the examiner should be aware that assembling data with respect to feelings may extend well beyond the boundaries of one or two sessions. A complete evaluation in this area includes information from five sources: the client's report; informal tests and observations; formal tests; physiological measures; and referral for psychological appraisal.

The client's report. The easiest and most direct way to determine how a person feels about something is to ask him. We find that we got better responses from clients who stutter by *leading into* questions about feelings. Instead of asking directly about how he feels—a generic question he may find difficult to answer, we commence with queries like these: What is he aware of in the process of stuttering—before, during and right after it occurs? Is he more aware of the reactions of his listeners or his own internal state? What bothers him the most about stuttering? The least? What are his major satisfactions, hopes, deprivations?

It may be easier for the client to write his responses. In this case, the diagnostician can use an inventory, such as the *Fear Survey Schedule* devised by Brutten and Shoemaker (1974); this device contains fifty-one items to which the stutterer can respond employing a five-step rating scale. Some clinicians prefer to have the stutterer prepare an autobiography or prepare a vignette in which he describes himself as if he were a character in a play. Whatever method is used, the diagnostician attempts to delineate the range of emotions, arrange them into thematic content categories, and begin the process of establishing rankings or hierarchies.

Like normal speakers, persons who stutter vary in their ability to verbally *express* their feelings. The key word is *express,* since many stutterers learn to hide their disorder, to pretend that it doesn't bother them, to wear a mask of indifference. Genuine expression of feelings is discouraged for coverup, image-making, or retreating behind a facade. Perhaps we are too harsh, but it is hard to ignore the extreme popularity of encounter groups, pop psychology fads, and telephone-listening services. It seems apparent that something is lacking in our day-to-day relationships.

The point we are making is this: strong forces augur against a person talking openly about his hopes and fears, and we may have to help the client learn to accept and express his feelings in relation to his problem of stuttering. There are several techniques for assisting the person to get in touch with himself. First, the clinician should consult the large body of information about enhancing self-awareness (Stevens, 1971). The adjustment inventories and self-inspection checklists published by Fox and Connelly (1970) and Chapman (1959) are also useful, especially when the results are analyzed in a group setting. Finally, we often ask our clients to keep daily logs of their moods in relation to their stuttering and listener reactions. This provides a body of information which is useful for counseling.

Informal tests and observation. A significant amount of information about the client's personality and emotional adjustment can be obtained by direct observation, interviews with his relatives, scrutiny of documents in his school file, and the administration of various indirect and non-standardized testing procedures. From these data, the diagnostician tries to assemble answers to the following questions:

1. What are the salient features of the client's personality? Is he basically shy, aggressive, anxious, guilty, or do other adjectives apply? How does he confront problems? Are there special features of his personality—phobias, obsessive-compulsive behavior, nervous tics, eneuresis, etc.—which may confound treatment? What are the client's major assets and liabilities?

2. How does the client perceive himself relative to his stuttering problem? That is, how salient is his problem in regard to his self-image and day-to-day functioning? We have seen some clients whose stuttering problem completely dominates their life; it dicates their occupation, their friends, even their choice of a marriage partner. There are several ways, all very limited in their scientific rigor, to gain some insight into a client's self-view: the use of free drawing (Bar, 1969), open-ended sentences (Griffith, 1969) and queries such as, "What would you do differently if you woke up in the morning and no longer stuttered?". How might the diagnostician use word association tasks or the W-A-Y (Who are you?) technique (Zelen, Sheehan and Bugental, 1954) to gain additional information?

3. How does the client handle the moment of stuttering? Although there are no significant personality differences between stutterers and the rest of the population, when the stutterer is struggling in a block he feels very different from everyone else:

> What is it like to stutter? Think of yourself on a highway. It's dark. You're in a hurry. No traffic. You squeeze on the gas. Suddenly, out of nowhere, directly in front of you, looms the terrifying back of a huge truck. Horror! Slam on the brakes, spin the wheel, swerve, pray. Anything to keep from colliding. The truck is the word that looms ahead of a stutterer. You can't always tell what word it will be. But suddenly you see one that could spell trouble.

Each moment of stuttering is a miniature crisis (Goraj, 1974). Fear and panic flood the person's consciousness; the autonomic nervous system is triggered into action, increasing pulse rate and blood pressure; the individual feels trapped, helpless, and disoriented. Some stutterers actually "tune out" from their surroundings temporarily.

Is there any meaning in the way a client goes about his stuttering (Crahay, 1973)? Is the act of stuttering revealing of self? Some stutterers feign bewilderment; others an uneasy amusement; some appear to whimper and moan; a few stutter in an aggressive, hostile manner, while others remain inert, frozen until the panic passes. At present, all our attempts to read the meaning of how a person "chooses" to stutter are highly speculative.

Formal tests. There are several personality inventories which purport to assess several facets of an individual's psychological adjustment. We believe that, for the most part, these inventories are of limited value in the evaluation of an adult stutterer. The *Minnesota Multiphasic Personality Inventory,* and *Bell Adjustment Inventory* and the *Eysenck Personality Inventory* are probably the most useful for clinical purposes (Ellis, 1946; Wiener, 1947; Eysenck and Eysenck, 1963).

Physiological measures. Another method of identifying emotional reactions to stuttering is to measure indices of autonomic arousal. The palmar sweat index, galvanic skin response, blood pressure and pulse rate changes, and variations in respiration are all useful if the clinician has access to the equipment.

Referral for psychological appraisal. Although very few stutterers require psychological appraisal, from time to time such a referral is indicated. (See Chapter 3 for general guidelines.) Be sure to inform the client *at the outset* of a diagnostic session that it may be necessary to look at his problem from many perspectives, including the psychological. A consultation of our clinical files revealed a number of reasons for referral of individual stutterers: conflicting information (the client says that stuttering doesn't bother him and yet restricts his life severely because of the disorder); presence of other problems (marital, academic, familial); repeated failures in professional treatment programs; and a significant amount of secondary gain (pity, excuse for failure, attention) derived from the disorder.

Appraisal of Mental Constructs

In this final section we are concerned with how the client *thinks* about his stuttering problem: what type of mental images does he have about oral communication in general and disfluent speech in particular?

To a great extent, humans process the universe and direct their behavior by reference to mental constructs or analogs of reality. Through the use of language symbols, we create cognitive models which filter or mediate between the environment and ourselves. The meaning of an experience for a person, and the intent and nature of his responses, can be understood more clearly by examining his mental images.

A person's images can be altered significantly by an anomalie. Criminals, alcoholics, and obese individuals not only *act* and *feel* different; they also come to *think* in different ways. In order to help them change their behavior, it is also necessary to modify their mental constructs. The same situation prevails in dealing with the stutterer (though we are *not* saying that stuttering is the same type of problem as obesity or alcoholism); repeated failures in oral communication creates a host of negative images which hamper his ongoing performance. He comes to believe that there are certain things he must do in order to speak, and his intentions become new obstacles. Gradually, the stutterer's self-image as a talker becomes almost totally infiltrated with these abnormal mental schema. At this point, stuttering is perpetuated because he becomes highly skilled at it:

> No wonder the stutterer keeps on exercising this skill of his. He knows how to relate to people when he stutters but they are a mystery to him when he does not (Fransella, 1972: 70).

We maintain that a form of treatment which identifies and alters cognitive components of stuttering—as well as overt speech behavior and emotional reactions—is far more effective than those which focus on only one aspect. We could cite many others, but a single example will illustrate: desensitization, a popular form of therapy for negative emotion, is far more potent when rational elements are included (Kazdin and Wilcoxon, 1976; Moleski and Tosi, 1976).

Diagnostically, we explore four dimensions of a client's mental constructs regarding stuttering: his theory about his stuttering, his attitude, his motivation, and the type of adjustments he has made to the disorder. To illustrate the scope of activity in assessment of these four dimensions, we include a memorandum prepared by a diagnostic team:

> There is, of course, a great deal of overlapping in the four areas we will explore with the client. In addition, you should have some good clinical hunches regarding the answers to the questions posed in each area on the basis of other contacts with the client. Here are some guidelines for the assessment.
>
> *The client's theory.* We are interested in his theory about the onset and nature of his stuttering because it influences his personal and social adjustment, propels him to undertake certain forms of self-therapy, and may interfere with the treatment program we devise. (Johnson, 1955: 325–334). How does he talk about his stuttering? Does the way in which he talks reflect personal responsibility for his behavior, or does he infer that stuttering is somewhere inside him, that words won't come out (Williams, 1957)? Does he confuse the consequences of stuttering—nervousness, excitement, etc.—for what causes it? Do his assumptions about his problem compound it; for example, does he worry that he is psychologically disturbed? What can be discerned about his *intent* or purpose when he uses various mannerisms during speech attempts? Does he believe he can improve? What does he think he needs to do in order to improve?
>
> *Attitude.* The client's attitude toward his disorder—a composite of both emotional and cognitive elements—is pivotal to his recovery (Guitar, 1976). To a significant extent, a stutterer's attitude about his problem may reflect attitudes of the non-stuttering population toward the disorder. A strong, unfavorable stereotype does

exist and apparently it is unaffected by exposure to stuttering (Woods and Williams, 1976); there is even evidence that speech clinicians share this negative image of stutterers (Tracy and Hood, 1976).

There are two popular inventories of a stutterer's attitude. The *Iowa Attitude Scale Toward Stuttering* (Johnson and Ammons, 1944) samples a client's reaction to questions like, "A husband who stutters should try to have his wife answer the doorbell or telephone." The respondent indicates his degree of agreement or disagreement by circling one of five scale values. If the Iowa Scale is used, look for the following things: the intensity of the client's reactions, the relationship between scale scores and his observed behavior, evidence of projection or paranoid responses, and whether his responses are equivocal.

The instrument devised by Erickson (1969) is a more objective measure of attitude. The final form of his thirty nine-item *S-Scale* evaluates the extent to which a stutterer's communication attitude deviates from those of non-stutterers. Andrews and Cutler (1974) analyzed the relationship between speech-fluency changes and attitude using a short version of the Erickson scale. They found that the subjects' attitudes did not change after they achieved fluency, and conclude that "it may be important that successful treatment requires not only that stutterers speak normally but also that they believe themselves to be as effective as normal speakers in their interaction with others." (Andrews and Cutler, 1974: 317)

Motivation. How much does the stutterer want to get better—what is he willing to sacrifice in terms of time, expense, energy, and temporary discomfort? Is he being pushed into treatment by others (fiancé, parent, employer)? Can various forms of resistance (denial, intellectualization, and so forth) be seen during the diagnostic session (Starkweather, 1974)?

To broaden the concept of motivation, use the following paradigm. Prepare a chart with three categories, *motivation, opportunity* and *capacity,* and then list as many factors as possible under each category. Try to assign a weight or priority ranking to the factors. See if you can extend upon this heuristic model:

Motivation	*Opportunity*	*Capacity*
utility of the speech change	family cooperation	personal adjustment
cost to the client	frequency of therapy	social adjustment
self-estimate regarding probability of success	distance to be traveled for therapy	severity of problem
history of achievement		
current level of aspiration	others	attitude
secondary gains derived from defective speech		general health and vitality
others		others

Adjustment to the disorder. We need to determine the degree to which the client has adjusted to the problem of stuttering. For a number of adults, stuttering becomes a way of life, a familiar means of structuring responses to his social environment. When he is uncertain or anxious about a particular situation, he can gain a measure of self-control—in the sense that the results are predictable—by returning to old habits of disfluency (Fransella, 1972). But habits are like fences: they provide a modicum of protection but limit an individual's range of freedom. We have seen stutterers who had considerable difficulty adjusting to fluency; speech without stuttering was not a facet of their personal system of mental imagery. Almost without exception, the stutterers who achieved lasting improvement in their speech also underwent significant changes in their life style.

Now, more specifically, seek answers to the following questions in the diagnostic-therapeutic sessions:

1. What does he do because he stutters? In what respects does he narrow or limit his life, his choice of roles? One client reported that he waited outside a coffee shop every morning until a particular waitress to whom he could speak freely came on duty. Another said he always ordered fish in fast-food restaurants because that is what he could say fluently.

2. How realistic is the client's view of his potential as a person if he acquires fluent speech? Many stutterers harbor a Demosthenes fantasy: if only they were fluent speakers, they could do mighty deeds. A few even seem to look at life as if it were a dress rehearsal and believe that someday they will have a chance to replay it over again. It is sometimes difficult to relinquish a dream for the demanding labor that speech therapy requires.

3. What advantages accrue to the client because he stutters? Does he use his speech problem as a ready excuse for failure? Does he use it as an excuse to get out of responsibility? To what extent is stuttering an attention-attracting device for the client? Does he use his problem as a badge or ornament?

A more formal testing technique for assessment of the cognitive dimensions of stuttering is the *Role Construct Repertory Test* (Fransella, 1972). This instrument evaluates the nature of an individual's adjustments to a disorder by tapping his responses to queries regarding social interaction, forcefulness, self sufficiency, and other aspects. The client is asked to rate himself "when he is stuttering," "when he is fluent," and "as others see me."

One final admonition: remember that most everyone's adjustment is relatively fragile; do not attempt to break through a client's protective shell too soon or too forcefully.

Prognosis

Making a prognosis of success and failure in stuttering therapy is a little like predicting next season's fashions—even though the territory to be covered has finite limits, the possible variations make precise forecasting impossible. In the past decade, we have seen over two hundred adult stutterers, and for each client we made a private prognosis about the outcome of treatment. Our accuracy is only slightly better than 50 percent, which, interestingly enough, corresponds almost exactly with our ratio of therapeutic success. Some of our most disabled clients have made startling recoveries, often despite an awesome array of negative environmental factors. On the other hand, stutterers with an impressive number of personal advantages have failed to make a significant shift in their behavior. Even more confusing, many clinicians have been startled, as we have been, when a stutterer with whom we had only minimal success later returns and, talking easily, offers his thanks for our help. [For a fascinating account of success and failure in stuttering therapy, see the Speech Foundation booklet edited by Luper (1968)] But perhaps we have overstated the dangers of prophecy in clinical work with stutterers; there are, in fact, a number of considerations which therapists find useful in predicting a client's potential for treatment.

The following is an incomplete and heuristic list of factors which help in making prognoses. The items are presented in random order, for we at present have no data that would allow us to assign weight to them.

Severity. Paradoxically, the more severe stutterers, other factors being equal (which they seldom are), seem to make better progress than do milder stutterers. Perhaps the reason is that contemporary therapy is especially designed for the more involved cases. The only way they have to go is up; they have nothing to lose but their blocks. The mild stutterers, on the other hand, do get by, and it is difficult for them to relinquish their symptoms for the dubious sanctuary of "fluent stuttering."

Motivation. You can lead a client to the therapy room, but you can't make him follow the plan of treatment. Motivation is, of course, a most significant variable in all types of therapy.

Timing. A client's motivation for treatment is often related to crucial life experiences; stutterers who have reached a critical stage and feel blocked by their disordered speech, barred from job advancement, education, or marriage, and voluntarily seek therapy have a more favorable prognosis.

Age. Adolescents, particularly between the ages of thirteen and sixteen, are especially resistant to therapy. Similarly, clients over forty tend to do poorly in treatment, probably because older individuals are more rigid, and somehow, they may have made an accommodation with stuttering.

Sex. Women seem to be more difficult to treat in stuttering therapy than men. Our own records show not a single therapeutic success with adolescent girls.

Non-stuttered speech. The more well-integrated the client's non-stuttered speech (in terms of prosody), the better the prognosis.

Type of stuttering. Predominantly repetitive stutterers make more rapid progress than do predominantly fixative stutterers; clients who feature escape reactions are easier to work with than chronic avoiders. Interiorized stutterers—especially those manifesting laryngeal blocking—are very resistant to therapy.

Attitude. The better the client's pre-treatment attitude, the more successful will be the outcome of treatment (Guitar, 1976).

Organic or neurotic concomitants. Clients presenting organic complications (sensory impairment, motor slowness) or neurotic symptoms (compulsions and conversion symptoms) require more prolonged treatment and do less well than stutterers who do not have those characteristics.

Identification. The interpersonal relationship is crucial in stuttering therapy; the stutterer and clinician must come to share a common set of values, at least regarding the solution of the fluency problem. Clients who exhibit unusual life styles tend to see participation in therapy as an act of submission.

Prior therapy. It is far worse to have tried and failed than never to have tried at all. Clients with a history of therapeutic failure have a poor prognosis.

False fluency. Sudden, dramatic fluency early in treatment—we have even seen the phenomenon in trial therapy—is a poor prognostic sign (Prins, 1976). It rarely lasts and the client is often devastated upon the return of his symptoms. A rapid "flight to health" is generally attributed to suggestion.

The stutterer's environment. The prospects for successful treatment are enhanced by a supportive environment (Tharp and Wetzel, 1969). However, be wary of relatives or friends who say, when change is discussed, "But we love him just the way he is now. We don't notice the stuttering." Secondary gains—benefits from being a stutterer—are tough therapeutic competitors. In some instances, clients with good social adjustments find it more difficult to change than persons who are socially maladjusted (Prins and Miller, 1973).

Inconsistency. Variability in the client's stuttering pattern and fluctuation in his self-concept (Van Riper, 1971) are good prognostic signs. Clients who exhibit cycles in the frequency and severity of their stuttering seem to make better progress than those who do not. Perhaps they can see the possibility for change.

Assets and liabilities. Except in cases of overcompensation, clients who have acknowledged expertise or talent in some area make better progress than individuals with an excess of liabilities.

Intensive therapy. Token treatment is worse than no treatment at all. When intensive therapy (minimal daily contact of at least one hour) is available and the client can participate in a comprehensive program, the prospects for recovery are significantly more favorable.

PROJECTS AND QUESTIONS

1. Contrast and compare the classification systems of stuttering offered in the following references; separate them into two categories: types of stuttering at *onset* and types in *adults*:

ANDREWS, G., and M. HARRIS (1964). *The Syndrome of Stuttering*. Clinics in Developmental Medicine No. 17. London: William Heinemann Books, Ltd., Pp. 31–32.

BLOODSTEIN, O. (1960a). "The Development of Stuttering: I. Changes in Nine Basic Features." *Journal of Speech and Hearing Disorders*, 25: 219–237.

————— (1960b). "The Development of Stuttering: II. Developmental Phases." *Journal of Speech and Hearing Disorders*, 25: 336–376.

————— (1961). "The Development of Stuttering: III. Theoretical and Clinical Implications." *Journal of Speech and Hearing Disorders*, 26: 67–82.

DOUGLASS, E., and B. QUARRINGTON (1952). "The Differentiation of Interiorized and Exteriorized Secondary Stuttering." *Journal of Speech and Hearing Disorders*, 17: 377–385.

EISENSON, J. (1958). "A Perseverative Theory of Stuttering." In *Stuttering: A Symposium*, ed. J. Eisenson. New York: Harper & Row, Publishers, Pp. 246–259.

FRANSELLA, F. (1969). "The Stutterer as Subject or Object?" In *Stuttering and the Conditioning Therapies*, eds. B. Gray and G. England. Monterey, Calif: Monterey Institute for Speech and Hearing.

FREUND, H. (1966). *Psychopathology and the Problems of Stuttering*. Springfield, Ill.: Charles C Thomas, Pp. 136–152.

GLASNER, P. (1962). "A Holistic Approach to the Problem of Stuttering in Young Children." In *Psychological and Psychiatric Aspects of Stuttering*, ed. D. Barbara. Springfield, Ill.: Charles C Thomas.

HUTCHINSON, J. (1975). "Aerodynamic Patterns of Stuttered Speech." In *Vocal Tract Dynamics and Dysfluency*, eds. L. Webster and L. Furst. New York: Speech and Hearing Institute, Pp. 71–110.

LEITH, W., and H. MIMS (1975). "Cultural Influences in the Development and Treatment of Stuttering: A Preliminary Report." *Journal of Speech and Hearing Disorders*, 40: 459–466.

LUCHSINGER, R., and G. ARNOLD (1965). *Voice-Speech-Language*. Belmont, Calif.: Wadsworth Publishing Company, Pp. 746–751.

PRINS, D., and E. LOHR (1972). "Behavioral Dimensions of Stuttered Speech." *Journal of Speech and Hearing Research*, 15: 61–71.

QUARRINGTON, B., and E. DOUGLASS (1960). "Audibility Avoidance in Nonvocalized Stutterers." *Journal of Speech and Hearing Disorders*, 25: 358–365.

ROBINSON, F. (1964). *Introduction to Stuttering*. Englewood Cliffs, N.J.: Prentice-Hall, Inc., Pp. 80–102.

SCHWARTZ, M. (1976). *Stuttering Solved*. J. B. Lippincott Company: Philadelphia. Pp. 69–72.

VAN RIPER, C. (1971). *The Nature of Stuttering*. Englewood Cliffs, N.J.: Prentice-Hall, Inc., Pp. 101–117, 249–264.

WYATT, G. (1969). *Language Learning and Communication Disorders in Children*. New York: The Free Press, Pp. 300–301.

2. What practical applications of delayed auditory feedback can you find in this article:

McCORMICK, B., (1975). "Therapeutic and Diagnostic Applications of DAF." *British Journal of Communication Disorders*, 10: 98–110.

3. Search through the following two books for information which may be useful for evaluating the cognitive dimension of stuttering:

GALLWEY, W. (1974). *The Inner Game of Tennis*. New York: Random House.
————. (1976). *Inner Tennis*. New York: Random House.

4. Review the following publication for information relevant to differential diagnosis of fluency disorders:

JAFFE, J., S. ANDERSON and R. RIEBER (1973). "Research and Clinical Approaches to Disorders of Speech Rate." *Journal of Communication Disorders*, 6: 225–246.

5. Investigate the types of roles that the speech handicapped play in various forms of mass media-films, television, comic strips. What impact might these role portrayals have upon the self-esteem of a stutterer?

BIBLIOGRAPHY

ADAMS, M. (1976). "Some Common Problems in the Design and Conduct of Experiments in Stuttering." *Journal of Speech and Hearing Disorders*, 41: 3–9.
———— (1977). "A Clinical Strategy for Differentiating the Normally Nonfluent Child and the Incipient Stutterer." *Journal of Fluency Disorders*, 2: 141–148.

ANDERSON, E. (1970). *Therapy for Young Stutterers*. Detroit: Wayne State University Press.

ANDREWS, G., and J. CUTLER (1974). "Stuttering Therapy: The Relationship Between Changes in Symptom Level and Attitude." *Journal of Speech and Hearing Disorders*, 39: 312–319.

————, and M. HARRIS (1964). *The Syndrome of Stuttering*. Clinics in Developmental Medicine No. 17. London: William Heinemann Medical Books, Ltd.

BAR, A. (1973). "Increasing Fluency in Young Stutterers versus Decreasing Stuttering: A Clinical Approach." *Journal of Communication Disorders*, 6: 247–258.

————, and I. JAKAB (1969). "Graphic Identification of Stuttering Episodes as Experienced by Stutterers," in *Art Interpretation and Art Therapy*, ed. I. Jakab. New York: S. Karger.

BLOODSTEIN, O. (1975). *A Handbook on Stuttering*. Chicago: National Easter Seal Society for Crippled Children and Adults.

———— (1977). "Stuttering." *Journal of Speech and Hearing Disorders*, 42: 148–151.

BOLLER, F., M. ALBERT and F. DENES (1975). "Palilalia." *British Journal of Disorders of Communication*, 10: 92–97.

BRUTTEN, E. (1975). "Stuttering: Topography, Assessment and Behavior Change Strategies," in *Stuttering: A Second Symposium*, ed. J. Eisenson. New York: Harper & Row.

———— and SHOEMAKER, D. (1974). *The Southern Illinois Behavior Check List*. Carbondale, Illinois: Southern Illinois University.

CHAPMAN, M. (1959). *Self-Inventory*. Minneapolis: Burgess.

COOPER, E. (1971). "Reflections on conceptualizing the Stuttering Therapy Process from a Single Theoretical Framework." *Journal of Speech and Hearing Disorders*, 36: 471–475.

———— (1972). "Recovery from Stuttering in a Junior and Senior High Population." *Journal of Speech and Hearing Research*, 15: 632–638.

———— (1973). "The Development of a Stuttering Chronicity Prediction Checklist: A Preliminary Report." *Journal of Speech and Hearing Disorders,* 38: 215–223.

———— (1977). "Controversies about Stuttering Therapy." *Journal of Fluency Disorders,* 2: 75–86.

CRAHAY, S. (1973). "The Emotional Meaning of Stuttering," in *Neurolinguistic Approaches to Stuttering,* ed. Y. Lebrun and R. Hoops. The Hague: Mouton.

DOUGLASS, E., and B. QUARRINGTON (1952). "The Differentiation of Interiorized and Exteriorized Secondary Stuttering." *Journal of Speech and Hearing Disorders,* 17: 377–385.

EGOLF, D., et al. (1972). "The use of Parent-Child Interaction Patterns in Therapy for Young Stutterers." *Journal of Speech and Hearing Disorders,* 37: 222–232.

————; G. SHAMES; and J. BLIND (1971). "The Combined Use of Operant Procedures and Theoretical Concepts." *Journal of Speech and Hearing Disorders,* 36: 414–421.

EISENSON, J. (1975). *Stuttering: A Second Symposium.* New York: Harper & Row.

ELLIS, A. (1946). "The Validity of Personality Questionnaires." *Psychology Bulletin,* 43: 385–440.

EMERICK, L. (1970). *Therapy for Young Stutterers.* Danville, Ill.: Interstate Printers and Publishers.

———— (1970). *With Slow and Halting Tongue.* Marquette, Mich.: Guelff.

————, and C. HAMRE (1972). *An Analysis of Stuttering.* Danville, Ill.: Interstate Printers and Publishers.

————, and A. TEIGLAND (1965). "Pediatricians and Speech Disorders." *Central States Speech Journal,* 16: 290–294.

ERICKSON, R. (1969). "Assessing Communication Attitudes Among Stutterers." *Journal of Speech and Hearing Research,* 12: 711–24.

EYSENCK, H., and S. EYSENCK (1963). *The Eysenck Personality Inventory.* London: University of London Press.

FARMER, A. (1975). "Stuttering Repetitions in Aphasic and Non-Aphasic Brain-damaged Adults." *Cortex,* 11: 391–396.

FOX, D., and E. CONNELLY (1970). *Exiting the Circle.* Houston, Tex.: University of Houston.

FRANSELLA, F. (1972). *Personal Change and Reconstruction.* London: Academic Press.

FREUND, H. (1966). *Psychopathology and the Problem of Stuttering.* Springfield, Ill.: Charles C. Thomas.

GAUTHERON, B., et al. (1973). "The Role of the Larynx in Stuttering," in *Neurolinguistic Approaches to Stuttering,* ed. Y. Lebrun and R. Hoops. The Hague: Mouton.

GAVIS, L. (1946). "Bombing Mission No. 15." *Journal of Abnormal and Social Psychology,* 41: 189–198.

GENDELMAN, E. (1977). "Confrontation in the Treatment of Stuttering." *Journal of Speech and Hearing Disorders,* 42: 85–89.

GORAJ, J. (1974). "Stuttering Therapy as Crisis Intervention." *British Journal of Communication Disorders,* 9: 57.

GOVEN, P., and VETTE, G. (1966). *A Manual for Stuttering Therapy.* Pittsburgh: Stanwix House.

GREGORY, H. (1973). *Stuttering: Differential Evaluation and Therapy.* Indianapolis: Bobbs-Merrill.

GRIFFITH, F. (1969). "Use of the Sheehan Sentence Completion Test in Speech Therapy for Stuttering." *Journal of Speech and Hearing Disorders,* 34: 342–349.

GRINKER, R., and J. SPIEGAL (1945). *War Neuroses.* Philadelphia: Blakiston Company.

GUITAR, B. (1976). "Pretreatment Factors Associated with the Outcome of Stuttering Therapy." *Journal of Speech and Hearing Research,* 19: 590–600.

HEISTAD, M. (1977). *Stuttering and Respiration*. Brandon, Vermont: Brandon Gap Publishing Co.

HOFFER, E. (1969). *Working and Thinking on the Waterfront*. New York: Perennial Library.

HUTCHINSON, J., and K. BURKE (1973) "An Investigation of the Effects of Temporal Alterations in Auditory Feedback Upon Stutterers and Clutterers." *Journal of Communication Disorders*, 6: 193–205.

———— (1975). "Aerodynamic Patterns of Stuttered Speech." in *Vocal Tract Dynamics and Dysfluency*, ed. L. Webster and L. Furst. New York: Speech and Hearing Institute.

INGHAM, R. (1975). "A Comparison of Covert and Overt Assessment Procedures in Stuttering Therapy: Outcome and Evaluation." *Journal of Speech and Hearing Research*, 18: 346–354.

————; R. MARTIN; and P. KUHL (1974). "Modification and Control of Rate of Speaking by Stutterers." *Journal of Speech and Hearing Research*, 17: 489–496.

JOHNSON, G. (1961). "Environmental Reorganization in Primary Stuttering." Unpublished manuscript.

JOHNSON, W. (1955). *Stuttering in Children and Adults*. Minneapolis: University of Minnesota Press.

———— (1959). *Toward Understanding Stuttering*. Chicago: National Easter Seal Society for Crippled Children and Adults.

————, and R. AMMONS (1944). "Studies in the Psychology of Stuttering: XVIII. The Construction and Application of a Test of Attitude Toward Stuttering." *Journal of Speech Disorders*, 9: 39–49.

————; F. DARLEY; and D. SPRIESTERSBACH (1963). *Diagnostic Methods in Speech Pathology*. New York: Harper & Row.

KASPRISIN-BURRELLI, A.; D. EGOLF; and G. SHAMES (1972). "A Comparison of Parental Verbal Behavior with Stuttering and Non-Stuttering Children." *Journal of Communication Disorders*, 5: 335–346.

KAZDIN, A., and L. WILCOXON (1976). "Systematic Desensitization and Nonspecific Treatment Effects: A Methodological Evaluation." *Psychology Bulletin*, 83: 729–758.

KLEVANS, D., and G. LYNCH (1977). "Group Training in Communication Skills for Adults Who Stutter: A Suggested Program." *Journal of Fluency Disorders*, 2: 11–20.

LASSERS, L. (1945). *Eight Keys to Normal Speech and Child Adjustment*. San Francisco: Lassers.

LEBRUN, Y., and R. HOOPS (1973). *Neurologinguistic Approaches to Stuttering*. The Hague: Mouton.

LEITH, W., and H. MIMS (1975). "Cultural Influences in the Development and Treatment of Stuttering: A Preliminary Report." *Journal of Speech and Hearing Disorders*, 40: 459–466.

LUCHSINGER, R., and G. ARNOLD (1965). *Voice-Speech-Language*. Belmont, Calif.: Wadsworth Publishing Company.

LUPER, H., ed. (1968). *Stuttering: Successes and Failures in Therapy*. Memphis, Tenn.: Speech Foundation of America.

MADISON, D., et al. (1977). "Communicative and Cognitive Deterioration in Dialysis Dementia: Two Case Studies." *Journal of Speech and Hearing Disorders*, 42: 238–243.

MANNING, W., and L RIENSCHE (1976). "Auditory Assembly Ability of Stuttering and NonStuttering Children." *Journal of Speech and Hearing Research*, 19: 777–783.

MARTYN, M.; J. SHEEHAN; and K. SLUTZ (1969). "Incidence of Stuttering and Other

Speech Disorders Among the Retarded." *American Journal of Mental Deficiency,* 74: 206–211.

MOLESKI, R., and D. TOSI (1976). "Comparative Psychotherapy: rational and emotive therapy versus systematic desensitization in the treatment of stuttering." *Journal of Consulting Psychology,* 44: 309–311.

MULDER, R. (1960). *Tangled Tongues.* Monmouth, Oreg.: Educational Materials Production.

MURPHY, A., ed. (1962). *Stuttering: Its Prevention.* Memphis, Tenn.: Speech Foundation of America.

NATION, J., and ARAM, D. (1977). *Diagnosis of Speech and Language Disorders.* St. Louis: C.V. Mosby.

NOVAK, A. (1975). "Results of the Treatment of Severe Forms of Stuttering in Adults." *Folia Phoniatrica* 27: 278–282.

PENNINGTON, R. (1955). *For Parents of a Child Beginning to Stutter.* Danville, Ill.: Interstate Printers and Publishers.

PERKINS, W. (1973). "Replacement of Stuttering with Normal Speech: I. Rationale." *Journal of Speech and Hearing Disorders,* 38: 283–294.

———, et al. (1974). "Replacement of Stuttering with Normal Speech: III. Clinical Effectiveness." *Journal of Speech and Hearing Disorders,* 39: 416–428.

PEROZZI, J. (1970). "Phonetic Skill (Sound-Mindedness) of Stuttering Children." *Journal of Communication Disorders,* 3: 207–210.

———, and L. KUNZE (1969). "Language Abilities of Stuttering Children." *Folia Phoniatrica,* 21: 386–392.

POLOW, N. (1975). *A Stuttering Manual for the Speech Therapist.* Springfield, Ill.: Charles C. Thomas.

PRINS, D. (1970). "Improvement and Regression in Stutterers following Short-term Intensive Therapy." *Journal of Speech and Hearing Disorders,* 35: 123–135.

———, and M. MILLER (1973). "Personality Improvement and Regression in Stuttering Therapy." *Journal of Speech and Hearing Research,* 16: 685–690.

QUARRINGTON, B. (1956). "Cyclical Variations in Stuttering Frequency and Severity and Some Related Forms of Variation." *Journal of Psychology,* 10: 179–183.

RIEBER, R.; S. BRESKIN; and J. JAFEE (1972). "Pause Time and Phonation Time in Suttering and Cluttering." *Journal of Psycholinguistic Research,* 1: 149–154.

———; R. BRUBAKER; and L. GELDER (1977). "The Problem of Stuttering: Theory and Therapy." *Journal of Communication Disorders,* 10: 1–206.

RILEY, G. (1972). "A Stuttering Severity Instrument for Children and Adults." *Journal of Speech and Hearing Disorders,* 37: 314–322.

ROBINSON, F. (1960). *Children Who Stutter.* Oxford, Ohio: Miami University Press.

RYAN, B. (1969). *Behavior Modification Techniques with School Age Children Who Stutter.* Tulare County, Calif.: Scicon School.

SANDER, E. (1959). "Counseling Parents of Stuttering Children." *Journal of Speech and Hearing Disorders,* 24: 262–271.

SAVAGE, A. (1970). *Straight Talk: A Manual for Use by Therapists in Working with Elementary School Age Stutterers.* Pittsburgh: Stanwix House.

SCHUELL, H. (1949). "Working with Parents of Stuttering Children." *Journal of Speech and Hearing Disorders,* 14: 251–254.

SCHWARTZ, M. (1974). "The Core of the Stuttering Block." *Journal of Speech and Hearing Disorders,* 39: 169–177.

——— (1976). *Stuttering Solved.* Philadelphia: J. B. Lippincott Co.

SHAMES, G., and D. EGOLF (1976). *Operant Conditioning and the Management of Stuttering.* Englewood Cliffs, N.J.: Prentice-Hall, Inc.

SHEARER, W., and J. WILLIAMS (1965). "Self-Recovery from Stuttering." *Journal of Speech and Hearing Disorders,* 30: 288–290.

SHEEHAN, J. (1969). "Cyclic Variation in Stuttering." *Journal of Abnormal Psychology,* 74: 452–453.

——— (1970). *Stuttering: Research and Therapy.* New York: Harper & Row.

———, and M. MARTYN (1970). "Stuttering and Its Disappearance." *Journal of Speech and Hearing Research,* 13: 279–289.

———; M. MARTYN; and K. KILBURN (1968). "Speech Disorders in Retardation." *American Journal of Mental Deficiency,* 73: 251–256.

SILVERMAN, E. (1972). "Generality of Disfluency Data Collected from Preschoolers." *Journal of Speech and Hearing Research,* 15: 84–91.

SILVERMAN, F. (1970). "Concern of Elementary-School Stutterers about Their Stuttering." *Journal of Speech and Hearing Disorders,* 35: 361–363.

——— (1974). *Bibliography of Literature Pertaining to Stuttering in Elementary School Children: Tentative Edition.* Milwaukee: Marquette University.

———, and D. WILLIAMS (1972). "Prediction of Stuttering by School Age Stutterers." *Journal of Speech and Hearing Research,* 15: 189–193.

SIMPSON, B. (1966). *Stuttering Therapy: A Guide for the Speech Clinician.* Danville, Ill.: Interstate Printers and Publishers.

STARKWEATHER, C. W. (1972). *Stuttering: An Acount of Intensive Demonstrative Therapy.* Memphis, Tenn.: Speech Foundation of America.

STARKWEATHER, W. (1974). *Therapy for Stutterers* Memphis, Tenn.: Speech Foundation of America.

STENNETT, N. (1967). *A Workbook for Stuttering.* Chicago: King Company.

STEVENS, J. (1971). *Awareness: Exploring, Experiencing, Experimenting.* Moab, Utah: Real People Press.

THARP, R., and R. WETZEL (1969). *Behavior Modication in the Natural Environment.* New York: Academic Press.

TRACY, K., and S. HOOD (1976). "An Investigation of Responses from Speech Clinicians and Lay Public to the Concept 'Typical Adult Stutterer'." *Ohio Journal of Speech and Hearing,* 12: 58–68.

VAN RIPER, C. (1971). *The Nature of Stuttering.* Englewood Cliffs, N.J.: Prentice-Hall, Inc.

——— (1963). *Speech Correction: Principles and Methods.* Englewood Cliffs, N.J.: Prentice-Hall, Inc.

——— (1961). *Your Child's Speech Problems.* New York: Harper & Row.

———, ed. (1964). *Treatment of the Young Stutterer in the School.* Memphis, Tenn.: Speech Foundation of America.

——— (1973). *The Treatment of Stuttering.* Englewood Cliffs, N.J.: Prentice-Hall, Inc.

———, and L. GRUBER (1957). *A Casebook in Stuttering.* New York: Harper & Row.

VIOLON, A. (1973). "In Regard to a Case of Stuttering in the Child: Methodologic and Therapeutic Aspects." in *Neurolinguistic Approaches to Stuttering,* ed. Y. Lebrun and R. Hoops. The Hague: Mouton.

WALLE, E. (1974). *The Prevention of Stuttering: I. Identifying the Danger Signs.* (a film) Memphis, Tenn.: Speech Foundation of America.

——— (1975). *The Prevention of Stuttering: II. Parent Counseling and Elimination of the Problem.* (a film) Memphis, Tenn.: Speech Foundation of America.

——— (1977). *The Prevention of Stuttering: III. SSStuttering and Your Child. Is it Me? Is it You.* (a film) Memphis, Tenn.: Speech Foundation of America.

WEBSTER, L., and L. FURST (1975). *Vocal Tract Dynamics and Dysfluency.* New York: Speech and Hearing Institute.

WEBSTER, R. (1977). "Concepts and Theory in Stuttering: An Insufficiency of Empiricism." *Journal of Communication Disorders,* 10: 65–71.

WEISS, D. (1964). *Cluttering.* Englewood Cliffs, N.J.: Prentice-Hall, Inc.

WIENER, D. (1947). "Individual and Group Forms of The Minnesota Multiphasic Personality Inventory." *Journal of Consulting Psychology,* 11: 104–106.

WILLIAMS, A., and C. MARKS (1972). "A Comparative Analysis of the ITPA and PPVT Performance of Young Stutterers." *Journal of Speech and Hearing Research,* 15: 323–329.

WILLIAMS, D. (1957). "A Point of View about Stuttering." *Journal of Speech and Hearing Disorders,* 22: 390–397.

———— (1971). "Stuttering Therapy for Children." in *Handbook of Speech Pathology,* ed. L. Travis. New York: Appleton-Century-Crofts.

———— (1974). "Evaluation." in *Therapy for Stutterers,* ed. C. Starkweather. Memphis, Tenn.: Speech Foundation of America.

WILLIS, B., ed. (1965). *A Speech Therapy Workbook for the Child Who Stutters.* Chicago: Board of Education.

WINGATE, M. (1964). "Recovery from Stuttering." *Journal of Speech and Hearing Disorders,* 29: 312–321.

———— (1976). *Stuttering: Theory and Development.* New York: Irvington Publishers, Inc.

WOODS, C., and D. WILLIAMS (1976). "Traits Attributed to Stuttering and Normally Fluent Males." *Journal of Speech and Hearing Research,* 19: 267–279.

WOOLF, G. (1967). "The Assessment of Stuttering as Struggle, Avoidance, and Expectancy." *British Journal of Disorders of Communication,* 2: 158–171.

WYATT, E. (1969). *Language Learning and Communication Disorders in Children.* New York: The Free Press.

ZELEN, S.; J. SHEEHAN; and J. BUGENTAL (1954). "Self-Perception in Stuttering." *Journal of Clinical Psychology,* 10: 70–72.

8

The Assessment
Of Aphasia in Adults

Aphasia is the most common order of communication resulting from brain injury. The adult client with aphasia does not have a *speech* problem, but rather a more basic interference with his comprehension and use of *language*. The linguistic code, the substance of messages shared interpersonally, is deficient. Aphasia, then, is a disturbance in the very attribute that is so uniquely human, a person's ability to symbolize. More specifically, aphasia is a syndrome of language impairment resulting from destruction of cortical tissue, and is characterized by one or more of the following symptoms:

1. Disturbance in receiving and decoding symbolic materials via auditory, visual, or tactile channels. Although the individual can still hear and see, he has difficulty deciphering the learned associations of messages.
2. Disturbance in central processes of meaning, word selection, and message formulation.
3. Disturbance in expressing symbolic materials by means of speech, writing, or gesture.

Rarely is a client totally impaired in the use of language, and hence the term *dysphasia* may be more appropriate. Indeed, there is a rather wide range of disturbance extending from the mild impairment suffered by former President Eisenhower (1965) to the almost total loss of language described by McBride (1969). In keeping with traditional writing, however, we shall use the term aphasia to refer to this total range of impairment.

It is important to remember that the impoverishment of language observed in aphasia is not due to loss of mental capacity, impairment of sensory organs, or paralysis of the speech apparatus. Aphasia is not, however, simply a loss of words. It can generally be shown clinically—by the use of open-end sentences, oral opposites, or other forms of cueing—that even severe aphasics are capable of uttering words. The problem seems to be in *retrieving* words—that is, translating internal idiosyncratic symbols into conventional language forms. The more common a word, the more probable that it will be retained. For example, an aphasic may understand or use the words "kiss" or "rain" but not "osculation" or "precipitation," even though all four might have been in his premorbid vocabulary. Words more frequently used, such as special occupational vocabulary items, have a greater number of associations and hence greater probability of recognition or recall.

In addition to the language impairment, the individual may also have difficulty in the mechanical production of speech sounds due to paralysis or weakness of the oral area. This is termed *dysarthria*. Another curious disorder, *apraxia*, is sometimes associated with aphasia: it is a disturbance in voluntary muscle control, but without paralysis or weakness; although the individual may have no difficulty with reflexive or vegetative functions, he may exhibit partial or complete inability to execute the purposeful sequence of movements involved in speaking. For example, the client may be observed to lick his lips while eating an ice cream cone, but be unable to duplicate the act upon command. At present it is uncertain whether apraxia is a language-dependent disorder or simply a disturbance of skilled movements (Ettlinger, 1969; Atens, Johns, and Darley, 1971).

Early students of aphasia concerned themselves with an elaborate taxonomy based upon symptomatology. There was a compulsion to name and classify every possible phenomenon, even to the last anosmia. A host of isolated subtypes of aphasia disturbance was identified, accorded an appropriately obscure Latin or Greek term, and localized to specific sites on the cortex (Kerteiz, 1977). In our judgment, the many classifications and recategorizations tend to confuse rather than clarify. At any rate, despite the different terms employed, the various classification systems are essentially alike (Eisenson, 1971).

More recently, theoretical models have been devised (Schuell, Jenkins, and Jimenez-Pabon, 1964; Wepman et al., 1960; Osgood and Miron, 1963) to account for the linguistic, neurological, and behavioral manifestations of brain injury. Although there is some controversy as to whether the language disturbance in aphasia is uni- or multidimensional (Jones and Wepman, 1961; Schuell and Jenkins, 1962), careful clinical assessment of patients fails to reveal subtypes with isolated linguistic deficits (Smith, 1971); in fact, aphasics typically show some degree of disturbance in all areas of language usage. Aphasia is a multi-modality language impairment. For additional information about the nature of aphasia, see the work of Keenan (1968) and others (Goodglass and Kaplan, 1972; Halpern, 1972; Sarno, 1972; Brookshire, 1973; Eisenson, 1973; Sarno, 1974; Sies, 1974; Jenkins et al., 1975; Darley, 1977).

When evaluating aphasic clients, we prefer to simply describe what the client can and cannot do with respect to language. Instead of using esoteric labels, the clinician can delineate the client's ability to talk, listen, read, and write. However, the diagnostician should be familiar with the traditional terminology, for it is used by members of the medical and paramedical professions.

In our zeal to identify the psycholinguistic dimensions of aphasia, it is possible to forget that brain injury is a grave health problem. The individual has suffered a major life crisis which has profound medical, psychological, and social consequences. In addition to the language impairment, the client may present paralysis or paresis of the extremities (generally the right side, sometimes including the face), sensory abnormalities, and behavioral disturbances. There seems to be little, if any, relationship between these difficulties and the extent of the language impairment. Above all, the diagnostician must remember that aphasia is both a personal catastrophe and a family crisis, as Buck (1968) so eloquently points out.

DIFFERENTIAL DIAGNOSIS

The clinician is called upon occasionally to distinguish between aphasia and a number of other conditions involving abnormality in language. We include below a brief discussion of five disorders that might be confused with aphasia; laymen frequently misidentify aphasia as one of the first three listed, often with harmful consequences for the client. However, it should be kept in mind that impairment of symbolic functioning can coexist with any of these anomalies.

Mental Retardation

The most frequent interpretation of aphasia by laymen, in our clinical experience, is that the patient has become hopelessly retarded. Because of the stigma of brain damage, even educated persons have told friends or colleagues that their spouse has suffered a heart attack, rather than a stroke. Consider the impact of these impressions upon the aphasic:

Mr. Vernon Nelson, a forty-three-year-old former teamster and self-educated amateur archeologist, resided in a grim nursing home surrounded by old people. Following a stroke almost a year before our consultation, his relatives insisted upon aamitting him, claiming that he was senile and incapable of handling his affairs. Like many aphasics, Mr. Nelson on superficial observation, did seem infantile; he lacked expressive language; he cried easily and appeared apathetic and withdrawn. He used one phrase over and over again: "I can't think." He, too, was convinced of his mental incapacity. On testing, we found that he indeed could think; he scored in the 90th percentile on a test of recognition vocabulary and showed good auditory comprehension for short, simple messages. It took a great deal of supportive counseling and demonstration therapy before he agreed to enter treatment; but once he did, Mr. Nelson made excellent progress. He later took a seasonal position as a receptionist in a local museum that featured an extensive collection of American Indian lore.

It is sobering to speculate how many untested and untreated aphasic individuals are languishing in nursing homes or occupying some dim corner in private residences on the mistaken premise that they are mentally defective.

Although persons afflicted with senile dementia may also have a language disorder, their behavior patterns are distinct from aphasics: they are inattentive to their environment, do poorly on nonlanguage tasks, and may show profound personality changes.

Psychosis

Although it is rather easy for the professional to distinguish aphasia from psychosis, it is understandable why laymen are often confused. The aphasic may say "yes" when he means "no," use obscenities and other antisocial language or gestures freely, laugh or cry often, lapse into euphoria, deny his symptoms, or withdraw into severe depression and despair. The distinguishing features of psychosis are, however, rather obvious: severe personality decomposition—not just frustration or emotional overflow when trying to comprehend or speak—and distortion of, or loss of contact with, reality. The vast majority of aphasic patients do not show evidence of mental deterioration or gross disturbances in processing reality. Additionally, the aphasic generally will try hard to communicate with others, while for the psychotic interpersonal contact is irrelevant.

Considering all the frustrations aphasics encounter, we have often wondered why they do not behave in a more abnormal manner than they do. Indeed, their demeanor and social interaction, aside from the language impairment, are remarkably normal. Nevertheless, some individuals with aphasia do experience psychotic episodes, particularly periods of severe depression (See Hodgins 1964 for a personal account of an involutional depression following aphasia).

Paralysis of Tongue or Vocal Folds

Many relatives assume that the patient's language impairment stems from paralysis of the tongue or larynx. Even trained and experienced nurses will hand a pen to the adult aphasic and request that he write the message he cannot utter. Aphasia is a *breakdown of symbolic functioning*—the content (language) of messages is disturbed regardless of the modality attempted—while individuals with dysarthria or laryngeal paralysis present a disturbance in the mechanical production (speech) of language forms. Some clients will, of course, have difficulty with both aspects following a stroke or other type of brain injury.

Voluntary or Hysterical Mutism

The clinician will see a certain number of persons who feign an inability to talk when no organic impairment exists, or who exaggerate a problem that does exist. A few individuals may be trying to work out a psychological conflict by unconsciously embracing speechlessness. This is called a conversion neurosis. Three features distinguish nonorganic mutism from aphasia. First, an aphasic almost always has difficulty with comprehending; the hysterically mute will generally understand everything said to him, even complex instructions. Secondly, the brain damaged patient will exhibit concern over his language barrier; the psychologically disturbed individual, on the other hand, doesn't seem to mind his inability to talk because his "impairment" is a solution to his anxiety. Finally, the hysterically mute will be too silent, too speechless. Even profoundly impaired aphasics exhibit some automatic speech such as swearing, counting, and ritual social language; many respond to open-ended statements ("The flag is red, white, and ————"), and some can even repeat words after the examiner.

Language Confusion

Persons suffering generalized brain damage manifest language aberrations which, on cursory appraisal, might be confused with aphasia:

> Delver Lespi, age fifty-seven, was referred to us for evaluation in a veterans' hospital. His medical record revealed a diagnosis of multiple brain lesions (lead inhalation), bilateral weakness of the lower extremities, and disorientation. When we examined him, Mr. Lespi was confused and disoriented. Although his message was inappropriate to the situation, his sentence structure was normal. He frequently interrupted the testing situation to relate, in a rambling, fragmented manner, some tale of his early years as a lumberman. In general, his responses were slow, occasionally bizarre; at times he would begin to answer a query, stop, stare into space, and then lapse into a one-sided conversation with someone from his past.

Additional material on the differential diagnosis of aphasia may be found in Darley (1964) and others (Williams, 1970; Halpern, Darley, and Brown, 1973; Jenkins et al., 1975; Groher, 1977). For material regarding right hemispheric and bilateral brain lesions see Project 1.

INCIDENCE AND ETIOLOGY

Aphasia is always caused by damage to the brain. Brain damage, however, will not *always* result in aphasia. Automobile accidents in which head injury is incurred, infectious diseases (such as meningitis), tumors, or certain degenerative diseases are all possible sources of cortical damage and aphasia. The most frequent cause of aphasia, however, is a disturbance of the blood supply to the brain, commonly called a stroke. The cerebral vascular accident (CVA) is a relatively common illness that affects approximately a million persons each year. In the United States, stroke now stands in third place as a cause of death, outdistanced only by heart disease and cancer. No one knows precisely how many surviving stroke victims are left with language impairment; estimates suggest at least a quarter of a million or more individuals present some degree of aphasia that warrants treatment.

Information regarding the etiology of aphasia may be found in the following sources: Buchanan, 1957; Netter, 1958; Page et al., 1961; Grinker and Sahs, 1966; Chusid and McDonald, 1967; Vick, 1976; Adams and Victor, 1977.

CASE EXAMPLE

In order to portray the nature and scope of the clinician's involvement in the evaluation of adults with language impairment, we now present an extensive case example. The account is chronological and delineates our role from the moment we were first alerted by the physician until a treatment plan was devised.

A comprehensive evaluation of an adult aphasic includes several clinical tasks: 1) a review of pertinent medical information and the sequence of events leading up to the referral; 2) a preliminary interview with the client's spouse or other close relative; 3) a case history, including information about the impact of brain injury upon the client; 4) an inventory of the client's language performance; and 5) observation and related testing—oral peripheral examination, hearing test, a vocabulary measure, and, if indicated, specific assessment of speech fluency and auditory abilities.

Prologue

A series of events transpired prior to our entry into the case, and the following account was pieced together only after we began to work with the client—from limited fragments Mr. Tenhave could tell us, descriptions offered by his wife, and hospital records. Compare the following account with those by Hodgins (1964), Whitehouse (1968), Moss (1972) and Wulf (1973).

> Roy Tenhave arose abruptly at 11:30 P.M. soon after retiring, muttering something about an idea he must write down or he would surely forget it. His wife, familiar with her husband's late flashes of insight, turned over and dozed. Padding through the darkened house and into his study, Mr. Tenhave noticed that his right leg was somewhat stiff and felt a tingling and creeping numbness as if his limb were going to sleep. Turning on his desk lamp, he found his notebook and selected a pencil. Mr. Tenhave had been working on a manuscript dealing with bird migration in Upper Michigan, and just as he was drifting off to sleep, he had suddenly divined a novel way to illustrate flight routes. (Later, Mr. Tenhave could not recall the idea; that page of his notebook contained only an illegible scrawl.) As he bent over his desk and started to write, he felt dizzy and watched in curious fascination as the pencil slid

slowly out of his hand. Then the room became a fuzzy blur, and he felt himself cascade over the swivel chair and crash to the floor in a grotesque heap. "This is silly," he thought; as he was struggling to arise, he discovered that his right arm and leg stubbornly refused to function. After several unsuccessful attempts to get up, he called for his wife—at least, he meant to call—but all he heard was a strange vowel sound, almost like an animal bleating. In that instant, Mr. Tenhave knew what was happening to him: he was having a stroke. Mrs. Tenhave immediately summoned the city ambulance and alerted her husband's physician, Dr. Roger Wilson, a specialist in internal medicine. In the emergency room, the resident physician worked swiftly to insure the patient could breathe easily, carefully measured his blood pressure, and administered antibiotics.

Early Intervention

We entered the case five days later, on January 25, when Dr. Wilson's nurse called and requested consultation. A note from Dr. Wilson followed:

Roy Tenhave, fifty-two-year-old high-school biology teacher, suffered a moderately severe CVA on January 19. Left cerebral hemisphere, clinically diagnosed as thromotic. Right hemiplegia: the leg is responding to physical therapy but, though it is early yet, the arm is doubtful. He may also have a visual field cut on the right—his responses are inconsistent. A neurological workup is being done, and the results will be in his record when you get to the hospital. He is having a great deal of difficulty communicating. I talked briefly with his wife, but she needs more information about aphasia.

We cannot overemphasize the critical importance of early intervention in the clinical management of aphasic clients; this position becomes obvious when we consider the broader definition of aphasia as a personal and family catastrophe (Buck, 1968). A little bit of early support and counseling is much more effective than a great deal of help later. By prompt involvement, we do not necessarily mean initiating language therapy, although if accomplished indirectly in the form of general stimulation, it is certainly a wise recommendation. Rather, we refer to the following: (1) Nurses and others who work with the patient should receive inservice training. Hospitals in smaller, isolated communities are not geneally equipped or staffed to deal adequately with aphasic patients during the primary stage of recovery (Twamley and Emerick, 1970). (2) There should be information-sharing and planning conferences with professional team members —the physician, physical therapist, occupational therapist, social worker, and others concerned with the rehabilitation of the patient. Consult the work of Leutenegger (1975) and Haynes and Greenberg (1976) for useful material for in-service training. (3) Supportive monologue interviews with the aphasic patient should be conducted to provide release of feelings and to reassure him that a professional worker is concerned and attempting to do something about his language problem. (4) Finally, family counseling is most important: The maintenance of a supportive, non-threatening environment for the brain-injured patient is crucial to his recovery.

In order to adequately understand the aphasic patient, it is necessary to understand something about the people close to him, their prior relationships with him, their present fears and reactions, and their hopes for the future. Families are confronted with a crisis when an adult member is suddenly afflicted with a deadly, often mysterious illness that results in such profound physical and psychological alterations. A serious illness disrupts communication patterns, dissolves or shifts roles, and forces family members to assume unfamiliar responsibilities. The resolution of the crisis situation, the manner in which members reorganize the family structure, will have profound implications for the patient and the prospects for his rehabilitation. (Taylor and Myers, 1952). See Project 2.

As we planned our initial counseling session with Mrs. Tenhave, we reviewed the many difficulties with which the family of an aphasic must cope—often, unfortunately, without professional guidance (Derman and Manaster, 1967; Porter and Dabul, 1977):

> In terms of life-cycle, at what stage is the family? Are there young or adolescent children? Is it a middle-aged couple, now alone and with leisure and peak earning power? What premorbid marital problems existed? Will they be exacerbated or will the family unit draw more closely together to meet the threat? Does the spouse have health problems? How does the family handle the fear of recurring strokes? Are there financial difficulties? Is there any guilt? How are they coping with the communication impairment? What are their impressions of the physical changes?

We arranged to meet Mrs. Tenhave in the speech clinic, assuming that she had become satiated with the aseptic atmosphere of the hospital during her prolonged vigil. On January 26, she arrived early for the interview, a petite, attractive woman in her late forties. She was well dressed and groomed but looked haggard and worn. Despite her subdued manner, however, we sensed almost immediately her basic strength of character.

We directed Mrs. Tenhave to a comfortable chair and offered her a cup of coffee. Recalling Derman and Manaster's (1967) advice that relatives of aphasics need information, reassurance, and an outlet for frustration, we invited her to tell us about her husband's illness. We began by acknowledging quietly that the past few days must have been very difficult for her. She seemed to welcome the opportunity to pour out some of her pent-up thoughts and fears:

> Yes, it certainly was a shock. Roy was perfectly well and then, suddenly, he was struck down like this. At first I was terrified he was going to die; then, when I saw he was paralyzed and couldn't talk, I found myself praying that he would. That made me feel so terribly guilty—but an active life means so much to him. What will he be able to do now? If only I would have insisted that he see Dr. Wilson earlier when he had the dizzy spells and the tingling in his arm and leg; I just attributed it to arthritis and the fact that he had been working so hard on his bird migration manuscript. I feel so . . . so alone. No . . . (she raised her hand to politely reject our murmur of reassurance), I don't mean to play the little housewife in a quandary. I have taught elementary children for almost twenty years. I mean, Roy and I did so much

together—hikes, I edited all his writing, went on field trips with his students, I even went hunting with him. Now I don't know what will happen. The doctor talks about brain damage . . . but will he be normal? What can I expect? What will he be able to do? Here I am feeling sorry for myself when I should be thinking about him. He must be so upset.

At this point Mrs. Tenhave began to weep softly. We gently suggested that it was good to let the tension and uncertainty come out, that we understood how she felt, and that it was certainly normal to have the feeling she reported. When she recovered her composure, Mrs. Tenhave was full of questions:

Dr. Wilson said that Roy is aphasic. I looked that up in the dictionary and found it meant loss of power to use and understand speech. But how much can he understand? Can he write? I gave him a pencil the other day when he was trying to tell me something, and he just pointed to his right arm and shook his head. What can I do to help him? A colleague of mine at school gave me a child's first alphabet book and suggested I start teaching Roy with it. She said that it had helped her father when he had a stroke. When I tried with Roy, he threw the book and knocked over a vase of flowers. He never was a violent man. He swears so much now and cries so easily. He was always such a reserved and quiet person and now he seems so exposed. Perhaps that's why he doesn't want to see any of his colleagues or students. They come to the hospital, but I can tell Roy is terribly embarrassed. How can I make his friends understand when I don't myself?

Mrs. Tenhave had much more to say during this intial interview; we have included only a portion to show some of the concerns she reported. In many respects, she was an unusually easy respondent. Often we have had to be much more directive and reassuring with less educated and perceptive spouses. By the end of the hour, she was eager to receive the information we provided:

Aphasia is more than a disturbance in speech. It is an impairment of language that is coded and stored in the brain. When a person has a stroke, a portion of the brain dies. Initially, because of the swelling that occurs around the specific area of injury, the patient shows more disturbance in language and other respects than he will later. No one really knows how much recovery will take place spontaneously, or how long it will continue. Usually, however, spontaneous improvement occurs within the first three months after the stroke. The pamphlet I will give you at the end of our chat will explain this more fully.

I wanted to mention a bit more about language. As you know from teaching elementary children to read, language is an elaborate system of symbols. The word "cow," for example, stands for, or is used as, a shorthand way of identifying a Holstein or Hereford. It would be impossible to run out in the pasture and lead in a furry, lactating quadruped every time we wanted to use the word "cow." We use symbols, as you know, in four basic ways—talking, listening, reading, and writing. Usually an aphasic patient has difficulty in all four areas, although he generally seems to have more trouble generating language—that is, speaking and writing. So, Mr. Tenhave's reluctance to write may not just be due to his paralyzed arm. Often people think that the aphasic person seems to understand everything spoken to him. But it usually can be shown that the patient indeed cannot understand everything but rather detects certain nonverbal cues or makes some socially proved gestures that give the impression of accurate listening. As Mr. Tenhave seems to, many aphasics have some oral expression that we can call automatic speech. They may be able to count, recite letters of the alphabet (and other items occurring in a series), swear, and repeat memorized prayers and poems. It is important to remember that this language is mostly involuntary, it does not involve the conscious search for and use of words. Some patients can even imitate words uttered by others. This, too, is not true language. Most aphasics have a low threshold of frustration—and a horde of frustrations! Small wonder that they cry so frequently. What should you do when this happens? The best response is to acknowledge his feelings, let him know you understand, and then divert his attention to something else.

We advised Mrs. Tenhave to avoid the role of teacher with her husband; he needed her support and affection, not tutoring. We explained that children's books are insulting to aphasics who, even though severely retarded in language usage, retain an adult outlook. It is essential, we added, that people continue to deal with the aphasic on an adult level; it is infantilizing enough to be physically helpless, to have lost the power of speech, and to be utterly dependent upon others for satisfaction of all one's needs. Finally, we stressed the importance of maintaining lines of communication with her husband. Human contact and simulation appear to be vital deterrents to withdrawal and depression (Buck, 1968; Farrell, 1969; Knox, 1971). We concluded:

> Keep talking to him, even if the responses are negligible. In some cases, because the patient is more or less silent, the persons surrounding him cease to talk. They assume that because he does not verbalize, he does not want to hear conversation. It is obvious, of course, that no one should talk *about* Mr. Tenhave in his presence. Don't bombard him with questions that demand a response, for this will only serve to point up his lack of verbal ability and further frustrate him. Experiment with different ways to communicate with him—gestures, printed cards, anything (Eagleson, Vaughn, and Knudson, 1970). I plan to give your husband a brief screening test soon, and then we can get together again to discuss the best ways of communicating with him.

In order to further her understanding of Mr. Tenhave's problem, we loaned her a copy of a well-known pamphlet on aphasia (Taylor, 1958) and promised we would meet at a later date to discuss its contents. There are several other excellent publications written for relatives of adult patients with aphasia (Horowitz, 1962; American Heart Association, 1965; Longerich, 1955; Boone, 1961; Peterson and Olsen, 1964). The book by Griffith (1970) describes a rather complete home treatment plan.

Thinking she might need additional support, as well as an emotional outlet, we gave Mrs. Tenhave the phone number of the wife of a former patient who had recently started a discussion group for relatives of adult aphasics. The clinician can also refer relatives to a local or regional stroke club (McCormick and Williams, 1976) for information and guidance on how to deal with persons who have suffered brain injury.

The Screening Test

On January 28, we went to St. Luke's Hospital to make a preliminary appraisal of Mr. Tenhave's language problem. Although he had been in the hospital only eight days, his physical recovery, according to Dr. Wilson, had been remarkable. Mr. Tenhave now sat up in a chair twice daily for almost an hour, had regained bowel and bladder control, and seemed alert and responsive to his environment. We questioned the nurses on the floor, and they revealed that although he was still swearing and labile when he tried to communicate, he appeared to understand short, simple sentences, responded with a reliable "yes" or "no," and was using more words spontaneously. He also manifested considerable "reactive language"—words and short phrases that seemed to be prompted by the situation or a verbal stimulus but which he could not repeat voluntarily.

Checking Mr. Tenhave's medical file, we noted the neurologist's report:

> This alert, oriented adult male suffered a CVA on 1/19/70. Expressive-receptive aphasia. Right hemiplegia. Babinski sign on the right. Gross motor functioning of involved leg is returning; arm and hand are doubtful. Electroencephalography revealed a focal lesion in the left parietal-temporal region. Site of lesion confirmed by brain scan and angiography. Right side astereognosis. Right hemonymous hemianopsia.

This report told us several important things about the patient: the brain damage was apparently localized and was not widespread; the aphasia was probably not transitory since lesions in the region cited generally result in more persistent language impairment; he could not identify objects by touch when they were placed in his right hand, and he could not see in the right field of vision. This last anomaly would require that we present testing materials from the patient's left side. Information assembled by the neurologist is, of course, very useful to the clinician. In addition to the size and locale of the lesion, the nature of the injury may be pertinent diagnostically. Patients incurring traumatic brain injury often experience a different course of recovery than persons suffering vascular episodes. The clinician should be familiar with the terms and tests employed in a neurological examination—EEG, brain scan, angiography, and others. The work of Brookshire (1973) and others (Cobb, 1959; Merrit, 1970; Walshe, 1970; Jenkins, 1975; Walton, 1975) will be helpful in this regard.

Administering the screening test. An adult aphasic, especially during the primary stages of recovery, has little or no means of communication. He is, in a very real sense, isolated. Investigations in sensory deprivation have shown what a frightening and devastating experience isolation can be; in aphasia it can lead to profound depression and withdrawal as well as nonverbal habits that make subsequent therapy difficult. Therefore, by early testing, we must discover ways to establish bonds of communication with the client. In order to rapidly assess a client's language capacity, a short screening test was devised (Emerick and Coyne, 1972).[1]

This instrument is designed to swiftly evaluate a patient's language abilities prior to the administration of a more lengthy inventory. It assesses a patient's

---

[1]Shortened versions of published language inventories may be used for early screening (Eisenson, 1954; Sklar, 1963; Taylor, 1963; Wepman and Jones, 1961; Schuell, 1957; Porch, 1967.) See also the work of Orgass and Poeck (1969) and Spellacy and Spreen (1969).

communicative abilities in two broad areas, *input* (or the evaluation of stimuli from an external source) and *output,* the generation of verbal responses. Although patients change rapidly during the first month following brain injury, it is important that the workers in the helping professions have some preliminary notion of the individual's communicative abilities so they can: (1) advise relatives about the best means of communicating with the patient; (2) assist other professional workers in the management of the patient; and (3) chart the patient's progress or lack of progress during the early stages of recovery (prognostically, of course, early improvement is a good sign).

> It is not *necessary* to use a "test" at all; some clinicians prefer to rely on observation of the client in his natural environment. The *Functional Communication Profile* (Taylor, 1963) and the informal assessment tasks prepared by Ultaowska et al., (1976) are useful in providing a structure for observing the client's communicative abilities in real situations.

When I entered his room, Mr. Tenhave was sitting up in bed, looking idly out the window; his right arm lay useless in his lap. Approaching from his left side, I extended my hand and introduced myself as a speech clinician. He pointed to his paralyzed arm and shook his head in a gesture of futility. I sat down next to his bed, opened the kit of testing materials, and immediately came to the point.

> I would like to find out in what ways you are having difficulty talking and understanding. I will ask you some questions and have you look at some pictures. Some of the tasks will be simple; others will be more difficult. Just answer the best you can. Okay?

I talked slowly and distinctly, pausing often and watching carefully for any signs of confusion. Mr. Tenhave looked curiously at the testing kit, pointed to his mouth, and made a motion that seemed to say, "Let's get on with it." Testing need not be traumatic if the patient is approached in a friendly, humane, and adult manner. In fact, as Schuell, Jenkins, and Jimenez-Pabon (1964) point out, most aphasics expect that the clinician will want to determine what they can and cannot do with regard to language. We prefer not to refer to the tasks as "tests," but rather encourage the patient to explore his problem with us so we can determine where to begin helping him.

Rather than beginning directly with the items on the screening test, we decided to check Mr. Tenhave's auditory comprehension by using several verbal disparities (Snidecor, 1955). This procedure would allow him time to "tune-up" his input circuits and also permit us to check the reliablity of his "yes" and "no" responses. Keeping in mind Buck's (1968) advice that it is important to provide links with a client's former life, and remembering that Mr. Tenhave was an accomplished ornithologist, we named several real birds and some imaginary ones, and asked him to indicate which were real by nodding or answering.

We then turned to the screening kit and, starting with the input tasks (why do we begin with the input portion?), moved through the various items. The completed test protocol form is included (Figure 8.1) in order to show the type of tasks

SCREENING TEST OF APHASIA

Test Protocol

by

Lon Emerick, Ph.D.
J. Michael Coyne, M.D.

| Roy O. Tenhave | January 4, 1918 | January 28, 1970 |
| patient | date of birth | date |

I. INPUT

A. Auditory (to be answered "yes" or "no" or in some
manner of signaling affirmative and negative)

1. Disparities:

a. Is your name Mr. (use incorrect name)   "yes"
b. Are you in the hospital? "yes"--disgusted look
c. Are you 20 years old? shook head "no," smiled
d. Is this the year 19 "yes" "yes"
e. Do you take a bath in a teacup? "no," emphati-
cally, waved as if wishing to move to more
difficult tasks.

2. Commands (the patient is instructed to point to
appropriate objects and pictures after hearing a
verbal cue): Card I

a. match	+	f. bed	+
b. coin	+	g. pencil	+
c. key	+	h. knife	+	swift, certain
d. pen	+	i. chair	+	responses
e. books	+	j. hammer	+

3. Understanding multiple commands (avoid gestures
that reveal the appropriate response):

a. Put the key on the bed picked up the key--asked
for repetition
b. Put the pen on the table   +
c. Put the coin in my hand put the coin on the table
d. Put the match on the table   +

Figure 8.1 Screening Test Protocol: Mr. Tenhave.

B. Visual (matching tasks):

1. Matching identical objects (The objects--pens, keys, coins, and matches--are arrayed in random fashion on the table before the patient, and he is instructed to place like objects together.) The examiner can demonstrate if necessary.

_____+_____ _____+_____
all correct--swift
certain responses

_____+_____ _____+_____

2. Matching pictures and written words (tne patient is instructed to place the word cards on the corresponding picture): Card I, Card Series Ia

a. books	+	d. car	+	
b. pencil	+	e. bed	+	All correct
c. knife	+	f. hammer	+	

II. OUTPUT

A. Automatic speech (have the patient perform the following tasks):

1. Count from 1 to 10 _____+_____
2. Say the letters of the alphabet _stopped at "m,"_ _refused to continue_
3. Repeat the days of the week _when cued_
4. Does the patient exhibit other forms of automatic language, for example, swearing? _yes_
5. Does the patient use gestures? _points; expressive_ _gestures (wave of dismissal; shoulder shrug);_ _no complex pantomime_

B. Simple repetition (have the patient repeat after the examiner):

1. Say "methodist episcopal"   "methdist piscopal"
2. Say "ah"   +
3. Say "puh"   +   no abnormality noted
4. Say "tuh"   +
5. Say "iuh"   +
6. Say "puh-tuh-kuh" several times _____refused_____

Figure 8.1 (Cont'd)

C. Repetition of words (have the patient repeat after the examiner):

1. car   "drive"   4. paper   "write"
2. snow   "snow"   5. rake   "rake"
3. clock   "time"   6. leaves   "rake"

7. Winter is cold "it's winter" (looked out window)
8. In fall the leaves turn many colors "leaves turn . . ."
9. She had a face that launched a thousand ships "Troy!"

D. Open-end sentences (have the patient complete the sentences):

1. You pound nails with a "wood, no, no, pound . . ."
2. You chop wood with a "ah, ah, oh, shit, no, wood-- chop--axe!"
3. You read a "book"
4. When you want to stop a car you step on the "pedal"
5. Don't change horses in the middle of the "...shit"
6. Don't put all your eggs in one (no response)

E. Spontaneous speech (the patient is asked to name objects that the examiner points to about the room):

1. bed   "sleep"   4. light   "lamp"
2. table   (no response)   5. door   (no response)
3. window   "window"   6. chair   "sit"

F. Self-formulated responses: (not tested)

1. Is it good to get an education? Why or why not?
2. What is democracy?
3. What does it mean to say "one swallow doesn't make a summer?"

Comments: visual field cut; lots of struggle behavior; self-correction attempts noted. See attached report.

Figure 8.1 (Cont'd)

employed and the patient's response to them. The total test took less then ten minutes to administer, but even that brief period of concentration left Mr. Tenhave somewhat fatigued.

As I thanked him and collected my things to leave, Mr. Tenhave seemed to be upset. He pointed to the testing kit and then his mouth; his eyes glistened with tears and his chin quivered slightly. Sitting down again beside his bed, I realized my error: aphasic patients need closure like any other client. Remembering that monologue interviews are often helpful in providing an outlet for language-impaired adults (Anders and Emerick, 1963), I began to verbalize his feelings, speaking slowly and carefully:

> This is tough for you. You have words inside and you can't seem to get them out. Some people talk down or too loudly; some talk too fast and don't give you a chance to understand. It's booming and buzzing; your own language is like a foreign one. You get mad and want to fight, but your arm and your leg are holding you back. You swear and sometimes can't stop crying. But it is going to get better. I am encouraged by how you did today. Oh, sure, the tasks were simple ones, but the point is, you could do them. You recognized false bird names; you matched pictures and words; you were even able to repeat some words when I provided the model. These are all good signs, especially so soon after the stroke. I also like the way you are able to tell when you do make a mistake. I am going to talk to Dr. Wilson and arrange to come back again.

During this brief monologue, Mr. Tenhave signed, nodded, and appeared to relax considerably.

Before leaving the hospital, we wrote this short note to Dr. Wilson:

> The results of the screening test are encouraging. Mr. Tenhave has good auditory recognition (pointing to objects and pictures when named) and his comprehension for auditory materials is good within his limited auditory memory span. His listening is accurate for simple, short messages. He seems to understand more than he really does because he is alert, well oriented, and he picks out a crucial word in a sentence. He has a good supply of automatic (counting, emotional language) and reactive speech. He frequently gives associations when asked to name objects or pictures; for example, he said "pedal" for "brake." His gestures are not more complex than his verbal output. We did not ask him to write at this time, but it is my impression that his language deficit cuts across all modalities. No dysarthria was observed, although he did "simplify" complex words such as "Methodist." He is making a great many attempts at self-correction. On balance, then, I would say that he has a good prognosis.

The Case History

Language therapy for an adult aphasic has to be very personalized. Therefore, we need to know as much as possible about the individual when planning a program of treatment. What sort of person was he before the stroke? How did he meet his problems? What educational level did he achieve? What was his occupation? His avocations? What changes in his behavior, if any, have occurred following the brain injury? The style, pace, and content of therapy will be based upon the answers to these and many other questions.

Unfortunately, the aphasic patient himself is in no position to provide the kind of detailed information we seek. In some instances, official records (educational tests, military records) and personal documents (diaries, letters) are helpful. Usually, however, we must rely on the accuracy and veracity of informants who presumably are familiar with the patient. The most common method of assembling information about the language-impaired individual is a case-history form that is filled out by a spouse or other close relative. Ideally, the clinician also interviews the respondent to clarify any ambiguities in the written information and to permit additional questioning. Keep in mind, however, that a long-term marriage partner typically sees the client as less impaired than objective language testing may show (Helmick, Watamori and Palmer, 1976); Holland (1977) points out, however, that acontextual tests of language do not measure communication and the client may, in fact, perform better in a "real" setting.

> In addition to a case history, the diagnostician may wish to prepare an index that reflects the severity of the client's total disability. The clinician can choose from three published scales, *The Maryland Disability Index* (Wylie, 1964), *Communication Status Chart* (Wisconsin Division of Health, 1966) and the *Functional Life Scale* (Sarno and Sarno, 1973). We prefer the latter device since it provides a quantitative measure of the individual's ability to participate in all phases of daily activity—in the home, outside the home, and in social interaction.

On the basis of our initial contact with Mrs. Tenhave, we decided that she would be a detailed and objective reporter. We therefore gave her an aphasia case-history form and simply requested that she answer the various queries to the best of her ability. The entire form follows (see Figure 8.2).

We then had a rather detailed description of the salient aspects of Mr. Tenhave's premorbid personality, health history, and social orientation. We knew a lot about the man he had been, but what impact had this sudden illness wrought? How much change could we expect, and in what areas? Would his responses to the language impairment and physical disabilities merely be an exaggeration of earlier behavior patterns?

There are only limited answers to these questions. We suspect, however, that the nature of the illness, the treatment the patient receives, and his interpretation of both these aspects (as well as premorbid factors) are all crucial in determining the impact of the problem upon the individual. Understandably, the literature is limited in this area (see Project 3). Some workers refer to the aphasic's altered behavior patterns with handy labels, for example: "egocentricity," "catastrophic response," "concretism." It is often inferred that these nonlanguage "deviations" are a direct product of the brain damage. The designation of "organicity" then excuses the clinician from identifying any further the dynamics behind the labels.

We do not deny that many aphasics become obsessed with themselves and

General Information

Name Roy O. Tenhave   Birthdate Jan. 4, 1918   Sex M

Address 211 Radisson   Phone 226-3801

Person filling out this form Mary Tenhave (wife)
                              (name and relationship to client)

Address -----   Phone ----- Date Feb. 3, 1970

Person(s) or agency who referred you to the Clinic
                Dr. Roger Wilson

Personal and Family History

Marital status: single __ married X separated __
                 divorced __ widowed __ remarried __.

Spouse's address   Phone

Children: Names: Addresses: Ages:
          Raymond   APO San Francisco   28
                       (in Viet Nam)

Grandchildren: Number -----   Ages

Father's Name: Ogden Tenhave   Living ____   Deceased x

If deceased, give cause of death heart disease

Mother's name: Bertha Trezona Tenhave Living ___   Deceased x

If deceased, give cause of death cancer

Medical Information

Date of injury (accident, illness, stroke) January 19, 1970

What caused the injury? C.V.A.

Was the client unconscious? Yes   If yes, for how long?
       less than two hours

Was the client paralyzed? yes   Describe right arm and leg

Did the client have convulsions? no   Have they been
       controlled? _____

Does the client complain of dizziness, fainting spells,
headaches? did have several dizzy spells prior to the stroke

Figure 8.2 Aphasia Case History: Mr. Tenhave

Does the client have any visual or hearing problems?
  Myopia, corrected

Has the client been treated for other illnesses? _____
  heart condition ___ stroke ___ others Skin disorder
  (herpes zoster), kidney stones, arthritis

Name and address of physician Dr. Roger Wilson, Ishpeming,
  Michigan

Has the patient been seen for any of the following services:

	DATE	PERSON/AGENCY	ADDRESS
Speech Therapy			
Psychological counseling or testing			
Vocational counseling			
Physical Therapy	Presently	St. Luke's Hospital	Marquette
Occupational Therapy			

Speech and Language Information

Describe what the client's speech was like at the onset of
the problem couldn't say anything but "ah"

How has it changed? says some words

Check the appropriate column as it applies to the patient
now. Add comments on the right if needed to qualify the
answers.

CAN CANNOT

CAN	CANNOT		
x		Indicate meaning by gesture	some
	x	Repeat words spoken by others	
x		Use one or a few words over and over	swearing
x		Use emotional speech (swear words); (count or use other words that occur in a series, days of week, prayers)	
x		Use some words spontaneously	bird names
	x	Say short phrases	
	x	Say short sentences	
x		Follow requests and understand directions	

Figure 8.2 (Cont'd)

___	_?_	Follow radio and television speech
_?_	___	Read signs with understanding
_?_	___	Read numbers with understanding
_x_	___	Read single words
___	_x_	Read newspapers, magazines
_?_	___	Tell time
___	_x_	Copy numbers, letters
___	_x_	Write name without assistance
___	_x_	Write single words
___	_x_	Write sentences, letters
___	_x_	Do simple arithmetic
___	_x_	Personal care (dressing, shaving, etc.)
___	_x_	Handle money

How did the client react when he discovered that speech was difficult? very frustrated

What was your reaction? thought it was temporary, then concerned

What do you do when the client cannot answer or when he tries to talk? try to give him a "yes - no"

How does the client react when he cannot say what he wants to? swears; tries to use signs or gestures; scribbles with left hand

How does the client respond to personal contacts other than family members (friends, associates)? he does not seem to want to see them--or have them see him like he is.

Personal and Social Information

A. Before the injury:

Where did the client spend his childhood? Upper Peninsula, White Pine, L'Anse

Where did he go to school? L'Anse, Michigan

How far did he go in school? M.A. degree, plus extra course work

What is his occupation? biology teacher
Did he like his work? yes, very much

Figure 8.2 (Cont'd)

How long has he worked at this job? <u>24 years</u>
What other work has he done?
 <u>naturalist in summers at state parks (11 summers)</u>
    (give dates and length of time)

What is the client's native language? <u>English</u>
Does he speak any other? <u>some Finn</u>

What hobbies or special interests does he have? <u>bird</u>
 <u>study; photography; hiking and canoeing; hunting and</u>
 <u>fishing</u>

What did he like to read? <u>all types--ecology, philosophy,</u>
 <u>biographies</u>

Which television programs did he enjoy? <u>movies; news</u>
 <u>programs</u>

Did he do much writing (if so, what **kind**)? <u>yes; pamphlets,</u>
 <u>a science unit</u>

Which hand did he prefer? <u>right</u>

Describe the client's personality A. <u>Before the injury</u>:

Nervousness <u>not especially</u>

Shyness <u>basically a private person although he liked</u>
 <u>small groups</u>

Moods <u>no</u> Getting along with others <u>good</u>

Meeting problems: gave up easily ___ kept on trying <u>x</u>
other <u>he always tried to approach things rationally</u>

B. <u>After the injury</u>:

How has the client reacted to the injury? <u>very frustrated.</u>
 <u>I think he feels that his body is letting him down.</u>

What seems to bother him the most? <u>can't make himself</u>
 <u>understood</u>

What personality changes have you noted? <u>he is so</u>
 <u>emotional now</u>

What is his attitude toward speech therapy? <u>I don't know</u>

Has the physician talked to you about the client's
speech difficulty? <u>briefly</u>

Any further information which may aid in the examination?
 <u>Roy always prided himself in his ability to think and</u>
 <u>reason. He is a skilled naturalist, especially in the</u>
 <u>area of ornithology. He is an expert in bird calls,</u>
 <u>and he has written a widely used pamphlet on attracting</u>
 <u>birds. He was an excellent teacher, and his students</u>
 <u>seem to have great respect for his quiet strength and</u>
 <u>wry humor.</u>

Figure 8.2 (Cont'd)

their situation, that they often respond emotionally to even seemingly minor barriers, or that they have difficulty dealing with abstractions. However, it is our position that *an aphasic's behavior is largely a product of his drastically altered life experience, not merely a result of damaged brain cells* (Wepman, 1951). Further, we contend that if the experience of being aphasic is carefully examined, the basis for many of the so-called nonlanguage deviations becomes evident. Let us consider briefly two important interrelated factors: *isolation* and *infantilization*.

The parallels between the experience of sensory (and perceptual) deprivation and aphasia are startling. It is surprising, then, that to the best of our knowledge, the results of research dealing with subjects' responses to isolation have not been applied to the situation of the adult aphasic. Consider this sampling of findings from sensory deprivation studies (Solomon, 1961; Zubek, 1969):

1. Subjects show regression in perception and cognition to more primitive modes.
2. Subjects manifest a marked reduction in motivation.
3. Subjects tend to create internal images, experience hallucinations.
4. Subjects, after adjusting to a severely restricted environment, may exhibit severe emotional reactions to increments in sensation.

Now, consider again the aphasic patients: there is an abrupt reduction in sensory stimulation; the sensory input they do receive may be severely distorted or lack variety; their physical activity is restricted; there are prolonged periods of enforced rest in quiet, darkened rooms. Several publications that describe the recovery of adults with aphasia stress the importance of continued stimulation, especially during the primary stage of recovery.

The bland, dependent existence of the aphasic tends to be INFANTILIZING. There are at least four overlapping factors responsible:

The nature of the disorder. Aphasia generally has a very sudden onset; the individual has no chance to prepare himself for the experience. The illness destroys or alters drastically those attributes most critical to human functioning—communication, control of body functions, and physical ability. Abruptly, the person is stripped of his identity, and without identity an individual is without humanity.

Holmes and his associates (Holmes and Rahe, 1967) have prepared a scale which assigns an "impact value" to the relative amount of adjustment required to cope with life events. For example, loss of a work role is rated at 47 points; personal injury or illness, 53 points; change in eating habits, 15 points. The more life-change units a person experiences in a given period of time, the greater the impact in terms of his biological, psychological, and social functioning. Behavior patterns break down as the individual attempts to cope with the changes. According to Holmes, change—either good or bad—causes stress to a person and leaves him more susceptible to disease.

The sick role. Minor illness is a socially acceptable excuse for the tempo-rary abandonment of normal adult decorum and responsibilities. The gravely ill person, such as the aphasic adult, is exempted from all his former role require-ments and demands—work, family responsibilities, and social obligations. Since he is not responsible for his condition (although one middle-aged aphasic patient who suffered a stroke while shoveling snow, an activity forbidden by his physi-cian, was severely and continually blamed for his condition by his family), he cannot be held accountable for anything except being a "good patient." A good patient submits without question to the hospital routine and treatment program; he forfeits reliance upon his family and follows orders given by strangers; his existence is passive, and he is always in a horizontal posture; he must not complain about his lost roles or the rules of the institution. In short, many hospitalized persons manifest EPB—environment pleasing behavior.

The hospital routine. Another closely related source of regression is the hospital experience (Coser, 1956). Note the possibilities for infantilization in this vivid description of the hospital experience by Duff and Hollingshead (1968: 269):

> Between admission to and discharge from the hospital, the patients were subjected to orders of the staff. They were separated from their families. Their street clothes were shed. They were assigned beds, given numbers, and dressed in bedroom apparel. They had to permit strangers access to the most intimate parts of their bodies. Their diet was controlled, as were the hours of their days and nights, the people they saw, and the times they saw them. They were bathed, fed, and ques-tioned; they were ordered or forbidden to do specific things. *As long as they were in the hospital they were not considered self-sufficient adults.* (Italics ours.)

In some hospitals, nurses and aides are instructed to call patients by their first names, apparently to simulate personal involvement. It is ludicrous and an insult to his dignity when a fifty-two-year-old biology teacher is referred to as "Roy" by a twenty-year-old student nurse. Consider, finally, the impact upon a seriously ill and profoundly frustrated patient of the determined cheerfulness and casual bonhomie which often seem to be the main features of nurses' professional character armor. One of our colleagues who suffered a moderately severe cerebral vascular episode and has experienced a good recovery made this comment:

> Whenever I tried to find out something about myself, the nurses just smiled benignly and, using the title without an article, suggested that DOCTOR will let *us* know how everything is going. That's the worst cut of all, that dreadful hospital "we." "How are *we* today?" "How is *our* patient?" "Time for *our* bath." My wife told one nurse's aide that only the Pope and people with tape worms should use the pronoun "we." She just smiled and said that *we* were following doctors orders.

The style of interaction. But perhaps the most devastating and pervasive source of infantilization the aphasic experiences comes with the altered style of interaction—verbal and nonverbal—used with impaired individuals. Persons do not (indeed, often cannot) talk to the patient the same way they did before the language disturbance:

1. They talk more loudly, more precisely.
2. They ask simple, obvious questions.
3. They frequently answer their own queries.
4. They talk around the person to others.
5. They may talk about the person in his presence.
6. They may overrespond to his infrequent verbalizations or minor communicative successes.

Note that each instance is a typical (but even so, unfortunate) mode of communicating with a child.

Physically, the aphasic patient is often dependent upon others (Henrich and Kriegal, 1961; Smith, 1967; Dallas and Ratcliffe, 1973; Skelly, 1975; Porter and Dabul, 1977). His wife, or someone else close to him, must help him bathe, dress, perhaps even eat. It is easy to slip back into childhood when one is hovered over, insulted, and guarded.

> And I had seen so many begin to pack their lives in cotton wool, smother their impulses, hood their passions, and gradually retire from their manhood into a kind of spiritual and physical semi-invalidism. In this they are encouraged by wives and relatives, and it's such a sweet trap. Who doesn't like to be a center for concern? A kind of second childhood falls on so many men. They trade their violence for the promise of a small increase in life span. In effect, the head of the household *becomes the youngest child* (Steinbeck, 1961: 19). (Italics ours.)

But is all of this discussion relevant to the assessment of an adult aphasic patient? We think it is. Any information about the individual is important since it might bear upon the responses to the examiner and to the tests employed. What does it mean if a client fails to respond to a test item? A simple minus designation? A scoring category value of one? Rejection of the task? Fear of failure, anxiousness? Severe depression/Hostility? Auditory comprehension difficulty? Reduced auditory memory span? Perhaps a combination of any or all of these?

The point is that we must attempt to understand the person and what has happened to him as completely as possible; the more time spent in this regard, the better a diagnostician we become. Otherwise, it is dreadfully easy to be seduced by a particular diagnostic tool to the point that we come to see aphasia and the aphasic solely through a test. Indeed, if it is worth forty hours of study to acquire proficiency in scoring a patient's language responses according to a multidimensional scale (Porch, 1971), then certainly it is worth at least as much time trying to appreciate the impact of aphasia upon an individual's humanity. A patient is more than a neat array of carefully charted profiles, as significant and desirable as those measurements may be. We must not mistake *measurement* for understanding (Siegel, 1975).

Mr. Tenhave was discharged from the hospital on February 16. He wore a brace on his lower right leg and walked with the aid of a tripod cane; his right arm was held up in a sling. Each day he returned to the hospital as an outpatient for physical and occupational therapy. Although he was using some voluntary speech, including a few short phrases, his attempts to communicate were still extremely frustrating.

In order to devise a plan of treatment for Mr. Tenhave, as well as to predict the probable course and outcome of treatment, we would need a comprehensive appraisal of his present language abilities: Where is he having difficulty? Which modalities are working best? How does he make his errors? Are there discernible patterns to his errors? To answer these and other questions, we had to administer a language inventory.

The clinician has several published tests of aphasia from which to choose:

Examining for Aphasia (Eisenson, 1954)

Language Modalities Test for Aphasia (Wepman and Jones, 1961)

Minnesota Test for Differential Diagnosis of Aphasia (Schuell, 1965)

The Orzech Aphasia Evaluation (Orzech, 1966)

Aphasia Evaluation Summary (Sklar, 1966)

Porch Index of Communicative Ability (Porch, 1967)

Boston Diagnostic Aphasia Examination (Goodglass and Kaplan, 1972)

Aphasia Language Performance Scales (Keenan and Brassell, 1975)

These instruments have been reviewed by Brookshire (1973) and others (Halpern, 1972; Eisenson, 1973; Perkins, 1971; Leutenegger, 1975; Nation and Aram, 1977) and there is no need to duplicate their efforts here (see Project 4). Some diagnosticians prefer to select portions of many different tests and, in an eclectic manner, assemble a comprehensive battery. Eisenson (1971) describes the efforts of several workers from different countries to devise a composite international diagnostic instrument which hopefully would provide a common basis for understanding among aphasiologists.

Beginning clinicians often ask which aphasia inventory they should select for examining clients. We prefer not to advocate any particular instrument but instead ask the clinician to specify her purposes in testing. What does she want the test to show? If she wants to be able to predict the course of the client's recovery, the *PICA* (Porch, 1967) is the instrument of choice; if she is more interested in the site of the lesion, the *Boston Examination* (Goodglass and Kaplan, 1972) is indicated; if she wishes to identify how the client performs on basic language functions, then the *Minnesota Test* (Schuell, 1965) is the best choice. In the hands of a skilled and perceptive clinician who is thoroughly familiar with the materials, any of the tests cited above will provide a detailed description of an aphasic's language disturbance.

Most diagnosticians prefer to administer a battery of tests rather than limit themselves to one particular instrument. Each sample of a client's performance permits another glimpse of his underlying language competence. None of the extant tests—except the checklist devised by Taylor (1963)—elicits genuine communication:

> The PICA, or any other aphasia test, to the best of my knowledge makes no claim for measuring how a person communicates; it claims rather to address his or her ability to perform on a set of fairly stereotyped tasks which have only a tangential relationship to give and take of everyday communicative interaction (Holland, 1977: 307).

Several workers (Wepman, 1972; Vantreen, 1975; Bliss, Guilford and Tikofsky, 1976) advocate a method of assessment and treatment which focuses on more real language functioning; Ultaowska et al. (1976) devised a technique which samples a client's communicative ability in his natural environment.

As we pointed out in Chapter 3, a test is only a tool, a way to help the examiner make relatively precise observations of a particular client. None of the published aphasia inventories is pure, none is sacrosanct, not even the three most popular tests, the Boston, the Minnesota and the PICA.

> The PICA is perhaps the most popular tool at present for evaluating adult aphasics. It is a good test, very well-constructed and features a thorough scoring system employing a 16-step scale. The instrument allows the examiner to make precise observations and accurate predictions. It is not, however, the Holy Grail of aphasiology that some overly zealous diagnositicians impugn it to be. For example, we dislike the rigidity with which the test is used; we feel that the so-called standard procedure breaks down the client-clinician relationship, inhibits the client, and creates "noise" in his system. We agree with Keenan and Brassell, (1975: 36) that "a badly presented item is a minor error, far less important than an impersonal or mechanical response to the patient." Additionally, we find that starting the examination with the most difficult task often overwhelms the aphasic and disturbs his subsequent performance. Although we have often used the instrument, and find it extremely valuable, the PICA offers only limited information about a client's verbal ability: only four of the eighteen subtests elicit verbal behavior; only one of the four, "describing how objects are used," affords any insight into how the client talks. Finally, we don't feel that a diagnostician should abrogate his personal clinical responsibility for judgment by deferring to a test or the numerical scores it generates. Perhaps this reveals our disenchantment with the accountability fad—which has often been used as an accusation (Siegel, 1975)—but we believe it is a poor trade to lose the richness in descriptive detail for the convenience that comes to manipulation of numerical data.

Nation and Aram (1977, p. 258) state the issue succinctly: "A good diagnostician relies on the feelings that have resulted as much as on the tools that were administered."

To evaluate Mr. Tenhave, we selected an instrument of our own construction (Emerick, 1971). The Appraisal of Langage Disturbance (ALD) was developed as a product of the senior author's clinical experience with aphasic patients in Veterans' Administration hospitals, private medical settings, and an active outpatient speech-and-hearing center.

The ALD is a clinical tool designed to permit the clinician to make a systematic inventory of a patient's communicative abilities both in the modalities of input and output and the central integration processes. It enables the worker to make a careful appraisal of all possible linguistic transmission factors—gesture to oral, aural to gesture—delineated in the research of Wepman and his associates (Wepman, et al., 1960; Jones and Wepman, 1961). In this manner, the clinician receives a precise description of the patient's capacity with respect to the various pathways for stimulation and response. In addition, tasks are arranged in an ascending order of linguistic complexity within each subtest assessing input and output factors; this permits the clinician to determine not only the nature of the dysfunction but also the extent of the problem. (The several open-end items included provide additional flexibility.) The ALD also includes a unit designed to assess central language processes and a final segment for evaluating areas of functioning peripheral to symbolic language such as tactile recognition, arithmetic abilities, and the oral area (Emerick, 1971: 1).

We arranged to administer the language inventory to Mr. Tenhave at an early morning appointment when he was most alert and rested. On March 3, we met Mr. Tenhave sitting impatiently in the clinic waiting room. Ushering him into a quiet, plainly furnished office, we offered him coffee and made him comfortable at a long table. The clinician positioned himself on the patient's left side. In order to give him time to adjust to the room and the communicative situation before starting the formal testing, we engaged Mr. Tenhave in casual conversation about the weather and the visitors to his bird-feeding station. We then carefully explained the purpose of testing and provided several examples of the types of tasks to be included. Mr. Tenhave nodded that he understood and motioned eagerly toward the testing materials.

We proceeded through the ten subtests in a casual manner, pausing often, commenting about specific items, and watching carefully for signs of fatigue. At one point Mr. Tenhave objected mildly to the wording of a particular sentence, and we reinforced his criticism; if a patient can criticize the test, he will not be threatened by it. The *ALD* is carefully designed to insure initial success by having the client begin with simple items. We agree with Toubbeh (1969) that failure, especially at the beginning of the language testing, can be devastating; indeed it may inhibit the patient's ability to focus on all incoming stimuli (Brookshire, 1972).

When administering a language inventory, the diagnostician should be alert for signs of auditory processing difficulty (Brookshire, 1973; Salvatore, 1972): 1) the client may miss the first part of a message due to "slow rise time"; (2) he may, as the test proceeds, experience "noise buildup"; (3) the instructions for a task, or the task itself, may overload the capacity of his input circuits; or, (4) his auditory system may shut off intermittently.

A portion (subtest I) of the *ALD*, containing Mr. Tenhave's responses, is included in Figure 8.3 to show the kind of tasks employed and to illustrate his responses. We subscribe to the view of Goodglass and Kaplan (1972) that subtests are "windows" which allow us to peer through a glass dimly at the patient's underlying language competence. The total time consumed by testing, including the brief

1. Aural to Oral

   In this subtest the examiner provides auditory stimulation
   and the patient responds with oral language.

   A. Automatic:
      1. ask patient his name "Roy"
      2. ask patient to count to 10 (the examiner may provide
         some stimulation to get the patient started)
      3. ask patient letters of the alphabet
      4. ask patient days of the week

   B. Imitative: the patient repeats the following words
      after the examiner; listen for articulation errors.

1. cat	6. scissors
2. hair	7. do you have a match
3. paper	8. very few have freedom
4. rock	9. judge not lest thee be judged
5. leaves	10. six times six is thirty-six

   C. Symbolic:
      1. oral opposites: have the patient supply the opposite
         orally.

a. thin	d. fast
b. man	e. living
c. strong	f. anarchy nR

      2. open end sentences: have the patient finish the
         sentence orally.
         a. you sleep on a ___"bed"___
         b. the boy picked up his bat and ball and went to
            play ___"ball"___
         c. please get me a drink of ___"milk"___
         d. a bird in the hand is worth two in the _____
         e. he who hesitates is ___N.R.___

      3. definitions: have the patient supply the word orally.
         a. something to read "book"
         b. a farm animal that gives milk "cow"
         c. a white cylinder of tobacco "don't smoke"
         d. something that registers the passage of time "watch"
         e. a black drink brewed from ground beans N.R.

      4. disparities: have the patient attempt to point out
         what is wrong with the following sentences.

         a. They filled the car with catsup.
         b. He spread his bread with butter and nails.
         c. She wrote a letter with paper and peanut butter.
         d. A penny saved is a penny burned.
         e. No man is an Ireland. smiled

Figure 8.3 Subtest I of ALD Showing Mr. Tenhave's Responses.

breaks and desultory conversation, was just over seventy-four minutes. We again chatted briefly with Mr. Tenhave at the end of the formal testing; we told him that although we would need to analyze the results carefully before starting therapy, we were encouraged by his responses.

The completed ALD provides a protocol that outlines the severity of a patient's language disturbance and the areas (modalities) of impairment. The test does not yield a classification system nor does it attempt to place aphasics into various categories. We agree with Buck (1968: 85) that "too often our diagnostic labels blind us to the true state of affairs and prevent further investigation." It is far more useful clinically to simply identify what the patient can and cannot do with language symbols. The ALD, however, does provide a summary form for collating data obtained from the patient on the ten subtests. Figure 8.4 shows the completed summary form for Mr. Tenhave.

The column on the left simply lists the ten subtests. Note the five columns enumerated 1 through 5 and labeled "rating." After administering the ALD we rated Mr. Tenhave's performance on each subtest utilizing the following crude scale:

1. All, or almost all, responses correct
2. Majority of responses correct
3. Approximately half the responses correct, half incorrect
4. Majority of responses incorrect
5. All, or almost all, responses incorrect

Thus, we have a summary profile of the patient's language abilities as manifested by his responses to the ten specific subtests.

It is also important to examine *how* the patient made his errors: Did he seem to perseverate? At what level of complexity did his responses break down? Did he give synonyms or associations for words when asked to name pictures or objects? Mr. Tenhave, for example, when asked to name a picture of a dollar bill, said, "Put it . . . pocket . . . wallet . . ." Obviously, his "error" is far better than a response of "soup" or "don't know." Was the patient attempting to correct his errors (Wepman, 1958)? Are his responses significantly delayed? How did he respond to various cueing techniques (Love and Webb, 1977)? What strategy does he use to attempt to retrieve words (Marshall, 1976)?

We summarized the test findings, together with our impressions and prognosis, in a detailed report:

Client: Roy Tenhave   *Date:* March 3, 1973

Test Findings. The Appraisal for Language Disturbance was administered and revealed the following information on each of the ten subtests:

I. *Aural-Oral* (client listens, responds with oral language). The client replied swiftly and accurately on tasks calling for automatic and imitative responses. His responses to symbolic items (oral opposites, open-end sentences, definitions) appear to be limited by reduced availability of less frequently used words. Auditory com-

ALD SUMMARY FORM

Lon L. Emerick, Ph.D.
Northern Michigan University

Transmission	Rating					Comments
	1	2	3	4	5	
I. Aural-Oral		x				limited by short auditory memory span
II. Aural-Visual	x					
III. Aural-Gesture	x					
IV. Aural-Graphic				x		used writing brace; spells phonetically
V. Gesture-Visual	x					
VI. Visual-Gesture	x					
VII. Visual-Oral			x			used association
VIII. Visual-Graphic			x			

IX. Central Language
    Comprehension   Rating: 1.5
    1. Matching   1 Peabody = 95%
    2. Sorting   2
    3. Manding   1

X. Related Factors   Rating:
   1. Tactile   5
   2. Arithmetic   1
   3. Oral Exam   1 normal

Observations: 1. Errors increase as length of material
                 increases.
              2. Mispronunciations are correctable by ear.
              3. Self-correction is evident.
              4. Visual field cut seems to have improved.

Roy Tenhave	71-493	March 3, 1970	E.
Patient	Number	Date	Examiner

Figure 8.4 ALD Summary Form for Roy Tenhave.

prehension is good within the limits imposed by a reduced verbal retention span. Recognizes disparities easily.

II. *Aural to Visual* (client listens and points). Auditory recognition for objects, pictures, and simple written words is intact. Mr. Tenhave's responses were rapid and positive.

III. *Aural to Gesture* (client listens and makes appropriate gesture). The patient can follow commands (shake hand, cough) with the appropriate gesture, point to body parts when named, and demonstrate complex gestures associated with writing, using a toothbrush, and throwing a ball.

IV. *Aural to Graphic* (client listens and writes). Mr. Tenhave was reluctant initally to attempt writing with his left hand; a Zaner-Bloser writing frame was offered, and he used it to complete the tasks.[2] Automatic items (his name, age) were accomplished easily. However, his attempts to write a series of dictated letters and numbers was limited by his reduced auditory memory span; he could retain three but not four or more digits or letters. No rotation of letters or confusion between them was noted. He missed over 50 percent of the total items included in this subtest. Several short words ("bird," "lamp") were written correctly, but in general his spelling tends to be done phonetically (e.g., "blu" for "blue," "nos" for "nose").

V. *Gesture to Visual* (clinician makes a gesture, client must select appropriate object, picture, or written word associated with the gesture). He responded accurately to each test item: he watched the clinician's gestures and selected the appropriate object, picture, and printed word from a series arrayed before him.

VI. *Visual to Gesture* (examiner shows an object, picture, or written word to the patient, and the patient makes a gesture typically associated with it). All items were done swiftly and correctly.

VII. *Visual to Oral* (client is presented a visual stimulus and is requested to read or name orally). Mr. Tenhave missed almost half of the items on this subtest. His oral vocabulary is reduced, and he frequently responded with words that were associated with the stimulus (e.g., "ring" for "bell," "eat" for "spoon," "Ford" for "car"). His reading rate is very slow; he labored over the test sentences and paragraph, pausing often to reread portions. His comprehension for reading material was good, but again, it was limited by a reduced verbal retention span. No dysarthria or apraxia was noted. He tends to mispronounce or simplify longer words; however, when he is instructed to listen carefully and is given an auditory model, he corrects his errors readily.

VIII. *Visual to Graphic* (client is presented a visual stimulus and responds by copying or writing). Mr. Tenhave had considerable difficulty with this subtest, missing more than half the items. He was able to copy letters, numbers, and written words accurately. However, he was able to identify in writing only two of the ten objects and pictures presented. When shown a drawing depicting several features, he simply enumerated three items and, after a long pause, put down the marking pen in obvious disgust. (Note: at this point the testing was stopped and the examiner and client relaxed over coffee; a respite should have been given before beginning this subtest. His concentration was so intense that it was difficult to discern when he was getting fatigued. This will have to be taken into account in therapy with him.)

IX. *Central Language Comprehension* (in this subtest, the client is given various tasks—matching, sorting, object assembly, recognition vocabulary—which more directly assess the status of the client's central sorting and integrative functioning). Matching (objects to silhouettes, pictures to pictures, objects to pictures), object assembly, and manding presented no difficulty to Mr. Tenhave. He scored at the 95th

---

[2]The Zaner-Bloser Company, 612 N. Park Street, Columbus, Ohio.

percentile on the Peabody Picture Vocabulary Test (Dunn, 1958). His errors involved sorting: he arranged the circle and squares according to color initially (note: check to see if he has a type of colorblindness—he seemed to confuse green and blue. It is rather peculiar, though, for a skilled ornithologist to be colorblind) and when the request was made to recategorize them, he was unable to do so.

X. *Related Factors* (in this subtest, areas of functioning peripheral to symbolic language are examined—tactile recognition, arithmetic ability, and motor speech behavior). Tactile recognition in the right hand is totally absent; he made two errors with his left hand. Simple arithmetic problems presented no difficulty for Mr. Tenhave; he requested several repetitions of the short story problem, however, before he could successfully complete it. This reflected his reduced verbal retention span. Oral examination revealed normal functioning.[3]

Prognosis. Excellent prospects for recovery. The patient's auditory recognition is intact, and his comprehension is good; both are essential to a favorable response to therapy. Another favorable sign is Mr. Tenhave's ability to detect his errors and, when provided with an auditory model, correct them. A determined attitude augers well for his continued efforts during treatment.

The language inventory permits the clinician to identify islands of ability the client retains. In some instances, it may be necessary to do additional testing in particular areas: *speech fluency*—length of utterance, grammaticalness (see Chapey, Rigrodsky and Morrison, 1976 for a procedure using divergent semantic behavior); *reading* (using graded material); and *auditory competence*. The integrity of the auditory modality is crucial prognostically: can the client detect, localize, retain, discriminate, and sequence items he hears? Consult the work of Berry (1976) and others (Needham and Swisher, 1973; Brookshire, 1973; Duffy and Ulrich, 1976) for information regarding in-depth testing of a client's auditory abilities.

PROGNOSIS

Selecting patients for treatment who have the best chance of recovery from aphasia is an unsettling task. Rather than abandon anyone, one's impulse is to attempt to work with every aphasic even though prospects for improvement in cases of severe language impairment are dim (Sarno, Silverman, and Sands, 1970). When there is little real progress, the patient's labors are like those of Sisyphus.

How then can the clinician identify aphasic clients with the best potential? A list of interrelated factors which we have found helpful for making a prognosis is presented below; however, we trust the reader's forecasting will be guided by three important maxims: (1) do not make a final prognosis on the basis of a single evaluation session—a period of trial therapy is always highly informative; (2) do

---

[3]Before starting therapy, Mr. Tenhave was given an audiometric evaluation; his hearing was within normal limits (see studies by Street, 1957; Miller, 1960; Needham and Black, 1970).

not make a prognosis solely on the basis of a single measure of behavior—e.g., the client's performance on a language inventory; and (3) be sure you understand the value of predictors—they can be potent self-fulfilling prophecies.

1. *Auditory recognition.* Patients who make errors (even a few errors—two or three out of ten items—are significant) when identifying pictures or common objects named by the examiner have an unfavorable prognosis; an impairment at this level is apparently irreversible (Schuell, Jenkins, and Jimenez-Pabon, 1964).

2. *Comprehension.* Patients who have marked difficulty in comprehending verbal messages make poor candidates for treatment. In fact, a reliable index of the severity of language impairment in aphasia is the degree of disturbance in comprehension (Smith, 1971).

3. *Self-monitoring.* Patients who are aware of their errors and attempt to correct them have a more favorable prognosis than those who do not. See the self-correction rating scale devised by Wepman (1958).

4. *Jargon.* The presence of jargon is a poor clinical sign, especially when it is coupled with lack of self-monitoring, euphoria, or denial (Cohn and Neumann, 1958).

5. *Primary stage of recovery.* The more untoward events (infantilizing, isolation, withdrawal, exposure to negative attitudes) that occur during the first few months after the brain injury, the poorer the patient's motivation will be to undertake treatment.

6. *Time elapsed since onset.* The longer the time elapsed since onset of aphasia and the beginning of treatment, the poorer the prognosis. Habits of dependence, withdrawal, and possible secondary gains accruing from a nonverbal role tend to defeat therapeutic intervention.

7. *Family response.* Patients whose families provide supportive understanding and appropriate stimulation and permit the individual to regain his role within the family unit have a more favorable prognosis.

8. *Age.* Generally, the younger the patient the better are the prospects for recovery. Aphasics in or near retirement often lack the energy and motivation to persist in a treatment program. In addition, the older patients may have more widespread cerebral damage due to arteriosclerosis.

9. *Presence of other health problems.* In our clinical experience, aphasic patients presenting health problems in addition to the brain injury (such as diabetes, systemic vascular disease, or kidney disease) often do poorly in therapy.

10. *Premorbid personality.* The more outgoing, flexible individual generally responds better to treatment than does an inhibited, introverted person (Eisenson, 1949).

11. *Intelligence and education.* The more intelligent, better educated patients make better candidates for therapy. Although this is generally true, a few of our most highly educated clients were so vivdly aware of the discrepancy between their premorbid abilities and their present condition, they simply withdrew in futility.

12. *Extent of the lesion.* The more extensive the brain injury, the poorer the prospects for recovery.

13. *Location of the lesion.* Damage occuring posterior to the Fissure of Rolando, especially at the junction of the parietal temporal lobe, tends to result in more persistent aphasia (Penfield and Roberts, 1959).

14. *Physical disability.* We have observed good language recovery in aphasics with severe hemiplegia. Generally, however, those patients without paralysis, or with

milder forms of paresis, made swifter and more complete improvement. Although we lack sufficient data to document this relationship, many of our aphasic patients have exhibited sudden spurts of progress in language as their physical condition improved.

The student will want to consult the following references for further information regarding prognosis in aphasia: Eisenson, 1949; Bourestom, 1967; Smith, 1971; Sarno, Silverman, and Sands, 1970; Culton, 1969; Keenan and Brassell, 1974.

PROJECTS AND QUESTIONS

1. What language-related functions are subtended by the right hemisphere? Spatial relationships? Body schema? Stimulus equivalence? What characteristics identify patients with bilateral brain damage? The references listed below will provide a beginning for your search for answers to these questions.

BONKOWSKI, R. (1967). "Verbal and Extraverbal Components of Language as Related to Lateralized Brain Damage," *Journal of Speech and Hearing Research*, 10: 558–564.

BROOKSHIRE, R. (1973). *An Introduction to Aphasia*. Minneapolis, Minn.: BRK Publishers.

———, and M. LOMMEL (1974). "Perception of Sequences of Visual Temporal and Auditory Spatial Stimuli by Aphasics, right hemisphere damaged, and non-brain damaged subjects," *Journal of Communication Disorders*, 7: 155–169.

COLLINS, M. (1976). "The Minor Hemisphere." In R. Brookshire, ed. *Clinical Aphasiology*. Minneapolis, Minn.: BRK Publishers.

FAGLIONI, P., H. SPINNLER, and L. A. VIGNOLO (1969). "Contrasting Behavior of R. and L. Hemisphere Patients on a Discriminative and a Semantic Task of Auditory Recognition." *Cortex*, 5: 366–389.

HELAEN, H., and M. PIERCY (1956). "Paroxysmal Dysphasia and Problems of Cerebral Dominance." *Journal of Neurology and Neuro Surgery*, 19: 194–201.

LAPOINTE, L., and G. CULTON (1969). "Visual-Spatial Neglect Subsequent to Brain Injury." *Journal of Speech and Hearing Disorders*, 34: 82–86.

PECK, L., L. SWISHER, and M. SARNO (1969). "Token Test Scores of Three Matched Patient Groups: Left Brain-Damaged With Aphasia; Right Brain-Damaged Without Aphasia; Non Brain-Damaged." *Cortex*, 5: 264–273.

2. The family's responses to aphasia: Why do some families draw together during a serious health crisis while others tend to become fragmented? What professional workers can assist families through the crisis period? Relate the problem of aphasia to the six basic functions of the family. Why would sexual relations be disrupted by aphasia and other sequelae of brain injury? Most of the literature assumes the husband is aphasic; can you identify any differences that might occur if it were the wife? Search for the answers to these questions in the references below:

ADLER M. (1962). "Hemiplegia and the Social Structure." Ph.D. dissertation, University of Pittsburgh.

ARTES, R. (1967). "A Study of Family Problems as Identified and Evaluated by the Wives of Stroke Patients." Ph.D. dissertation, University of Iowa.

BIORN-HANSEN, V. (1957). "Social and Emotional Aspects of Aphasia." *Journal of Speech and Hearing Disorders*, 22: 53–59.

BUCK, M. *Dysphasia*. Englewood Cliffs, N.J.: Prentice-Hall, Inc., 1968.

Committee on Family Diagnosis and Treatment. *Casebook on Family Diagnosis and Treatment*. New York: Family Service Agency.

DeFOREST, R., ed. (1966). *Proceedings of the National Stroke Congress*. Springfield, Ill.: Charles C. Thomas, P. 109.

DUFF, R., and A. HOLLINGSHEAD (1968). *Sickness and Society*. New York: Harper & Row, Pp. 25–340.

GARRETT, J., and E. LEVINE (1962). *Psychological Practices with the Physically Disabled*. New York: Columbia University Press.

JACOBSON, M., and R. EICHORN (1964). "Family Response to Heart Disease in the Husband-Father." *Journal of Marriage and Family*, 26: 166–173.

MABRY, J., (1964). "Medicine and the Family." *Journal of Marriage and Family*, 26: 160–165.

MALONE, R., (1969). "Expressed Attitudes of Families of Aphasics," *Journal of Speech and Hearing Disorders*, 34: 38–41.

McDANIEL, J. (1969). *Physical Disability and Human Behavior*. New York: Pergamon Press, Pp. 146–150.

PARAD, H., ed. (1965). *Crisis Intervention: Selected Readings*. New York: Family Service Association.

SCHUELL, H., J. JENKINS, and E. JIMENEZ-PABON (1964). *Aphasia in Adults*. New York: Harper & Row, Pp. 328–331.

3. The experience of being aphasic: what can you learn about the problem of aphasia by consulting the references listed below? What impact does aphasia have upon the individual? Which is worse, denial or depression? Does the aphasic have a reduced threshold of frustration, or is he simply faced with more frustrations? What can you learn about the impact of aphasia by consulting biographies of famous stroke victims such as Louis Pasteur, Samuel Johnson, Woodrow Wilson, H. L. Mencken, Walt Whitman, R. L. Stevenson?

BAY, E. (1969). "The Lordat Case and Its Import on the Theory of Aphasia." *Cortex*, 5: 302–308.

BIXBY, L. "Comeback from a Brain Operation." *Harpers Magazine* (November, 1952), pp. 69–73.

BRODAL, A. (1973). "Self-observations and Neuro-anatomical considerations after a stroke." *Brian*, 96: 675–694.

BUCK, M. (1968). *Dysphasia*. Englewood Cliffs, N.J.: Prentice-Hall, Inc.

——— (1963). "The Language Disorders: A Personal and Professional Account of Aphasia." *Journal of Rehabilitation*, 29: 37–38.

CAMERON, C. (1973). *A Different Drum*. Englewood Cliffs, N.J.: Prentice-Hall, Inc.

DALLAS, R., and J. RATCLIFFE (1973). *The Kennedy Case*. New York: G. P. Putnam's Sons.

DIKMEN, S., and R. REITAN (1974). "Minnesota Multiphasic Personality Inventory Correlates of Dysphasic Language Disturbance." *Journal of Abnormal Psychology* 83: 673–679.

EISENHOWER, D. (1965). *Waging Peace*. New York: Doubleday & Co., Inc., pp. 227–228.

FARRELL, B. (1969). *Pat and Roald*. New York: Random House, Inc.

FRANK, S. (July, 1967). "Patricia Neal: Suddenly I Wanted to Live." *Good Housekeeping*, p. 70.

HALL, W. (1961). "Return From Silence—A Personal Experience." *Journal of Speech and Hearing Disorders,* 26: 174–77.

HENRICH, E. and L. KRIEGEL (1961). *Experiments in Survival.* New York: Association for the Aid of Crippled Children.

HODGINS, E. (1964). *Episode: Report on the Accident in My Skull.* New York: Atheneum.

HYMAN, M. (1972). "Social Psychological Determinates of Patient's Performance in Stroke Rehabilitation." *Archives of Physical Medicine and Rehabilitation,* 53: 217–226.

KNOX, D. (1971). *Portrait of Aphasia.* Detroit: Wayne State University Press.

LURIA, A. (1972). *The Man With A Shattered World.* New York: Basic Books.

MCBRIDE, C. (1969). *Silent Victory.* Chicago: Nelson-Hall.

MELVIN, J., and N. SAAD. (1970). "Factors in Behavioral Responses to Impairment." *Archives of Physical Medicine and Rehabilitation,* 51: 522–557.

MOSS, C. (1972). *Recovery With Aphasia.* Urbana, Ill.: University of Illinois Press.

RITCHIE, D. (1961). *Stroke: A Diary of Recovery.* New York: Doubleday & Co., Inc.

ROLNICK, M., and H. HOOPS. (1969). "Aphasia As Seen by the Aphasic." *Journal of Speech and Hearing Disorders,* 34: 48–53.

ROSE, R. (1948). "A Physician's Account of His Own Aphasia." *Journal of Speech and Hearing Disorders,* 13: 294–305.

SIES, L., and R. BUTLER (1963). "A Personal Account of Dysphasia." *Journal of Speech and Hearing Disorders,* 28: 216–266.

SIMENON, GEORGES (1964). *The Bells of Bicetre.* New York: Harcourt, Brace and World.

SKELLY, M. (1975). "Aphasic Patients Talk Back." *American Journal of Nursing,* 75: 1140–1142.

SOLOMON, P., et al. (1961). *Sensory Deprivation.* Cambridge, Mass.: Harvard University Press.

ULLMAN, M. (1962). *Behavioral Changes Following Stroke.* Springfield, Ill.: Charles C. Thomas.

VAN ROSEN, R. (1963). *Comeback: The Story of My Stroke.* New York: Bobbs-Merrill.

WHITEHOUSE, E. (1968). *There's Always More.* Valley Forge, Pa.: The Judson Press.

WINT, G. (1965). *The Third Killer.* New York: Abelard-Schuman.

WULF, H. (1973). *Aphasia, My World Alone.* Detroit: Wayne State University Press.

4. Various methods of scoring responses are employed in the language inventories cited in this chapter. After consulting articles by Kaplan (1959) and others (Schuell, 1966; Sarno and Sands, 1970; Porch, 1971; Davis and Leach, 1972; Cohen et al., 1977; Stachowlak et al., 1977), review the most widely used tests of aphasia in light of the questions posed below:

   a. Which tests use plus-minus scoring? What is the rationale offered for the efficacy of this method of scoring?

   b. Which tests employ rating scales? How many categories are included? What might be the ideal number of steps in a rating scale—four, eight, sixteen? What is Schuell's rationale for including both a diagnostic and a severity scale? How might the concept of Occam's razor apply to the relative complexity of rating scales?

   c. Which tests yield a numerical score to summarize the patient's responses? What is measurement? Are there levels of measurement? Do any tests of aphasia employ measurement levels more precise than nominal or ordinal? In terms of statistical procedure, is it permissible to perform arithmetical computation (adding, computing means) an ordinal data?

   d. Which tests utilize psycholinguistic units for scoring responses?

e. The manuals of most aphasia tests present reliability data regarding the scoring system. Which include information on validity?

f. Do some aphasia inventories employ greater mathematical precision than the nature of the observations warrant?

BIBLIOGRAPHY

ADAMS, R., and M. VICTOR (1977). *Principles of Neurology*. New York: McGraw-Hill.

AMERICAN HEART ASSOCIATION (1965). *Aphasia and the Family*. New York: American Heart Association.

ANDERS, J., and L. EMERICK (1963). "Exploration on a New Frontier: The Social Worker in Speech Therapy." *Journal of Rehabilitation*, 29: 24–26.

ATENS, J.; D. JOHNS; and F. DARLEY (1971). "Auditory Perception of Sequenced Words in Apraxia of Speech." *Journal of Speech and Hearing Research*, 14: 131–143.

BERRY, W. (1976). "Testing Auditory Competence in Aphasia: A Clincial Alternative to the Token Test," in *Clinical Aphasiology*, ed. R. Brookshire. Minneapolis, Minn.: BRK Publishers.

BLISS, L.; A. GUILFORD; and R. TIKOFSKY (1976). "Performance of Adult Aphasics on a Sentence Evaluation and Revision Task." *Journal of Speech and Hearing Research*, 19: 551–560.

BOONE, D. (1961). *An Adult Has Aphasia*. Danville, Ill.: Interstate Printers and Publishers.

BOURESTOM, N. (1967). "Predictors of Long-term Recovery in Cerebral Vascular Disease." *Archives of Physical Medicine and Rehabilitation*, 48: 415–419.

BRODAL, A. (1973). "Self-observations and Neuroanatomical Considerations after a Stroke." *Brain*, 96: 675–694.

BROOKSHIRE, R. (1973). *An Introduction to Aphasia*. Minneapolis: BRK Publishers.

———— (1972). "Effects of Task Difficulty on Naming Performances of Aphasic Subjects." *Journal of Speech and Hearing Research*, 15: 551–558.

————, and M. LOMMEL (1974). "Perception of Sequences of Visual Temporal and Auditory Spatial Stimuli by Aphasic, Right Hemisphere Damaged, and Non-brain Damaged Subjects." *Journal of Communication Disorders*, 7: 155–169.

BUCHANAN, A. (1957). *Functional Neuro-Anatomy*. Philadelphia: Lea & Febiger.

BUCK, M. (1968). *Dysphasia*. Englewood Cliffs, N.J.: Prentice-Hall, Inc.

CHAPEY, R.; S. RIGRODSKY; and E. MORRISON (1976). "Divergent Semantic Behavior in Aphasia." *Journal of Speech and Hearing Research*, 19: 644–677.

CHUSID, J., and J. McDONALD (1967). *Correlative Neuroanatomy*. Los Altos, Calif.: Lange Medical Publications.

COHEN, R., et al. (1977). "Validity of the Sklar Aphasia Scale." *Journal of Speech and Hearing Research*, 20: 146–154.

COHN, R. and M. NEUMANN (1958). "Jargon Aphasia." *Journal of Nervous and Mental Disorders*, 127: 381–399.

COLLINS, M. (1976). "The Minor Hemisphere," in *Clinical Aphasiology*, ed. R. Brookshire. Minneapolis: BRK Publishers.

COMMUNICATION STATUS CHART (1966). Madison, Wisconsin: Division of Health.

COSER, R. (1956). "A Home Away from Home." *Social Problems*, 4: 3–17.

CULTON, G. (1969). "Spontaneous Recovery from Aphasia." *Journal of Speech and Hearing Research*, 12: 825–832.

DARLEY, F. (1964). *Diagnosis and Appraisal of Communication Disorders*. Englewood Cliffs, N.J.: Prentice-Hall, Inc.

DARLEY, F. (1972). "The Efficacy of Language Rehabilitation in Aphasia." *Journal of Speech and Hearing Disorders*, 37: 3–21.
——— (1977). "A Retrospective View: Aphasia." *Journal of Speech and Hearing Disorders*, 42: 161–169.
DAVIS, N., and E. LEACH (1972). "Scaling Aphasics' Responses." *Journal of Speech and Hearing Disorders*, 37: 305–313.
DERMAN, S., and A. MANSTER (1967). "Family Counseling with Relatives of Aphasic Patients." *Journal of American Speech and Hearing Association*, 8: 175–177.
DUFF, R., and A. HOLLINGSHEAD (1968). *Sickness and Society*. New York: Harper & Row.
DUFFY, R., and S. ULRICH (1976). "A Comparison of Impairments in Verbal Comprehension, Speech, Reading, and Writing in Adult Aphasics." *Journal of Speech and Hearing Disorders*, 41: 110–119.
DUNN, L. (1965). *Expanded Manual for the Peabody Picture Vocabulary Test*. Circle Pines, Minn.: American Guidance Service, Inc.
EAGLESON, H.; G. VAUGH; and A. KNUDSON (1970). "Hand Signals for Dysphasia." *Archives of Physical Medicine and Rehabilitation*, 51: 111–113.
EISENHOWER, D. (1965). *Waging Peace*. New York: Doubleday & Co.
EISENSON, J. (1971). "Aphasia in Adults: Basic Considerations." In *Handbook of Speech Pathology and Audiology*, ed. L. Travis. New York: Appleton-Century Crofts.
——— (1954). *Examining for Aphasia*. New York: Psychological Corporation.
——— (1949). "Prognostic Factors Related to Language Rehabilitation in Aphasic Patients." *Journal of Speech and Hearing Disorders*, 14: 262–264.
EISENSON, J. (1971). *Adult Aphasia*. New York: Appleton-Century-Crofts.
EMERICK, L. (1971). *Appraisal of Language Disturbance*. Marquette, Mich.: Northern Michigan University Press.
———, and J. COYNE (1972). *Screening Test of Aphasia*. Danville, Ill.: Interstate Printers and Publishers.
ETTLINGER, G. (1969). "Apraxia Considered as a Disorder of Movements that Are Language-Dependent: Evidence from Cases of Brain Bisection." *Cortex*, 5: 285–289.
FARRELL, B. (1969). *Pat and Roald*. New York: Random House, Inc.
GARDNER, H.; M. ALBERT; and S. WEINTRAUB (1975). "Comprehending a Word: The Influence of Speed and Redundancy on Auditory Comprehension in Aphasia." *Cortex*, 11: 115–162.
GOODGLASS, H., and E. KAPLAN (1972) *The Assessment of Aphasia and Related Disorders*. Philadelphia: Lea & Febiger.
———; J. GLEASON; and M. HYDE (1970). "Some Dimensions of Auditory Language Comprehension in Aphasia." *Journal of Speech and Hearing Research*, 13: 595–606.
GRIFFITH, V. (1970). *A Stroke in the Family*. New York: Delacorte Press.
GRINKER, R., and A. SAHS (1966). *Neurology*. Springfield, Ill.: Charles C. Thomas.
GROHER, M. (1977). "Language and Memory Disorders Following Closed Head Trauma." *Journal of Speech and Hearing Research*, 20: 212–223.
HALPERN, H. (1972). *Adult Aphasia*. Indianapolis: Bobbs-Merrill.
———; F. DARLEY; and J. BROWN (1973). "Differential Language and Neurological Characteristics of Cerebral Involvement." *Journal of Speech and Hearing Disorders*, 38: 162–173.
HAYNES, W., and B. GREENBERG (1976). *Understanding Aphasia*. Danville, Ill.: Interstate Printers and Publishers.
HELMICK, J.; T. WATAMORI; and J. PALMER (1976). "Spouses' Understanding of the Communication Disabilities of Aphasic Patients." *Journal of Speech and Hearing Disorders*, 41: 238–243.

HODGINS, E. (1964). *Episode: Report on the Accident in My Skull.* New York: Atheneum.

HOLLAND, A. (1977). "Comment on 'Spouses' Understanding of the Communication Disabilities of Aphasic Patients." *Journal of Speech and Hearing Disorders,* 42: 307–308.

HOLMES, T., and R. RAHE (1967). "The Social Readjustment Rating Scale." *Journal of Psychosomatic Research,* 11: 213–218.

HOROWITZ, B. (1962). "An Open Letter to the Family of an Adult Patient with Aphasia." *Rehabilitation Literature,* 23: 141–144.

JENKINS, J., et al. (1975) *Aphasia in Adults.* 2nd ed. New York: Harper and Row, Publishers.

JONES, L., and J. WEPMAN (1961). "Dimensions of Language Performance in Aphasia." *Journal of Speech and Hearing Research,* 4: 220–232.

KAPLAN, L. (1959). "A Descriptive Continuum of Language Responses in Aphasia." *Journal of Speech and Hearing Disorders,* 24: 410–412.

KEENAN, J. (1968). "The Nature of Receptive and Expressive Impairments in Aphasia." *Journal of Speech and Hearing Disorders,* 33: 20–25.

———— (1975). *A Procedure Manual in Speech Pathology with Brain-Damaged Adults.* Danville, Ill.: Interstate Printers and Publishers.

————, and E. BRASSELL (1974). "A Study of Factors Related to Prognosis for Individual Aphasic Patients." *Journal of Speech and Hearing Disorders,* 39: 257–269.

———— (1975). *Aphasia Language Performance Scales.* Murfreesboro, Tenn.: Pinnacle Press.

KERTEIZ, A., and J. PHIPPS (1977). "Numerical Taxonomy of Aphasia." *Brain and Language,* 4: 1–10.

KNOX, D. (1971). *Portrait of Aphasia.* Detroit: Wayne State University Press.

LECOURS, A., and F. LHERMITTE (1969). "Phonemic Paraphasias: Linguistic and Tentative Hypotheses." *Cortex,* 5: 193–228.

LEUTENEGGER, R. (1975). *Patient Care and Rehabilitation of Communication-Impaired Adults.* Springfield, Ill.: Charles C. Thomas.

LONGERICH, M. (1955). *Helping the Aphasic to Recover His Speech.* Los Angeles: College of Medical Evangelists.

LOVE, R., and W. WEBB (1977). "The Efficacy of Cueing Techniques in Broca's Aphasia." *Journal of Speech and Hearing Disorders,* 42: 170–179.

LURIA, A., and J. HUTTON (1977). "A Modern Assessment of the Basic Forms of Aphasia." *Brain and Language,* 4: 129–151.

MARSHALL, R. (1976). "Word Retrieval Behavior of Aphasic Adults." *Journal of Speech and Hearing Disorders,* 41: 444–451.

MCBRIDE, C. (1969). *Silent Victory.* Chicago: Nelson-Hall.

MCCORMICK, G., and P. WILLIAMS (1976). "The Midwestern Pennsylvania Stroke Club: Conclusions Following the First Year's Operation of a Family Centered Program," in *Clinical Aphasiology,* ed. R. Brookshire. Minneapolis: BRK Publishers.

MERRIT, H. (1970). *A Textbook in Neurology,* 4th ed. Philadelphia: Lea & Febiger.

MILLER, M. (1960). "Audiological Evaluation of Aphasic Patients." *Journal of Speech and Hearing Disorders,* 25: 333–339.

MOSS, C. (1972). *Recovery with Aphasia.* Urbana, Ill.: University of Illinois Press.

NEEDHAM, E., and J. BLACK (1970). "The Relative Ability of Aphasic Persons to Judge the Duration and Intensity of Pure Tones." *Journal of Speech and Hearing Research,* 13: 725–730.

NEEDHAM, L., and L. SWISHER (1973). "A Comparison of Auditory Comprehension for Adult Aphasics." *Journal of Speech and Hearing Disorders,* 37: 123–131.

NATION, J., and D. ARAM (1977). *Diagnosis of Speech and Language Disorders.* St. Louis: Mosby.

NETTER, F. (1958). *The Nervous System*. New York: Ciba.

ORGASS, B., and K. POECK (1969). "Assessment of Aphasia by Psychometric Methods." *Cortex*, 5: 317–330.

ORZECK, A. (1966). *The Orzeck Aphasia Evaluation*. Los Angeles, Calif.: Western Psychological Services.

PAGE, I., et al. (1961). *Strokes: How They Occur and What Can Be Done about Them*. New York: E. P. Dutton.

PARISI, D., and L. PIZZAMIGLIO (1970). "Syntactic Comprehension in Aphasia." *Cortex*, 6: 204–215.

PENFIELD, W., and L. ROBERTS (1959). *Speech and Brain Mechanisms*. Princeton, N.J.: Princeton University Press.

PERKINS, W. (1971). *Speech Pathology*. St. Louis: Mosby.

PETERSON, J., and A. OLSEN (1964). *Language Problems after a Stroke*. Minneapolis: American Rehabilitation Foundation.

PIZZAMIGLIO, L., and A. APPICCIAFUOCO (1971). "Semantic Comprehension in Aphasia." *Journal of Communication Disorders*, 3: 280–288.

PORCH, B. (1971). "Multidimensional Scoring in Aphasia Testing." *Journal of Speech and Hearing Research*, 14: 776–792.

———— (1967). *Porch Index of Communicative Ability*. Palo Alto, Calif.: Consulting Psychologists Press.

PORTER, J., and B. DABUL (1977). "The Application of Transactional Analysis to Therapy with Wives of Adult Aphasic Patients." *Journal of the American Speech and Hearing Association*, 19: 244–248.

SALVATORE, A. (1972). "Use of a Baseline Probe Technique to Monitor Test Responses of Aphasic Patients." *Journal of Speech and Hearing Disorders*, 37: 471–475.

SARNO, M. (1974). "Aphasia Rehabilitation." in *Communication Disorders*, ed. S. Dickson. Glenview, Ill.: Scott, Foresman and Company.

———— (1972). *Aphasia: Selected Readings*. New York: Appleton-Century-Crofts.

———— and E. SANDS (1970). "An Objective Method for the Evaluation of Speech Therapy in Aphasia." *Archives of Physical Medicine and Rehabilitation*, 51: 49–54.

SARNO, J., and M. SARNO (1973). "The Functional Life Scale." *Archives of Physical Medicine and Rehabilitation*, 54: 214–220.

SARNO, M.; M. SILVERMAN; E. SANDS (1970). "Speech Therapy and Language Recovery in Severe Aphasia." *Journal of Speech and Hearing Disorders*, 13: 607–623.

SCHUELL, H. (1965). *The Minnesota Test for Differential Diagnosis of Aphasia*. Minneapolis: University of Minnesota Press.

———— (1966). "A Reevaluation of the Short Examination for Aphasia." *Journal of Speech and Hearing Disorders*, 31: 137–147.

———— (1957). "A Short Examination for Aphasia." *Neurology*, 7: 625–634.

———— and J. JENKINS (1962). "A Factor Analysis of the Minnesota Test for Differential Diagnosis of Aphasia." *Journal of Speech and Hearing Research*. 5: 349–369.

————; J. JENKINS; and E. JIMENEZ-PABON (1964). *Aphasia in Adults*. New York: Harper & Row.

SCHUELL, H., et al. (1969). "A Psycholinguistic Approach to the Study of Language Deficit in Aphasia." *Journal of Speech and Hearing Research*, 12: 794–806.

SIEGEL, G. (1975). "The High Cost of Accountability," *Journal of the American Speech and Hearing Association*, 17: 796–798.

SIES, L. (1974). *Aphasia Theory and Therapy*. Baltimore: University Park Press.

SKLAR, M. (1966). *Sklar Aphasia Scale*. Los Angeles: Western Psychological Services.

SMITH, A. (1971). "Objective Indices of Severity of Chronic Aphasia in Stroke Patients." *Journal of Speech and Hearing Disorders*, 36: 167–207.

SMITH, G. (1967). *Care of the Patient With a Stroke*. New York: Springer Publishing Company.

SNIDECOR, J. (1955). "A Method of Disparities for Evaluating Aphasic Disturbance." *Journal of Nervous and Mental Disorders*, 122: 92–93.

SOLOMON, P., et al. (1961). *Sensory Deprivation*. Cambridge, Mass.: Harvard University Press.

SPELLACY, F., and O. SPREEN (1969). "A Short Form of the Token Test." *Cortex*, 5: 390–397.

STACHOWLAK, F., et al. (1977). "Text Comprehension in Aphasia." *Brain and Language*, 4: 177–195.

STEINBECK, J. (1961). *Travels with Charley*. New York: The Viking Press.

STREET, B. (1957). "Hearing Loss in Aphasia." *Journal of Speech and Hearing Disorders*, 22: 60–67.

TAYLOR, M. (1963). *Functional Communication Profile*. New York: New York University Medical Center.

——— (1958). *Understanding Aphasia*. New York: Institute of Physical Medicine and Rehabilitation.

——— and J. MYERS (1952). "A Group Discussion Program with the Families of Aphasic Patients." *Journal of Speech and Hearing Disorders*, 17: 393–396.

TOUBBEH, J. (1969). "Clinical Observations on Adult Aphasia." *Journal of Communication Disorders*, 2: 57–68.

TWAMLEY, R., and L. EMERICK (1970). "The Nurses' Role in Aphasia." *Today's Speech*, 18: 30–33.

ULTRAOWSKA, H., et al. (1976). "The Assessment of Communicative Competence in Aphasia." in *Clinical Aphasiology*, ed. R. Brookshire. Minneapolis: BRK Publishers.

VANTREEN, J. (1975). "Current Approaches to the Linguistic Assessment of Aphasic Speech." *British Journal of Disorders of Communication*, 10: 134–141.

VICK, N. (1976). *Grinkers Neurology*. 7th ed. Springfield, Ill.: Charles C. Thomas.

WALSHE, F. (1970). *Diseases of the Nervous System*. Baltimore: Williams & Wilkins.

WALTON, J. (1975). *Essentials of Neurology*. Philadelphia: J.B. Lippincott Co.

WEPMAN, J. (1958). "The Relationship Between Self-Correction and Recovery from Aphasia." *Journal of Speech and Hearing Disorders*, 23: 302–305.

——— (1972). "Aphasia Therapy: A New Look." *Journal of Speech and Hearing Disorders*, 37: 203–214.

——— (1976). "Aphasia: Language Without Thought or Thought Without Language." *Journal of the American Speech and Hearing Association*, 18: 131–136.

———, et al., (1960). "Studies in Aphasia: Background and Theoretical Formulations." *Journal of Speech and Hearing Disorders*, 25: 323–332.

———, and L. JONES (1961). *Studies in Aphasia: An Approach to Testing*. Chicago: Education/Industry Service.

WHITEHOUSE, E. (1968). *There's Always More*. Valley Forge Pa.: The Judson Press.

WILLIAMS, M. (1970). *Brain Damage and the Mind*. Middlesex, England: Penquin Books.

WINT, G. (1965). *The Third Killer*. New York: Abelard-Schumann.

WULF, H. (1973). *Aphasia, My World Alone*. Detroit: Wayne State University Press.

WYLIE, C. (1964). "Administrative Research in the Rehabilitation of Stroke Patients." *Rehabilitation Literature*, 25: 2–8.

ZUBECK, J. (1969). *Sensory Deprivation: Fifteen Years of Research*. New York: Appleton-Century-Crofts.

9

Voice Disorders

INTRODUCTION

> Todd and Clyde grudgingly left their sixth-grade classroom for the semiweekly
> session with the speech clinician. Todd had been taking this same route twice each
> week for the past five years, and Clyde had a similar dismal record for lack of
> correction of a distorted /r/. For two years now speech therapy had become a burden,
> and several of their ploys to get dismissed had failed. It was not until this morning
> that the fail-proof method was to be employed. "I think I have it," said Clyde
> feigning the most hoarse voice he could muster. "We will both begin talking like this
> to the speech clinician, and she is sure to drop us from therapy and put us on the
> waiting list with all those other voice cases."

Contrived, yes. Inaccurate? We are not so sure. For reasons we shall soon
enumerate, voice disorders are perplexing sources of failure for many speech
clinicians. Although disordered voices represent but a small percentage of our total
professional clientele, any individual whom we cannot deal with efficiently is one
too many.

Prevalence figures for voice disorders among school-aged children vary
considerably. Silverman and Zimmer (1975) report that 23.4 percent of the
primary grade children they evaluated possessed chronically hoarse voices while
Wilson and Rice (1977) postulate that 1 percent of the school age population need
voice therapy. From our experience it would appear that substantially less than 1
percent of the school aged children are presently receiving voice therapy. (See

Deal, McClain, and Sudderth, 1976). The practicing speech clinician, for a variety of reasons, is not identifying the number of voice cases that the experts predict exist.

Definition of Voice

The imprecision of labels, which is the bane of voice study, begins with the term "voice" itself. Some definitions restrict the term to the generation of sound at the level of the larynx, while others include the influence of the vocal tract upon the generated tone, and still others broaden the definition to ultimately include aspects of tonal generation, resonation, articulation, and prosody.

Definitions reflect our point of view, and as such they tend to fit the circumstances of the moment. The laryngologist will listen to the voice from a unique perspective and hear only the signals of vocal malfunction. A parent will hear a voice based primarily upon what she expects to hear, and a speech clinician, in some cases, may hear a voice relative to the type of client she is comfortable dealing with. For the purposes of this chapter, voice is defined as the end product of respiratory power, laryngeal valving and sound generation, vocal tract resonation and alteration of the tone, and it is categorized into pitch, quality, and loudness characteristics.

The meaning and intent of a message are primarily matters of semantic choice, syntax, prosody, phone accuracy, and in certain instances voice characteristics. There are, of course, instances where the voice does indeed alter the content of a spoken message. The total lack of voice (aphonia) is a far more serious handicap than an altered phoneme or two.

The imprecise definitions and the subsequent insecurity of speech clinicians are both related to several factors:

1. The voice is the product of muscle functions that are not readily observed and are difficult to control directly. Whereas in articulation an individual can be told to elevate the tongue tip and the success of this action can be observed and measured, the voice clinician cannot request the client to bring his arytenoid cartilages together. There is a mystique which surrounds the unobservable, and much of voice rehabilitation has been "mystical."

2. The voice is indirectly influenced by several body systems, including the respiratory, phonatory, resonatory, endocrine, and neural. With so many systems functioning, it is often difficult to determine just which potential etiological factor is responsible for any given symptom.

3. There are contradictory points of view on the relative influence of the physical and psychic factors of vocal production. The voice is said to be a bellwether of the psychological state and is subject to insidious and hard-to-detect influences.

4. There is no clear concept of just what normal voice is, since the influences of culture, age, sex, role, and specific activity alter the expected vocal output. Under certain circumstances, nearly any voice variation could be termed "normal."

5. The various parameters of voice are subject to continuous and flowing change at the whim of the speaker. Whereas it would be considered aberrant for a speaker to

abruptly alter his syntactical system or articulatory pattern, each of us continuously changes the pitch, loudness, and quality of his voice in keeping with the meaning of the spoken signal. Such instantaneous changes make voice characteristics rather difficult to define precisely.

6. The listener's perceptions of vocal characteristics are mediated through other aspects of the speech signal. For example, Sherman (1954) pointed out that the perception of nasality is partially dependent on articulatory patterns.

7. In the literature concerning voice there has been a tendency to confuse perceptual and physical characteristics. To state that the "natural *pitch*" of the adult male is approximately 125 Hz encourages confusion and imprecision.

8. There is no clear idea of the compensatory capabilities of the vocal tract in voice production. It is not known if the resonators can and do mask phonatory differences in some individuals or, on the other hand, if an increased exhalatory effort results in a compensating function of the vocal folds which in turn causes minimal signal change.

9. The study of voice has been divided between the "scientists" and the "practitioners." "Voice scientists" and "experimental phoneticians" have provided the discipline with much of the hard data upon which to assess clincial behavior, but there have been precious few who have been willing to make clinical suggestions from the laboratory findings. Similarly, the flow of information has not been reciprocal; clinicians have been remiss in collecting clinical data which can hold up under the critical eyes of the researchers.

10. The versatility of the vocal mechanism is exemplified by the number of uses it is put to. Speaking, singing, shouting, crying, laughing, whispering, moaning, sobbing, sighing, burping, yodeling, snoring, coughing, sneezing, hiccuping, and ventriloquism—all involve some portion of the respiratory, phonatory, or resonatory systems.

With this set of factors in mind, then, there is little wonder that some clinicians are poorly prepared to deal with the disordered voice. University classes in voice disturbance typically dwell on descriptions of the problem, classification systems, research data, and the like but somehow find little time for thorough discussions of the actual clinical practice with the voice patient. The difficult voice cases are rare and are coveted by a few staff members or graduate students. Worthley (1969) found in a survey of over 400 public-school speech clinicians that they rate their training in voice disorders poorer than in any other area.

Parameters of Voice and Vocal Disturbance

A framework to conceptualize voice and voice disturbance is shown by Figure 9.1. The auditory characteristics of pitch, loudness, and quality constitute one dimension of our paradigm. All of these are perceptual attributes of the voice and relate generally to the fundamental frequency, amplitude, and complexity of the signal.

Pitch that is too high, too low, too invariant, or inappropriately variant for the speaker or the circumstances constitutes a voice disorder.

The loudness of the speaking voice is usually judged according to the

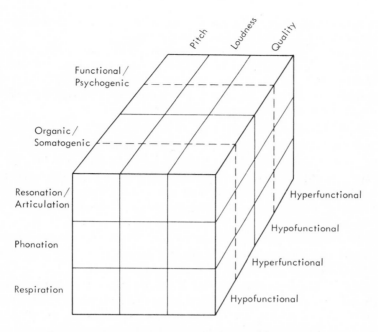

Figure 9.1 An Organizational Schema of Voice Disorders.

speaking circumstance, the aberrant ranging from the total lack of voice (aphonia) to the inappropriately loud. Inappropriate loudness indicates a lack of control of the phonatory system.

For our purposes the term quality refers to the perceived pleasantness, or appeal, of the voice. This perception is linked both to the phonatory and resonatory characteristics of the speaker.

The physical systems that most directly influence the vocal production are the respiratory, phonatory, and resonatory-articulatory systems. Although these systems have the most direct impact on the voice signal, they are not the only systems that influence the voice.[1]

The respiratory system provides the motive force for voice production, and ultimately the resultant airstream becomes the vibrator that embodies all of the characteristics which the ear eventually senses. That the airstream is important to vocal production is not really the issue at this point, but there is some question as to the influence of the respiratory mechanism upon the various vocal characteristics. It appears that the respiratory mechanism must be capable of the following:

1. Providing an adequate amount of air so that the speaker can sustain speech with ease to allow for natural phrasing and prosodic factors;

2. Providing adequate breath support so that the vibratory pattern can be established without undue laryngeal valving tension;

[1]Read Luchsinger and Arnold's (1965) account of the impact of the endocrine system on voice production.

309

3. Providing adequate control of the flow of air so that the mechanism can, when necessary, either initiate or arrest the speech signal;

4. Providing an airstream that is not so indebted to active muscle contraction that it encourages unnecessary muscle tension in the respiratory and phonatory mechanisms;

5. Providing an airstream that is instantly available upon demand and able to be sustained somewhat constantly for a sufficient length of time.

The physiology of the respiratory mechanism has been poorly understood. Early writings spoke of "breathing from the diaphragm," and stressed the "proper" inward movement of the abdomen during inhalation. Some clinicians still concentrate on the respiratory function when the disorder is clearly phonatory. If a tire loses air because of a leak in the air valve, one would not attempt to fix the leak by altering the pressure within the tire, one would attack the problem at the site of the breakdown.

A protracted discussion of the physiology of phonation is not within the scope of this text; however, some elements of laryngeal function are crucial in diagnostic evaluation. In order to be an efficient sound source, the larynx must perform a valving action upon the flow of air that establishes alternate, regular pressure changes within the body of air. In order to do this the vocal folds must:

(1) be capable of wide range valving actions, from keeping the passageway open and unrestricted to closed and totally restricted, and a wide variety of closures between those two points; (2) be able to valve fairly completely along their entire length; (3) be of approximately equal size and shape so that they can move in synchrony with one another; (4) close and open during phonation with just the right amount of firmness so that they are not subject to extremes of pressure during the closing phase; (5) be of appropriate size (length and mass) for the age and sex of the person; (6) be capable of natural movement that is free from superimposed and undue tension; and (7) be capable of small, subtle, instantaneous adjustments that must be made continuously to alter the various vocal characteristics. These adjustments must allow for a variety of cyclic variations in the potential time of glottal opening and closing. These range from the long closing time of the glottal fry to the short closing time of the falsetto voice.

The glottal tone is complex and rich in higher harmonics, but it is only through the resonant and damping effects of the vocal tract that the speech sounds achieve their identity. In order for the resonating chambers of the vocal tract to be efficient, they must be flexible in size, shape, texture, and relationship with one another. The effect of the resonators upon the laryngeal valve has been discussed by several writers (Curtis, 1968; Wendahl and Page, 1967), but the exact nature of this relationship has yet to be determined.

The term functional should imply more than the simple absence of measurable organic deviation; it should imply that the diagnostician has found some active agent of etiology and that that agent is nonorganic. We agree with Powers (1957) that the term functional has unfortunately come to mean diagnosis by default. We hope that the clinician will be encouraged to a more thorough search if he uses the more active definition of "functional." Voice disorders offer an interesting testing ground for the traditional organic-functional dichotomy. This separation does not stand up on almost any basis. Murphy (1964) points out the continuous nature of vocal-disorder etiologies, a concept with which we heartily agree.

Figure 9.1 identifies function/psychogenic and organic/somatogenic as clinically meaningful categories. The term functional refers to those disorders where the learned, psychic, or maladaptive behavior has resulted in faulty vocal production but not in physical alteration. If physical change has resulted from the functional cause, however, the proper designation is psychogenic. Similarly, if the original factor was physical or organic, then the term organic is justified; but if the physical difference results in behavioral change—i.e., emotional response or faulty compensatory adjustments—the term somatogenic is appropriate (Murphy, 1964).

The terms hyper- and hypofunctioning refer to an excess or insufficiency of laryngeal tension and, as such, could apply to a wide variety of organic or functional disorders.

The term voice disorder, then, refers to abnormal pitch, loudness, or vocal quality according to sex, age, status, temporary physiological state, purpose of the speaker, and elements of the speaking circumstance. Vocal disorders may be primarily organic or functional and may be affected by any of the primary systems that influence voice production such as the neurological and endocrine systems.

DIAGNOSTIC FORMAT

This chapter will not cover the anatomy and physiology of the mechanisms of vocal production. Moore (1971a), Zemlin (1968), Kaplan (1971), and others offer this information, and the student should study it carefully before undertaking voice diagnosis. We also cannot provide an elaborate description of each voice disorder type; this information is available to the student in several sources (Luchsinger and Arnold, 1965; Greene, 1964; and Boone, 1977). We shall not discuss pitch meters, sound spectrographs, respirometers, and the like. Most clinicians do not have a laboratory available and thus are forced to be inventive during the voice diagnosis. Hanley and Peters (1971) provide a complete discussion of the speech laboratory.

Our major focus will be on the actual thought, planning, preparation, and execution of voice diagnoses. Diagnosis is intended to define the parameters of the problem, determine the etiology, and outline a logical course of action.

The Presenting Complaint

The diagnostic process begins with a careful scrutiny of the original statement of the problem as provided by the referral source. Four perspectives guide our evaluation of this information: who, what, why, and when.

Who. It is important to know who presents the original complaint about the client's voice. We have found that the "best" source from a motivational standpoint is the client himself, but that any individual who might have a significant impact upon the client may be a satisfactory referral source. If the client and those around him do not consider his voice to be a problem, then in reality, there is none. With voice disorders, however, this may be dangerous because some minimal changes in voice quality may reflect anatomic changes. There is a circular pattern of cause and effect in voice disorders that is best treated early.

> Mrs. N. referred her husband to us with a pleading phone call. "He had his laryngectomy four months ago and the doctor says he will never talk again. Is there anything you can do?" For some unknown reason we resisted the urge to reassure Mrs. N. that her husband could indeed speak again, but we made an appointment for evaluation. When Mr. and Mrs. N. came into the office they had with them their newly purchased electrolarynx which was obtained at the insistence of their daughter. Much to our chagrin, it soon became evident why Mr. N. had been told he would not speak again. Not only had the surgeon removed the larynx, he had also excised the entire lingual structure. The fact that the referral came from the spouse rather than from our usually reliable laryngologist should have provided the first clue in this case. Although Mr. N. learned alternate means of communication, articulate speech was not an attainable goal.

An amazing number of people do not consider voice characteristics to be in the realm of speech disorders. One high-school sophomore who spoke in a falsetto voice was referred to us by his English teacher, who stated, "I don't think this kid really has a speech problem, but I don't know who else to send him to." The typical response is "Oh, that's just Jimmy's voice, he's always sounded like that." The implication is that the characteristics that determine a person's voice are genetically determined and cannot be changed by training or practice.[2] When our screening process determines that an individual has a significant vocal deviation, we take particular pains to present this information to the individual so that he will not be tempted to use hidden and ill-defined factors to rationalize the problem.

What. The description of the problem is important not only because it helps us to understand the problem better but also because it allows us to see the problem through the eyes (and ears) of another. When the statement comes from the person with whom we will be working, we listen not only to the actual words spoken, but also to the way in which they are presented. One of the best sources of information about the impact of the problem upon the individual is the way in which he describes it. Invariably, when interviewing the client we find it valuable to ask the following five questions: (1) "Describe your voice." Listen for the terms used, the factors which appear to alter the voice, other sources of variance in vocal charac-

---

[2]For an indication of the classroom teacher's efficacy in referral of children with voice disorders, see Diehl, C., and C. Stinnett, "Efficiency of Teacher Referrals in a School Speech-Testing Program," *Journal of Speech and Hearing Disorders*, 24 (1959): 34–36, or James, H., and E. Cooper, "Accuracy of Teacher Referral of Speech-Handicapped Children," *Exceptional Child*, 30 (1966): 29–33.

teristics, and subtle signs of concern. (2) "How do others react to your speaking voice?" Generally we attempt to judge this answer against reality as best we can. Very often the individual will respond that no one ever mentions his voice, and the diagnostician must take care not to reinforce such reactions, while on the other hand, not to strip the client of all his defenses. It is quite possible that there has been little environmental reaction and that the client is being quite honest in his reply, but we are concerned with the client's perception of other's reactions. Remember that you may be the first person to ask him such questions, and he should be given plenty of time to respond. (3) "How severe do you consider this problem to be?" Generally we give the client some sort of subjective rating scale upon which to judge. This is very useful baseline information and is directly related to the next question. (4) "How much does this problem bother you?" We have found that the degree of concern and the judgment of severity are not always directly related, but in any case we must know just how much this individual wishes to change his voice. The clinician must be careful in such discussions since the client may respond that he has no problem and he does not desire to change in the least. Although this is important diagnostic information, it is also important to the therapy process; and the diagnostician must be able to recover the initiative and put the client back on the track. (5) "What caused the problem?" Although generally the client claims ignorance, every once in a while we open a Pandora's box with this question.

> Following a rather benign discussion, Mrs. A. was finally asked just what caused her vocal hoarseness. Her response began cautiously enough, but soon she was describing her "second" visit to the state mental hospital (we had not known there was a "first" visit) and how the staff had resorted to electric shock treatments in an attempt to break the profound depression she was experiencing. From that point on, the discussion opened up and significant information was offered freely.

Murphy (1964: 92) presents a series of twenty questions to clarify the individual's self-concepts regarding his speaking voice. Such lists often provide a useful starting place for the diagnostician.

Why. The reason for referral to the voice clinician may vary from an impending trip ("I just have to sound better than this by the first of August") to fears of serious medical problems. In evaluating the reasons for referral, it is important to keep in mind that a referral to a speech clinician is often seen as psychologically safer than referrals to medical doctors or psychiatrists. This points up the importance of secondary referrals.

When. Three things are of major concern here. First, it is important to know when, in the sequence of events of the problem, the referral was made. Is this a problem of long standing that has only recently become serious, or is it a relatively new phenomenon that has been detected early? Second, what is this person's age and maturational level? Whereas certain vocal changes are to be expected before puberty (Curry, 1949) and would thus be considered normal, a similar vocal quality at a later maturity level is serious. Third, does his problem appear in cycles? Does the client suffer from this vocal quality only during "hay fever" season? The time of the year of the referral may provide some important diagnostic information.

Referral

In most cases of phonatory voice disorders some type of referral for medical or psychological evaluation will be necessary. Voice disorders may be caused by life-threatening situations such as carcinoma of the larynx or something as simple as vocal misuse. Structural changes such as ulcers, polyps, or nodules may be detected through laryngeal examination. Symptoms such as hoarseness or harshness of the voice should prompt the clinician to make referral, particularly if the hoarseness lasts beyond ten days.

A general medical evaluation or a specific neurological examination may be indicated in certain cases. When dysfunction of the peripheral or central nervous system appears to be a possible contributing factor to the voice disorder referral is indicated. For a comprehensive treatment of the various etiological categories for voice disorders and behavioral clues to indicate the need for referral see Luchsinger and Arnold (1965).

Historic Data

A general case-history form is provided in Appendix A of this text and in several other texts (Johnson, Darley, and Spriestersbach, 1963; Berry and Eisenson, 1956). Our purpose is to identify those specific aspects within each of the historical subcategories that have particular relevance to voice diagnosis. Discussions of case-history evaluation tend to be rather sterile if the relevance of each aspect is not made clear. The reader is encouraged to complete the project outlined in Appendix A, since it is exactly that type of study which makes the bland discussion of routine diagnostic tasks come alive.

Family data. Information regarding the parental occupation, number of siblings, history of family adjustment, other voice problems within the family, and general health pattern of the family tells us a great deal about the client's social and physical milieu. Generally, the following characteristics are considered danger signals: (1) too much or too little structure and organization to the home; (2) premium placed on verbal competition; (3) interparental friction; (4) unusual sibling competition; (5) history of voice disorders in others within the family; (6) poor parental adjustment; (7) history of extended or recurrent health problems within the family; and (8) general level of concern for physical and health problems within the family.

Onset of the problem. In many instances the nature of the onset of the voice problem will have great diagnostic significance. It is important to investigate not only the nature of the onset but the circumstances surrounding it. Physical or psychological trauma may have equally instant effects upon voice production. In some cases, extended questioning may be necessary because it is common for clients to repress uncomfortable incidents of the past. Unfortunately, physical trauma is often inextricably related to psychological trauma in a large number of cases; therefore, this information must be judged against all the other diagnostic data available. Just as the beauty of a painting is not appreciated through the microscope, individual bits of information only have meaning when viewed in broad perspective.

Although the abrupt onset of a vocal disorder is traumatic and startling, most voice disorders are of insidious origin. Many people cannot pinpoint the exact date of onset and tend to indicate when people first noticed or remarked about their voices. Since a gradual onset is not specific to organic or functional etiologies, the examiner must look to other data for final answers. Probably more important than the problem's rate of development is information on coincident factors such as the client's general health and emotional state.

Course of development. A careful description of the developmental stages of the voice disturbance may provide helpful diagnostic information. Not only are the developments themselves important, but also the sequence of events before and after.

> Mrs. F. was seen in the speech-and-hearing clinic three times in three years, each time with a similar complaint. Vocal fatigue and hoarseness characterized this first-grade teacher's voice. Medical examinations had been negative on each of the first two occasions, but on the third visit small vocal nodules were noted. Looking over our records, it was noted that Mrs. F. had been to the clinic in late March of 1968, early April of 1969, and late April of 1970. After some further discussion with Mrs. F., we determined that she was not only suffering from vocal fatigue but from teaching fatigue as well.

The course of the development of the voice disorder may be found to parallel a chronic medical problem, cumulating vocational stress, certain periods of physical maturation, changes in family relationships, or developing financial crises. The clinician will want to keep in mind that once a voice disorder has firmly been established only a minimal amount of tension, misuse, or abuse will be necessary to perpetuate the problem.

Social adjusting. Assessment of the personality characteristics of the individual may assist the diagnostician in interpreting other information. Formal personality testing, briefly discussed in Chapter 3, is not within the jurisdiction of the speech clinician, but each clinician is expected to be perceptive and sensitive to clues about the client's basic adjustment to life. The concept that the voice is closely related to the individual's self-concept and reveals inner conflict has been carefully examined by several researchers. Moses (1954) and Rousey and Moriarty (1965) present interesting views of the interaction of the personality and voice production. This relationship is seen in a wide range of examples from the hypernasal whine of a college freshman giving his first speech in "Speech I" to the deep-seated symptoms of the psychotic. Classification of voice characteristics with specific personality types has not provided overwhelming evidence; but the personality and the voice interact in a complex fashion and this results in many symptomatic characteristics both permanent and temporary.

The danger in taking a purely symptomatic approach to voice disorders has already been implied. The following example underscores the point:

> Ted, a strapping six-foot high-school sophomore, presented himself to our office upon the referral of his English teacher. Ted knew that his voice was "too high" and stated that he desired to change it. Within the first session Ted was phonating at an appropriate pitch level, and the postpubescent falsetto voice appeared to be an easy challenge. Within three weeks Ted was speaking in controlled sentences at the proper pitch level, and our purely symptomatic approach appeared to be satisfactory. In fact Ted habituated to the proper pitch within the academic semester. This is not an unusual occurrence, however.
>
> The following events, however, give reason to question the clinical approach. Ted was the younger of two sons and by far the "junior" in many respects. Ted's older brother was an excellent student, outstanding athlete, and class officer until he was killed in a hunting accident at the age of seventeen. Ted was twelve at the time of his brother's death, and his voice had already begun to change. Within a few weeks, however, Ted resorted to the falsetto voice and maintained that voice until he was seen for speech therapy some three years later. Early in our therapy Ted's mother was interviewed, and the tape of Ted's masculine voice was played. She immediately began to sob, relating that the voice was identical to that of the older brother. Fearful that we were forcing Ted to compete with the memory of his older brother, we nonetheless pressed our attack on his voice. By the end of the academic year, Ted appeared delighted with his progress and had established a close relationship to the clinician. The following fall Ted called the clinician to set up a partridge hunting trip. We felt this would afford an excellent opportunity to test the carryover of the voice, and the trip took place as planned. Ted's voice had remained normal, although curiously, his speech contained several articulatory errors that had previously not existed. The startling event, however, was not his improved voice or speech. During our last walk down a tote road, Ted, who was a good distance behind, accidently discharged his gun and sprayed pellets in our direction. Ted responded by laughing hysterically to the point where he could not be controlled for some time. There are several interesting interpretations of this event, but the most disturbing is that Ted may well have been unconsciously displaying his hostility toward the person who forced him to employ a voice and role his psyche had previously rejected.

Vocation. We are interested in the vocation of our voice client for two reasons. First, we must determine if the occupation demands a great deal of talking and if that talking is under adverse conditions. There is not only a boilermaker's ear but a boilermaker's voice as well. Not all teachers develop "teachers' nodules" however, and the vocation must be judged in relation to the person. Several writers have postulated that there is a personality type that develops vocal nodules (Jackson, 1941; Withers, 1961). We have found many of these people to be tense, energetic, high strung, and verbally aggressive. Place this type of person in an occupational setting that demands a great deal of speaking under tension, and a bit of poor judgment in choosing adaptive procedures, and the chances of finding an individual with vocal nodules are greatly enhanced.

A second factor in our evaluation of the vocation of an individual is the degree of satisfaction the person receives from his work. The task is not always easy, but clues may come from information on the person's interests, educational background, and qualifications, along with some measure of the rewards he receives from his work.[3]

Health. Realizing that the voice is influenced by many physiological systems, a complete medical history and examination are necessary in many instances. A history of the general health and physical development of the client should be obtained, along with information about specific illnesses, surgeries, and medication; the clinician should also obtain a familial health history and data concerning the general energy level and health-related habits such as smoking, drinking, and drug usage. Luchsinger and Arnold (1965) present a particularly comprehensive discussion of vocal disorders of organic etiology.

> Sherry was identified in the univeristy speech-and-hearing screening program. Her voice was described as breathy, low in pitch and volume, expressionless, and with varying degrees of nasality. The case history revealed the following information: low metabolic rate, rapid fatigue, and body temperatures generally below normal. Subsequent medical referral indicated specific muscle weakness and a medical diagnosis of myasthenia gravis. It should be noted that the speech clinician's alertness to the accumulation of medical danger signs in addition to the speech characteristics resulted in a proper referral and subsequent identification of the problem.

The Evaluation Process

The first step in the voice analysis involves simply listening to the client in an objective and yet analytical manner. We find it helpful to mentally rehearse the classifications of voice disorders while listening.

> During the initial interview, Mr. B. was requested to recount the events which brought him to our office. While he was speaking, the following mental notes were taken: Volume appears adequate with good variety and inflection; only problem in this area appears to be his lack of projection at the end of particularly long phrases:

---

[3]Approaches to the evaluation of job satisfaction are discussed in: Smith, P., Kendall, L., and C. Hulin, (1969) *The Measurement of Job Satisfaction in Work and Retirement; A Strategy for the Study of Attitudes,* Chicago: Rand McNally.

this should be evaluated. Before he leaves I will take him into a classroom and have him speak to me as if he were addressing a large gathering. His pitch sounds high, but this is difficult to judge since there is good variety and a strange low-frequency component I can't identify. He is an animated speaker with a lively gesture system accompanying his speech. In fact he continues to move and gesture when he is listening, almost as if he were saying what I was saying right along with me. As I listen to his speech, however, it is not the pitch that bothers me—the predominant feature is the hoarse vocal quality. I hear a breathy escape during phonation and a strained rough sound. I feel like clearing my throat with every sentence he speaks (and my throat felt tense when he left). Particularly noticeable was the manner in which he initiated sound—almost as if the pressure build-up was so great the folds were blasted apart with unusual force. He also had an unconscious mannerism of clearing his throat abruptly upon initiation of a statement. I'll bet he is not even aware of this. There are no articulation or resonatory problems, but his phrase structure bothers me. He appears to run short of air at odd places and strains to continue talking until he gets to a natural juncture. This doesn't work all of the time, however, and often he just stops and begins with that coup de glotte vocal onset again. I really shouldn't bias myself with a prediction, but I'm betting on vocal nodules.

Obviously, this listening process is largely judgmental; therefore, it may be helpful to use a checklist such as Table 9-1 in order to reduce subjectivity.

Respiration. The laboratory scientists have made clinicians appreciate the importance of the respiratory process in speech but have not provided many efficient and accessible means for measuring the variables of respiration. For this reason, and possibly others, speech clinicians have not paid enough attention to this function. Spirometers, pneumographs, and respirometers are not available to many public-school speech clinicians.

Our concern for the respiratory process involves both the vegetative processes and breathing for speech. There are six areas of concern for the diagnostician:

AIR VOLUME. The maximum amount of air which can be exhaled following maximal inhalation is called vital capacity (Wood, 1971). The relationship of vital capacity to speech production is somewhat a matter of conjecture at this point. Vital capacity is apparently related to several factors such as body size, physical condition, and sex (Gray and Wise, 1959; Van Riper and Irwin, 1958). There is little or no research to vindicate those who have worked to increase the vital capacity of their voice clients. On the other hand, it is logical to assume that an individual with an extremely small amount of air available would find it difficult to sustain phonation and would resort to increased laryngeal tension and forcing to maintain normal or near-normal phrasing. It is probably not so much the volume of air as it is the individual's ability to control the airflow (Hardy, 1961).

Although we have made futile attempts to devise a mechanism that will adequately measure vital capacity, there appears to be no satisfactory substitute for the spirometer. Clinically we have found that a vital capacity insufficient for normal speech purposes was so obvious from normal observation that further

Table 9-1 Checklist of Vocal Characteristics

1 = normal   7 = severely disordered

Pitch

1   2   3   4   5   6   7

Description	Severity						
—too high	1	2	3	4	5	6	7
—too low	1	2	3	4	5	6	7
—invariant	1	2	3	4	5	6	7
—pitch breaks	1	2	3	4	5	6	7
—diplaphonia	1	2	3	4	5	6	7
—repetitive pattern	1	2	3	4	5	6	7

Loudness

1   2   3   4   5   6   7

Description	Severity						
—excessive	1	2	3	4	5	6	7
—inadequate	1	2	3	4	5	6	7
—uncontrolled variation	1	2	3	4	5	6	7
—repetitive pattern	1	2	3	4	5	6	7
—invariant	1	2	3	4	5	6	7
—tremulous	1	2	3	4	5	6	7

Quality

1   2   3   4   5   6   7

Description	Severity						
—Hoarseness	1	2	3	4	5	6	7
—Harshness	1	2	3	4	5	6	7
—Breathiness	1	2	3	4	5	6	7
—Hypernasal	1	2	3	4	5	6	7
—Hyponasal	1	2	3	4	5	6	7
—Other (describe)	1	2	3	4	5	6	7

Overall Judgment of Voice

1   2   3   4   5   6   7

Judgment of Vocal Tension
   —Aphonia/whisper
   —Breathy phonation
   —Normal
   —Hypertension
   —Hypertension/intermittent phonation

formal testing was not necessary. Vital capacity measurements may be of particular concern in cases of emphysema, later stages of Parkinson's disease, and children with cerebral palsy.

RESPIRATION TYPE. The methods of respiration have been classically designated as clavicular, thoracic, and abdominal. The terms refer to the area of greatest excursion during inhalation. More precise and demanding categorizations have been proposed (Russell, 1931); however, there appears to be general agreement that respiratory type has little influence on vocal characteristics except in the case of extreme upper chest or clavicular breathing, which tends to encourage great laryngeal tension and insufficient intake of air volume.[4]

Observation appears to be the most satisfactory method of determining the type of respiratory process, although the enterprising public-school clinician may find that the science lab may have a kymograph, and such devices are easily altered for use as a pneumograph. Once again, our concern is not so much with the method employed in respiration as it is with the ease and efficiency of the operation.

While observing for the region of respiration, the clinician should also determine the coordination of the thoracic and abdominal regions. When the contraction of the thoracic muscles of inhalation coincides with the contraction of the abdominal muscles and the diaphragm, easy inhalation is impossible, and the reverse of this situation results in the inability to control the exhalation of air. This pattern may result in an insufficiency of air or uneven phonatory patterns due to varying degrees of subglottic pressure. McDonald and Chance (1964) point out that this respiratory pattern is seen among cerebral-palsied individuals. We generally make an attempt to determine the degree of respiratory control while the client is engaged in the following activities: maintaining a slow, gradual inhalation; maintaining a slow, gradual exhalation; producing an isolated vowel for a few seconds duration; producing controlled phrases and sentences; panting; and speaking while engaged in some extraneous motor activity.

RESPIRATORY RATE RATIO. Vegetative respiratory rate varies considerably depending upon the age and activity level of the individual. A rate of thirty to forty per minute is not uncommon in the very young infant, but beyond one and one-half to two years of age the rate should have stabilized in the low twenties. With some children the extremely high respiratory rate appears to interfere with contextual speech development, just as most people find it difficult to carry on a conversation while jogging. The continual interruption of the speech for respiratory purposes makes flowing speech difficult.

While observing the respiratory rate, it may be helpful to make note of the rhythm of respiration as well. Inconsistency in the rhythm of breathing may indicate neuromusculature problems and is quite typical in some cerebral-palsied individuals.

Respiratory patterns are altered significantly during speech. The inhalatory

---

[4]Diaphragmatic breathing has been a concept long held dear by many voice and elocution teachers. What is the function of the diaphragm during respiration? Is it possible to consciously control the contraction or relaxation of this muscle? What is a better term for diaphragmatic breathing? (See Van Riper and Irwin, 1958; Luchsinger and Arnold, 1965; and Cotes, 1965.)

phase is shorter in duration and generally the volume of air intake is greater, while the exhalation phase is more controlled and gradual, with pulses of air being released with each syllable. Whereas the ratio of inhalation to exhalation time is approximately equal in normal respiration, it now may vary around the ratio of 1 to 7. Just as too frequent inhalations may alter the flow of speech, so may inhalation patterns that take too long to accomplish. It is by no means an easy task to measure the temporal aspects of respiration without the aid of graphic representation. In those cases where there is some serious question regarding the respiratory ratio, it may be necessary to video- and audio-tape the person and make careful evaluation by using a stopwatch.

DURATION The maximum duration of sustained exhalation reveals the respiratory mechanism's ability to regulate the exhalatory factors (rib recoil, muscle relaxation, lung tissue pressure, gravity) so as to provide a continuous flow of air without the intervening variable of vocal-fold interruption. This durational characteristic is obviously also related to vital capacity. Ptacek and Sanders (1963) obtained a low but positive correlation between this measure and maximum phonation time. These writers also determined that there is a much greater variability in exhalation time when phonation is employed than under unrestricted conditions, which indicates that the laryngeal interruption of the airstream has a significant influence upon the ability to control exhalation. Although Ptacek and Sanders provide data on this measure for various flow rates for young adults, no satisfactory normative information is available to aid the diagnostician. The measure is nonetheless useful in indicating the individual's ability to control flow rate while maintaining a steady airstream.

ASSOCIATED TENSION. Exhalation for speech purposes involves more than just the controlled relaxation of the inhalatory musculature. There is also a seris of pulselike and sustained contractions of the thoracic and abdominal muscles. Although there is no clear experimental evidence to prove the point, we feel that there are some instances in which this process results in a musculature tension that has an overflow effect upon the laryngeal musculature. The resultant hypertension may result in faulty phonatory behavior. In examination we have found this is most evident upon sustained utterance; therefore, we have devised a series of run-on sentences which the individual utters without taking additional breaths. Several contaminating variables must be assessed, however, since once the person gets below his resting lung-volume level, additional musculature tension of both the respiratory and phonatory structures will be imperative in order to maintain sufficient subglottic pressure. What we are looking for is an inordinate amount of additional tension that can sometimes be "observed" by placing the fingers lightly on the individual's neck beside the thyroid cartilage.

ASSOCIATED SOUNDS. In the healthy structure the vegetative respiratory process is fairly silent. Unwanted noise upon inhalation or exhalation may be a critical sign of a wide variety of problems ranging from laryngeal polyps and enlarged adenoidal tissue to laryngeal webs, abductor paralysis, or various types of neoplasms. Inspiratory stridor should be medically investigated immediately.

Articulation/resonation. The juxtaposition of the terms articulation and resonation is common if confusing. We are far more familiar with the uses of the term articulation to refer not only to the alteration of the airstream through muscle contraction and structure movement but also the resultant effects of that movement upon sound production. The term resonation, however, has a vague and ill-defined quality to it. The texture of the cavities, the shape and relationship of those cavities, and the opening size all have some effect upon sound production but the exact nature of these factors is not clear to most clinicians. Most unresolved of all is the question of the resonators' influence upon the so-called phonatory vocal characteristics. How much influence do the resonators have on vocal-fold action, and what effect do the resonating chambers have upon the perceived quality of the voice.[5]

Auditory skills. Routine testing for auditory acuity is suggested for all voice cases. We often go beyond simple acuity measures to evaluate the individual's ability to discriminate various speech characteristics. It is generally most appropriate to include discrimination of pitch, loudness, and quality differences, but be sure to evaluate the individual's ability to identify his own voice characteristics.

> Dan was ten years old when we first evaluated him. Referred by his classroom teacher as having a "monotonous" voice with a strange, harsh quality, we planned the following sequence of measures to measure his auditory discrimination abilities. (1) Following a hearing test we used the audiometer to see if Dan could determine the louder of two tones presented continuously. Pure tones were presented for three-second durations, followed by a two-second time lapse and a second tone 5 db louder or softer. Since this was a rather easy and possibly not too relevant task, we also used the live-voice circuit and gave Dan sentences with one word emphasized. His task was to select the word that sounded "louder" in each sentence. (This procedure ended up being a better therapy than diagnostic technique.) (2) In order to determine Dan's ability to discriminate among various pitch levels, we used a toy xylophone and had him replicate with the xylophone the various pitch patterns we presented to him. This was followed by some more vocal gymnastics on our part, with the examiner humming various inflectional patterns and Dan indicating the direction of the inflection by pointing either up or down. This same task later involved phrases and sentences and eventually, several directional changes within the same utterance. Finally, we concluded by having Dan determine the acceptability of a given utterance by ranking its adequacy on a seven-point scale. The examiner then attempted to imitate Dan's inflexible voice (without the quality distortion) and introduced sentences spoken with a moderate and maximum amount of vocal variety. (3) The examiner was put to the test when he tried to evaluate Dan's ability to discriminate

---

[5]Hoops (1960) defines two types of "quality"—vocal and speech sound quality. How do these concepts relate to the present discussion?

various vocal qualities. A series of phrases was recorded on blank language master cards, and Dan was asked to categorize them into the following groups: normal, nasal, hoarse, and breathy. We used "hoarseness" in order to replicate Dan's own voice quality. Following this task, Dan was asked to tape-record a series of phrases which we then imitated, varying our degree of imitation from normal to close approximations of his voice. Upon playback Dan was asked to determine how close in quality the two voices were.

Motor skills. Some voice disorder types require an examination of general motor skills. The general procedures as described in Chapter 3 are sufficient, although it may be well to pursue this testing further to determine the client's general strength, stamina, and ability to sustain motor activity. The oral mechanism must be examined in certain cases of resonatory vocal disturbances. Oral-sensory discrimination skills as well as velopharyngeal functioning and basic reflexes should be investigated (see Chapter 6).

Evaluation of the vocal end product. It is generally advisable to evaluate each of the vocal characteristics—pitch, loudness, and quality—no matter which dimension is the primary contributor to the vocal disorder. The following discussion parcels the evaluation process into these three primary categories, although we generally try to evaluate as many aspects of vocal production at one time as possible.

LOUDNESS. Disorders of loudness are sometimes in the ear of the beholder.

Within a span of five weeks, Mrs. W., a diminutive, proper, and somewhat elderly seventh-grade language arts teacher referred six young girls to the speech clinician because, "They speak in such soft voices no one in the room can hear them." Our initial evaluation of the girls indicated that they were rather shy and reserved but apparently were able to speak up when necessary. Suspecting that this "epidemic" was peculiar to Mrs. W.'s classes, we sent out a notice inviting any teacher in the school who might wish to have his hearing tested to come to our office on any of the following Wednesday afternoons of the month. Sure enough, Mrs. W. was one of our first customers. Unfortunately amplification did little to aid her, but we did suggest preferential seating for those students with whom she had difficulty. The girls' "voice problems" soon disappeared.

Although some of the following measurement techniques are rather subjective, we have found them to he helpful when we analyze individuals with vocal disorders:

1. Determine the normal conversational loudness level of the individual under a variety of speaking situations. First, open the conversation with your client seated a few feet away and gradually move back until you are ten to fifteen feet away. In order to determine his ability to adapt his voice to the speaking circumstance, you may wish to then provide a background noise such as a radio or tape-recorded conversation. Generally, we are listening to the loudness level at this point, but we also observe such factors as undue tension, pitch, quality change, and inability to alter with the circumstance.

2. The ability to project the voice can be evaluated by bringing the client into a large lecture room or an auditorium. We try to make the procedure rather formal in order to put the speaker under a degree of tension.

3. The ability to vary loudness with changes in meaning can be evaluated by using vocal variety drills such as those in the drillbooks of Fairbanks (1960) or Hanley and Thurman (1970). We generally ask the client to read "with feeling" sentences such as the following:

Get out of here, get out of here!
I don't know, I said I don't know!
Wash your hands, Billy!
I need more money Dad, I'm broke!
Where did she go, I can't find her?
Will you cut that out!

4. The ability to produce isolated vowel sounds is examined under a variety of conditions. First, the examiner must generally determine if the client can produce front and back and high, mid, and low vowels at various loudness levels. We listen for steadiness of tone, improved volume with changes in the resonant characteristics of the vowel, and ability to project without concomitant changes in other variables such as quality or pitch. We also determine the ability to produce a steady, unwavering tone at various loudness levels. The maximum duration of phonation of vowels is apparently related to a number of variables such as the vowel used, the frequency level, the sound-pressure level, and others (Michel and Wendahl, 1971). This variable involves both the respiratory capacity of the individual and his ability to coordinate respiration with the sound-generating mechanism of the larynx. Restricted ranges appear to be primarily related to laryngeal pathology, coordination of onset of phonation and exhalation, and vital capacity. Although there is an interesting discrepancy in the literature between the minimum length of time an individual should be able to phonate an isolated vowel, clinically we become concerned when the client cannot sustain the vowel beyond fifteen seconds.[6]

PITCH. Pitch is a perceptual phenomenon that correlates directly with the valving rate of the vocal folds. Obviously the pitch level of most voices varies continuously and flowingly, and for this reason it is sometimes difficult to measure it precisely. As the clinician attempts to formulate a diagnostic format to evaluate pitch characteristics, he must be concerned with several factors. First, there is probably a most efficient pitch level for each speaking voice. Second, each voice has a range of pitch variation. Third, there is a pitch level around which each speaker speaks during his contextual speech, and this level may or may not coincide with his most efficient pitch level. Fourth, several factors have a direct influence upon the pitch level of a given voice.

Optimal pitch. The concept of optimal performance is attractive—indeed, it is enticing. The term implies efficiency and we always expect an optimum performance from everything from our car to our golf swing. As voice clinicians

---

[6]Compare the norms stated by Van Riper (1954), Fairbanks (1960), and Luchsinger and Arnold (1965).

we are concerned not only with the acoustic end product and its appropriateness, but with the vocal mechanism's operating efficiency as well. Performance at nonoptimal levels implies greater constriction and strain of the vocal mechanism with greater potential for abuse.

The term optimal pitch is somewhat of a contradiction in terms since optimal refers to the physical workings of the voice mechanism and pitch refers to the perceptual characteristics. Optimum frequency level would be a more accurate term. We will use the concept of optimal performance to mean optimal physical performance as measured through perceptual means.

The determination of optimal pitch is by no means precise. Several methods have been described in the literature; and generally, when pitch level is of paramount concern, we use a combination of measures.

The procedures for determining optimal pitch described by Fairbanks (1960), Murphy (1964), and Boone (1977) are most frequently used by speech clinicians. They include the following:

1. The procedure described by Fairbanks is widely used. It essentially requires the client to determine his total pitch range including falsetto in full musical steps. For the adult male the optimal pitch is one-fourth of the total range up from the lowest level and for the adult female it is considered to be two notes lower than one-fourth of the way up from the lowest note.

2. Murphy describes the following procedures: (a) The loud-sigh technique: take a deep breath and intone "ah" on expiration; (b) the grunt method: grunt "ah" or "o," gradually prolonging the utterances until a passage is chanted at the original grunt pitch level; (c) the swollen tone technique: stop up the ears, sing "ah" or hum "m" up and down the scale until the pitch level at which the tone swells or is loudest is identified; (d) cough sonorously on an "ee" sound. (95)

3. Boone adds two techniques to the above: First it is suggested that the patient yawn and sigh with the phonation of the sigh expected to be at or near the optimal level. Second the patient is asked to say "uh-huh" in an affirmative voice, and this utterance, made automatically may approximate the optimal pitch level.

The following is an abstract of the notes taken during an evaluation of a thirty-three-year-old male with vocal nodules.

A total pitch range was determined by first having Mr. N. clear his throat—phonation terminating in the /a/ vowel and then, using that tone as the starting point, phonating down the scale to the lowest tone possible. After he reached this point, he began back up the scale to the highest tone possible. He had some difficulty with this, but he produced an average of sixteen tones. Using the ¼ range suggested by Pronovost (1942) as a criterion for optimal pitch, it is interesting to note that Mr. N. could sing down four notes from that original starting point, indicating that the throat-clearing may have produced almost optimal pitch. Following Murphy's (1964) suggestions, we attempted to determine optimal pitch by having the client produce loud audible sighs. We found that we had to listen only to the onset of the sighs because the client tended to lower the pitch during the sound. We also had him cough and attempt to hold the tone of the cough at a constant pitch level. This appeared quite variable, but it seemed to agree with the other findings. We tape-recorded Mr. N.'s attempts to hum up and down the scale, but neither of us could hear a "more predominant" sound at any pitch level. The idea that the optimal pitch is more resonant and pronounced is theoretically valid, but we couldn't make it work. Similarly, we attempted to measure the increase in energy by placing our fingers on the client's face and nose while he hummed up and down the scale. Apparently we have an elephant's touch, since we were unable to detect any prominent area of resonation. All of this was complicated by the fact that Mr. N. couldn't carry a tune, but the overall conclusion from these several techniques was that Mr. N. should be speaking at a pitch level approximately four tones above his lowest tone.

Pitch range. The pitch range is determined in relation to the tests for optimal pitch level. Information about the client's pitch range tells us something about the health, flexibility, and control of his respiratory and laryngeal structures. Many clients will have great difficulty humming up and down the musical scale, and consequently they usually display pitch levels in conversational speech that are above or below the one displayed in testing. It may be helpful to have the person produce the highest and lowest tones possible; by using a pitch pipe or piano, the examiner can then calculate the total range (see Fairbanks, 1960: 122–126).

Habitual pitch. The pitch level around which a person's voice varies in contextual speech is termed his habitual pitch level. Obviously this level will vary from circumstance to circumstance, but our main concern is the chronic use of a pitch level too high or too low for the individual vocal mechanism. Once again this process is probably best done through instrumental analysis of the vocal signal; however, it is possible to train the ear to listen to the client's running speech and identify his fundamental pitch level. Probably the best method of doing this is to tape-record the client and concentrate on the pitch level while listening. Make every attempt to disregard content. Match the pitch level your ear hears on a pitch pipe. The client should be totally unaware of the fact that you are recording for the purposes of evaluating pitch level, because this may affect his performance.

Boone (1971) suggests taking a tape-recorded sample and stopping the recorder a number of times on the playback and determining the pitch level by matching it with a pitch pipe. The process then results in a modal pitch level, which is the level most frequently occurring in the sample, and this is usually interpreted as the habitual pitch.

Influencing factors. Mass, effective valving length, and tension of the vocal folds are among the physical variables that influence pitch level; however, our concern at this point is with the variables that affect these three conditions and thus modify pitch.

The following evaluation techniques are used to determine the degree of pitch control, as well as the factors that influence the pitch level:

1. Ability to carry a tune
2. Ability to follow inflectional changes

3. Ability to produce a given pitch
4. Ability to match pitch change with meaning
5. Ability to maintain a steady pitch level for ten seconds
6. Ability to speak at three or more distinct pitch levels
7. Influence on pitch of changes in loudness
8. Influence on pitch of changes in vocal quality
9. Influence on pitch of physical exertion
10. Influence on pitch of distraction, encouragement, or hostility
11. Influence on pitch of posture changes
12. Influence on pitch of pressure on larynx, change in head position, or abdominal pressure
13. Influence on pitch of "aggressively" chewing gum while speaking
14. Influence on pitch of trail relaxation techniques
15. Influence on pitch of exaggerated articulation
16. Influence on pitch of verbal suggestion
17. Influence on pitch of alterations in vocal attack varying from breathy to gradual to abrupt.

QUALITY. The most difficult vocal characteristic to evaluate is quality. Involving both phonatory and resonatory characteristics, quality is that component of the voice which gives primary distinction to a given speaker's voice when pitch and loudness are excluded from judgment. Quality variations are essentially limitless but become of concern to the speech clinician when the variations take on an unpleasant and distracting character or are the precursors of physical abnormality. The variables of pitch and loudness can be scaled according to both physical and perceptual attributes, but the quality variable is still fairly dependent upon an array of subjective terms.[7]

The diagnostician must give the quality a label and describe it, determine the impact of various variables, and identify associated characteristics of the individual's speech signal.

DESCRIPTION. Since quality disorders may be either phonatory or resonatory, one of the first tasks is to make this differential determination. Following this determination, it is useful to label the quality for purposes of communication as well as conceptualization. Since there is some agreement on the meaning of the terms hoarseness, harshness, breathiness, hypernasality, and denasality (see Moore, 1971), we feel fairly confident in using them.

The following is an example of our efforts to describe the vocal quality of a young client:

Fred's voice is classified as hoarse in quality with associated components of glottal fry and breathiness. The glottal fry is transient and increases in severity at the end of

[7]For a discussion of the various terms used to describe vocal qualities, the reader is directed to the writings of Moore (1971a: 5–11), Murphy (1964: 62–74), and Perkins (1971a: 279–288).

phrases. Breath escape was evident throughout the phonatory period. Laryngeal tension, or constriction, was evidenced in excessive forcing and a general strained character to the voice. The quality disorder deserves a five on our seven-point severity scale.

IMPACT OF RELATED VARIABLES. During this portion of the evaluation the examiner determines what effects various behaviors have upon vocal quality. We generally use the same kinds of examinations as were described previously for pitch analysis.

The following conclusions were made following the examination of a young lady whose mild degree of hypernasality we had attributed to functional causes:

> Mrs. V.'s hypernasality was significantly reduced or eliminated under the following conditions: when she was asked to shout or speak with great force as if to a large gathering; when speaking while squeezing a rubber ball or attempting to lift the table; when overarticulating; and when attempting abrupt glottal attack. The common denominator appears to be increased muscle tone. Increased hypernasality was noted when Mrs. V. was speaking at a higher-than-normal pitch and when the examiner cross-examined her in a hostile manner to induce a feeling of threat. It is a positive sign that the client is able to voluntarily modify her voice quality under controlled conditions.

ASSOCIATED CHARACTERISTICS. Three additional characteristics are investigated. The nature of the glottal attack in contextual speech is determined. This is sometimes a rather difficult attribute to identify, so we generally also have the person produce a series of vowels and consonants. We also listen for the method of phonatory termination, since we have heard several speakers who terminate phonation with an abrupt grunting sound.

Second, we investigate the degree of laryngeal constriction, or tension, in phonation. Many vocal-quality disorders are directly related to laryngeal hyperfunction. We depend primarily upon four measures to determine the degree of vocal tension: observation, primarily for visible signs of strain; auditory cues that indicate a greater-than-normal degree of laryngeal valving; placing the hand lightly on the neck while the individual is speaking; individual self-report on the degree and locus of tension within the speaking mechanism.

The third associated characteristic we investigate is the general communicative skill of the individual, which includes articulation, prosody characteristics, and language level.

> Mr. G. was a prospering insurance executive. He was fifty-four years old, married, and had three grown children. Our introduction to Mr. G. followed a referral note from a local laryngologist who stated: "You are going to enjoy working with this fellow. He has a unique and bizarre vocal quality which I can't describe. We have done a thorough laryngeal exam and find no pathology. Let me know what you think!" During the initial interview we obtained the following information. Mr. G. began to have some difficulty with his voice about eighteen years ago, and it had gradually become more severe over that time. No particular incident was associated with the onset, and Mr. G. stated that he felt he had no serious psychological problems. In fact, three years prior to our seeing him, his family physician had

referred him for psychiatric counseling. "We met twice every week for six months, and he finally said I was sound as a dollar. He claimed there was something neurologically wrong with me. How about that? The medical doctors say I'm emotionally sick, and the psychiatrist says I'm physically sick—sounds like buck-passing to me." (The psychiatrist sent the following information upon our request: "Mr. G. appeared to me to be a highly controlled, relatively stable individual. He is a bit prone to depression and worry, but I found no evidence that his voice problem was related to any psychoneurotic condition.")

Mr. G.'s voice was characterized by an irregular stoppage with a strained or strangled quality, relatively low monotonous pitch with some slight degree of harshness. He continuously cleared his throat in an abrupt manner, and his face contorted slightly during aphonic moments. The voice was like one subtype of spastic (or spasmodic) dysphonia. Once the voice quality was described and identified, it was our task to add any data we could in order to determine the etiology. We suspected both neurological and psychiatric factors. In analyzing the vocal quality, the following information was secured:

1. Mr. G. is able to prolong the /a/ vowel for six seconds, the /u/ for seven seconds, and the /i/ for five seconds.

2. The vowel sounds were intermittent in voicing, and showed some signs of tremor; and some air escaped during nonphonated periods, although the cessation of sound appeared to be related more to an increase in laryngeal pressure than to an abduction of the vocal folds.

3. Mr. G. was able to sustain nonphonated exhalation for seventeen seconds.

4. Examination for pitch range was incomplete because the client was unable to vary his pitch in the lower ranges. However, we discovered at that time that Mr. G. was able to phonate without any symptoms at the higher levels. He stated that he can sing in a high pitch quite well, and this was evident upon examination.

5. The disorder was noted to be quite variable; it improved noticeably when the client made casual comments ("oh, sure, I see, uh, uh") during the conversation.

6. When the examiner placed his fingers firmly on the side of the larynx and pushed with some force, the client was able to speak with hardly any symptoms. This same voice improvement was noted when the examiner placed his fingers lightly on the side of the larynx, or up to the neck but never touching the neck surface. This suggests that the improvement was due to suggestion rather than some anatomic change. This procedure was repeated on two different occasions with similar results.

7. Changes in the posture of the head did not affect the vocal quality.

8. Three methods of vocal attack were investigated; abrupt, gradual, and breathy. Mr. G. produced significantly improved voice with the gradual attack method but stated that he felt his voice was better with the abrupt attack method.

9. Alterations in pitch had a significant influence upon the voice. Higher pitch produced improved vocal quality. Upon later retests of this same phenomenon, it was found that there were still some symptoms in the higher pitch range but not as much as in the lower levels.

10. Vocal quality deteriorated during physical exertion, although the patient is an ardent jogger and stated that his voice is quite good when he is jogging and talking.

11. Exaggerated chewing and speaking produced some remission in symptom.

12. Mr. G. was asked to read a given passage four times and each time the vocal interruption occured almost at the same place.

The following signs appeared to point to some sort of psychological etiology:

1. Variability from one pitch level to another
2. Symptoms disappeared during certain types of utterance
3. Consistency in place of interruption
4. The impact of suggestion as exemplified by the hand placed upon the neck
5. The general attitude of the client—he was cooperative to a fault and yet did not follow up on suggestions. He appeared somewhat blasé about his problem, even though it made communication nearly impossible. Several factors also indicated the need for neurological examination:
   a. The gradual onset of the problem
   b. The lack of identifiable problems in life adjustment
   c. The lack of any major symptom of psychological disturbance

   Mr. G. refused to see a neurologist as suggested, and one year of speech therapy netted minimal improvement.[8]

Prognosis

There are several aspects to prognosis. First, there is the question of spontaneous remission of the presenting symptoms. Will this individual display an improvement in vocal quality without intervening voice therapy? Second, how much improvement can be expected following the prescribed clinical program? To what degree is the voice therapy as projected going to be effective? Third, how permanent are the gains shown in therapy going to be? Is the vocal quality of such a nature that continuous therapy will be necessary to maintain the optimal vocal performance? Finally, would some other clinical procedure be of greater benefit to the client?

A variety of factors have prognostic value in voice cases. Some of the variables are directly observable and subject to quantification, while others are much more subjective. The factors appear to fall into three broad categories: characteristics of the disorder, of the person, and of the environment. They include:

1. Duration of the problem. Generally disorders of long standing have greater resistance to clinical treatment.

2. Etiological factors. Two factors are relevant here: first, is the cause of the problem identifiable? Second, is the cause of the problem alterable? And if so, is the type of habilitating service required available?

[8]Spastic dysphonia is one of the most perplexing and fascinating vocal disturbances. Compare the findings of the following authors:

Aronson, A., J. Brown, E. Litin, and J. Pearson. "Spastic Dysphonia. I. Voice, Neurologic, and Psychiatric Aspects." *Journal of Speech and Hearing Disorders,* 33 (1968): 203–218.

———. "Spastic Dysphonia. II. Comparison with Essential (Voice) Tremor and Other Neurologic and Psychogenic Dysphonias." *Journal of Speech and Hearing Disorders,* 33 (1968): 219–231.

Robe, E., J. Brunlik, and P. Moore. "A Study of Spastic Dysphonia: Neurologic and Electroencephalographic Abnormalities." *Laryngoscope,* 70 (1960): 219–245.

Heaver, L. "Spastic Dysphonia: A Psychosomatic Voice Disorder." In *Psychological and Psychiatric Aspects of Speech and Hearing,* ed. D. Barbara. Springfield, Ill.: Charles C Thomas, 1960.

3. Degree of secondary psychological components. Generally, the greater the degree of physiological disturbance the poorer the prognosis.

4. Variability and general flexibility of the voice. Are there periods when the symptom seems to improve? Can the individual vary the pitch, loudness, and quality of his voice?

5. Ability of the individual to imitate various vocal characteristics.

6. Auditory skills. Ability of the client to hear his vocal disturbance and to discriminate it from other voices.

7. Impact, or degree, of the disability. The greater the impact of the voice difference upon the individual, the better the chances for cooperation. We have found this to be a real problem in children with vocal nodules, and have found that the "Weight Watchers" concepts of group pressure and encouragement are very helpful.

8. Cooperation of the family and environment.

9. Extrinsic motivational factors. Are there some factors in the environment that reinforce this pattern and encourage its continuance?

DIAGNOSIS OF THE LARYNGECTOMEE

Working with the laryngectomized patient is a most rewarding professional experience. Laryngectomees develop a loyalty to one another and to their speech clinician that is unmatched by any other group of speech-handicapped individuals. There are approximately 40,000 laryngectomees in the United States with an additional three to four thousand new patients each year. Although many laryngectomees never find their way to a speech clinician, those who do provide a challenge which we have found to be worth the effort in every respect.

Laryngeal surgery is primarily undertaken to preserve the life of the patient; however, the surgeon is continuously conscious of the need to provide as great a chance for continued vocal function as is possible. Surgery may include excision of the total larynx, half of the larynx, one vocal fold and part of the other, removal of the anterior section of the thyroid cartilage and both vocal folds, and various other combinations. It is important that the speech clinician know exactly what procedures were undertaken since the relearning process will vary relative to the amount and type of tissues remaining.

The exact nature of the diagnostic evaluation will vary depending upon when the client is seen. The preoperative evaluation will be markedly different from that of an individual who has been struggling to learn esophageal speech for some time. There are, however, three primary goals of the diagnostic process with the laryngectomee: to provide information, support, and release; to determine the speech potential; and to provide therapy direction.

Providing Information, Support, and Release

A preoperative visit by a speech clinician, skilled esophageal speaker, or both has potential for great value or harm. Even the most skilled clinician may find that he has done his client a disservice if the client simply is not emotionally or physically capable of dealing with the issues of this first meeting. Probably the physician is best qualified to make such judgments, and most speech clinicians depend upon the referral of the physician before working with the laryngectomee. The clinician must remember that he is dealing with an individual who is facing a trauma unparalled in his lifetime. Fears of death, loss of communication, loss of job and earning power, and social and marital adjustments plague him. The first confrontation is no social chat and may well demand all of the professional proficiency the clinician can muster. We have found on more than one occasion that the patient was not capable of dealing rationally with the topic immediately before surgery, and we terminated the discussion with assurance that we would be seeing them soon following their recovery.

One of the major goals of our first meeting with a laryngectomee is to provide some information about his operation and the implications for speech. Every attempt should be made to present a clear discussion of the anatomical changes. Charts and diagrams often are helpful. We generally use a demonstration tape of excellent esophageal speech or, if possible, have an exemplary esophageal speaker accompany us on this first visit. We stress that excellent esophageal speech is the major goal, but it is not the only one. Several options are discussed such as the electrolarynx, the Asai technique (with the physician's approval), and written communication.[9] Although there is still some controversy over the use of the electrolarynx, it is clearly the "treatment of choice" in some cases. We have found, however, that it is not always a particularly successful technique immediately after the operation, since the sublingual and cervical tissues tend to be extremely firm, which makes it difficult to get the generated tone into the resonating cavitites.

Although further information is sometimes provided in this first discussion, generally, it is best to deal with related problems after surgery, or as they arise. Many times even the discussion of the anticipated communication problem has little impact until after the patient has experienced muteness. Nearly every laryngectomee can recall the first time when he opened his mouth to say something only to be reminded of his plight.

Providing adequate information to the family can have far-reaching clinical implication. The spouse must understand the anatomy of the operation as well as the patient himself. The wife of one of our laryngectomees told of walking into her husband's room just in time to find a well-meaning friend attempting to feed the patient through his stoma.

Very often clinicians stress what the laryngectomee will be unable to do; and although this information is important, we feel that it is also important to stress to the family what the patient will be *able* to do. We generally attempt to have a frank discussion with the spouse about the typical reactions of the family. If a pattern can

----

[9]The Asai technique (see Miller, 1969) involves a series of three surgical techniques in which the patient's pharynx and trachea are connected by the neoglottis. Respiratory air provides the force for phonation, although the stoma must be blocked with finger pressure.

be identified before it develops, it may be easier to control. The tendency to dominate the silent mate (or parent) must be controlled, as must the inclinations to infantilize, overindulge, and pity. Very often we have to warn the family not to shout to the patient. Almost as if by instinct many people find themselves shouting at the laryngectomee as if he were deaf rather than voiceless. One of our laryngec- tomee friends had a sign posted at the foot of his hospital bed stating, "My hearing is fine—it's my voice that I've lost!" Many families readily admit to a feeling of repulsion because of the physical changes. Interestingly, this is easily conveyed to the laryngectomee, since many are extremely sensitive about their operation. The silent mate is often excluded from conversation and decision-making in many families. Some laryngectomees have reported feeling that there was a conspirato- rial mood in their house after the operation. The clincian must be sensitive to the fact that the spouse will have fears of his own. The fear of death, reduced income, new responsibilities, social changes, and changes in all facets of marital relation- ships may be topics for discussion.

One of the primary purposes of the clinician's first visit with the laryngec- tomee and his family is to let them know that he understands their feelings. The laryngectomized speech instructors we have worked with feel that they are more effective than speech clinicians in this area. "You can tell me how much you understand my feelings all you want, but unless I see that stoma shield on your neck I know darn well you don't really understand," stated one of our most astute friends. It is expected that the clinician will be warm, sincere, and insightful, but we resist the temptation to dictate any specific attitude beyond this because each patient will require a somewhat different approach. Some need to be dealt with gently, others straightforwardly and frankly. (We have several laryngectomee clients who learned to whistle soon after we told them that whistling was one of the things they could never do again.) Find the level and type of interaction your client responds to best and use it.[10]

Determining the Potential for Speech

A thorough case history is helpful with the laryngectomee, but two facets are particularly crucial. It is important to know the extent of the surgery, the degree of involvement of related structures such as the tongue or pharynx, general health of the client, and the medical prognosis. The second crucial area is the individual's vocation and interests. We find it most helpful to plan our clinical work about the client's interests and activities. One of our laryngectomees learned to produce esophageal sound while practicing his golf swing in our office, while another first produced the sound while slamming his cards on the table and exclaiming "gin."

[10]The following booklets may be helpful in your early work with the laryngectomee:

Lauder, E. *Self-Help for the Laryngectomee*. 1115 Whisper Hollow, San Antonio, Texas 78230. ($3.50)

Waldrop, W. and M. Gould. *Your New Voice*. Available free from a local American Cancer Society office.

It may also be necessary to examine the client's oral anatomy. Generally we evaluate the tongue, lip, and jaw mobility as well as the oral discrimination skills. Some information about the previous articulation, speech, and language pattern of the client is helpful, but this is not always available.

If the client has already begun to learn esophageal speech, some measure of his current performance level will be helpful. Wepman and his colleagues (1953) provide an objective measurement device. Berlin (1963: 42) presents the following guidelines:

1. Ability to phonate reliably on demand
2. Maintenance of a short latency between inflation of the esophagus and vocalization
3. Maintenance of an adequate duration of phonation
4. Ability to sustain phonation during articulation

Careful analysis should be made of the client's method of air intake and associated mannerisms. It is generally easier to prevent poor speaking habits than to correct them.

An assessment of the hearing acuity and auditory discrimination skills may prove helpful. Since a high percentage of laryngectomees are males above the age of fifty-five, it is common to find a degree of hearing loss. A moderate-to-severe hearing loss may make the learning process more difficult but not impossible.

No formal intelligence test is suggested for the laryngectomee client, but we do find it useful to assess the client's general understanding of our instructions. Generally, it is helpful to ask the client to rephrase your instructions to him, giving you some idea of his ability to understand and your ability to communicate. Similarly, the emotional state of your client should be appraised, although this is no time to administer formal tests, label, or judge. It would be difficult to know exactly what "normal" should be for such a client. Your task is to take note of the general tendencies and use this information for your work.

It is sometimes helpful to know something about the pre- and postsurgical habits of the client. Cigarette smoking and alcohol present two typical problems for these individuals. Although the sudden inability to smoke may contribute to further psychological upheaval, we have found that many previously heavy smokers claim almost no desire for cigarettes after the operation. This is a curious phenomenon and may be tied to the fact that inhalation smoking is obviously no longer possible, and the psyche had accepted this state of affairs with little struggle.

Trial Therapy and Therapy Direction

Once we have determined the performance level of the client, we must identify the most efficient method of air intake and sound production. We almost always begin by proving to the client that he can still make several speech sounds.

At this same time we emphasize methods for building up oral pressure for the voiceless consonants. This process serves to motivate the client by showing him that he can still make sounds while also stressing articulatory precision, oral pressure, and separation of breathing and speech. The plosive injection method of air intake has proven most successful for us and is used almost exclusively in our first session. We accept any port in a storm, however, and generally begin by having the client produce esophageal sound by any method he can. If this initial attempt is not successful, every available method of air intake and sound production is tried. It is relatively important that the client make some esophageal sound during that first session! Very often we even accept a "volunteer" (burp) as proof that something must be working to get air into the esophagus.

Little has been said in this discussion about the need to motivate the laryngectomee. Success in sound production is the best inspiration, and we have abandoned an earlier practice of pep talks, lectures, and cheer-leading in favor of direction, success, and reinforcement. A few intelligible words spoken by the client do more than our most eloquent speeches.

CLEFT PALATE

There is no such thing as cleft-palate speech. Granted, typical speech and language patterns can be identified within the cleft-palate population, but the clinician must be encouraged to assess the total communication ability of the child rather than analyzing a few identifying aspects. *Cleft palate is an etiological category, not a symptomatic denotation.* It is with some reservation, then, that we discuss "cleft palate" diagnosis, since we are actually diagnosing the child's oral communication skills, not his physical state. We cannot, however, simply select portions of the total diagnostic process and apply them to the cleft-palate child, since there are specific considerations unique to these children.

In cleft-palate diagnosis the speech clinician is a member of a team. The "cleft-palate team" (see Wells, 1971: 143–175) is a well-accepted clinical entity, and in many communities represents the ultimate in interdisciplinary cooperation. The speech clinician is expected to inform the team members about the child's speech, and predict the effects of contemplated rehabilitative procedures. In addition he is also to serve as a primary agent for change in the child's speech development. The dramatic growth in the development of surgical and other rehabilitative procedures for the cleft-palate child during the two decades from 1950 to 1970 (see Grabb et. al., 1971) has been encouraging. What is needed now, however, is not only new knowledge, but also a general dissemination of present knowledge to those responsible for the rehabilitation of the cleft-palate child. The cleft-palate teams throughout the world serve this second function nobly.

Diagnosis

The routine case-history data may need to be augmented for the cleft-palate child. Knowledge of the type of cleft the child was born with (see Harkins and others, 1962) as well as a description of the surgical, prosthodontic, orthodontic, and other rehabilitative procedures performed would be helpful. Some statement of the child's current medical status and plans for his future will also help direct the evaluative process.

Critical listening. Although the initial interaction between clinician and child should be free and relatively unstructured, the clinician has a most demanding task. Once the child is interacting and conversing in a spontaneous manner, the clinician must apply his critical listening abilities to assess the child's total communicative effectiveness. The first task involves systematically shifting perceptual sets from one aspect of the child's speech to another. First, the clinician should listen for the degree of nasality and the type. Although trained judges are able to identify nasality fairly adequately, the clinician may wish to tape-record the child and play the tape backwards (see Sherman, 1954; Spriestersbach, 1955) to isolate the nasality from the articulation. After noting the degree of nasality or denasality, preferably on some scaling device, the clinician should listen to the general articulatory pattern without recording actual errors. What influence does the articulation pattern have on the total judgment of the child's speech? Is there an obvious preponderance of a particular type of error (glottal stops, pharyngeal fricatives)? Does the articulation appear to alter with differing communication situations, rates, stress patterns? Next, he should listen to the language of the child, and check for appropriate word choice, sentence complexity and structure, and other grammatical aspects. The rate and rhythm of the child's speech should be evaluated. Lass and Noll (1970) found that cleft-palate speakers used a slower rate of speech. How does one judge the child's speaking rate? What other vocal quality characteristics are evident? Finally, what particular mannerisms attract your attention? Is there a facial grimace, constriction of the nares, or any other behavior which detracts from the child's total effectiveness? At this same time we generally note several particularly appealing characteristics of the individual. It is important not to fabricate, but to select the positive attributes. Later in the therapy process we will want to accentuate the positive, and now is the time to get started.

Articulation testing. Standard articulation-testing procedures may be satisfactory for cleft-palate children, but there are several special considerations.

First, the examiner must ask himself a critical question. Why would a child with a cleft palate have articulation problems? Certainly all of the functional, perceptual, and sensory factors which affect the normal child could be active, but what other factors unique to these children may be investigated? Most important are the degree of velopharyngeal closure and the resultant airflow and intraoral pressure.[11] The deviant geography of the oral cavity may also contribute to this problem, which is also complicated by the fact that the oral structure may well have undergone several architectural changes within the first few years of life. The diagnostician must keep in mind that this child has been trying to produce "standard" sounds with a nonstandard structure, and under these conditions he may have made unique compensatory adjustments. He may have increased the airflow in order to build up adequate oral pressure, or minimized it to lessen nasal escape. It is entirely possible that the habits developed before the final surgical adjustments may persist, even though he can now make the correct articulatory movements.

Articulation errors may be related to an existant or prior hearing loss, parental overprotection, general immaturity, or distortion due to concomitant nasal escape of air. Bzoch (1971) has devised an *Error Pattern Articulation Test* which may help categorize errors and systematize the search.

During articulation testing with cleft-palate children the following deserve particular attention:

1. Certain sounds have a higher probability for error than others. Be sure to listen carefully for the affricates, fricatives, and plosives. Modify the test to get a thorough sample of them.

2. Since articulation involves dynamic and overlapping movements, be sure to test for articulation errors with isolated sounds, sound groupings, words, and context testing. Make a careful analysis of blend production. Why would the dynamic nature of articulation be a more important consideration in cleft-palate children?

3. Certain types of errors, not often found with other children, are common among the cleft-palate population. Listen for glottal stops and pharyngeal fricatives and distortions involving nasal escape of air.

4. Group the sounds in error according to manner of production. This may give you a clue to the nature of the problem.

5. Listen for alterations in articulation accuracy with variations in rate and force of speaking.

6. Listen for weak consonants with a light articulatory contact and inadequate plosive pressure.

7. Stimulability testing may be most efficient if it includes stimulability for the acoustic characteristics and the articulatory placement of the stimulus sound. Jacobs and others (1970) developed the Miami Imitative Ability Test to test stimulability.

8. It is imperative to analyze the dynamics of the articulation errors in cleft-palate children. What specific anatomical adjustments is this child making in order to produce this sound? Make a careful kinetic analysis. It should come as no surprise that these children are selecting improper places and manners of production for very good reasons; normal methods simply result in too much nasality and nasal escape. It

[11]Subtelny and others (1970) noted a significant decrease (50 percent) in articulation errors following pharyngeal flap surgery. What indicators would you use to determine the need for such an operation? Look into the following: (1) type of articulation errors, (2) degree of nasality and nasal escape of air associated with velopharyngeal closure, and (3) intraoral breath pressure. Do you agree with the premise put forward by Alley (1965)?

is important to listen to the sound production in its various phases. What happens as the pressure builds up in the implosion stage of plosive production? Is there nasal escape or facial contortion?

Nasal resonance. Resonatory voice disorders are generally described as variations of two types: hyper- and hyponasality. Hypernasality is generally the results of inadequate velopharyngeal closure, which in turn may be related to functional factors such as tension and fatigue or organic factors such as bulbar polio or cleft palate. Listener evaluation of the nasality of a speaking voice is apparently related to such factors as articulation adequacy as well as the actual resonant characteristics (Lintz and Sherman, 1961). Although there is some controversy, trained judges can reliably measure nasality by playing tape-recorded stimuli backwards (Spriestersbach, 1955).

Many clinicians at one time felt that tongue carriage, oral opening, and articulatory precision were the primary factors in nasal quality and saw velopharyngeal closure as only a subordinate factor. (No doubt, some clinicians felt that they had more direct control over such factors as articulation and tongue carriage.) Now, however, it is evident that velopharyngeal closure is absolutely necessary to produce speech that is not hypernasal, although the exact nature of the relationship has not been determined.

Once the examiner has identified nasality in the voice, he must first determine the variations of nasality within the vowels. A careful study of vowel production may indicate a general pattern—i.e., low vowels are more nasal than high (Lintz and Sherman, 1961). Exaggerated articulation, force, light contact speech, strongly stimulated speech, and rate and tension variations—all will influence nasality.

Nasality is no longer a universal characteristic of the speech of the cleft-palate child. Current surgical procedures are having a positive impact on this component of speech, and nasality is no longer seen as the primary communication problem with most cleft-palate children.

Velopharyngeal closure. Velopharyngeal closure not only detemines the ultimate degree of nasality in the speaking voice, but also articulatory accuracy. The child must be able to *dynamically* close and open the velopharyngeal port to produce intelligible speech, and the assessment of this ability has been a source of concern and consternation for speech clinicians for some time. Objective measurements through X-ray procedures are not always possible, and the clinician must find some way to evaluate this crucial function. The oral manometer measures intraoral breath pressure, which is related to the ability of the velar port to close; however, this action is rather static and may not be related to actual speech production. Morris (1966) indicates the need to supplement manometric results with other diagnostic information. A similar complaint could be made of measures using blowing, as McWilliams and Bradley (1965) point out; speech may require a type of velopharyngeal action other than blowing.

Examination of the oral mechanism may be helpful but is very susceptible to error. We attempt to observe the movement of the pharyngeal walls and velum during production of the /a/ vowels as well as the length, width, and mobility of the palate and the general size of the oropharynx.

Fox and Johns (1970) describe a technique for measuring static closure whereby the child is required to maintain intraoral pressure by puffing up his cheeks. If this is accomplished, then he is asked to stick his tongue out and then puff up his cheeks. The examiner holds the child's nostrils while this is done to aid in impounding pressure. If no air escapes when the nostrils are released, it is assumed that velopharyngeal closure is adequate. (Why would it be necessary to have the child stick his tongue out while puffing up his cheeks?)

Morris, Spriestersbach, and Darley (1961) developed the Iowa Pressure Articulation Test to measure velopharyngeal closure. The test includes primarily fricative, plosive, and affricate productions and compares favorably with more objective tests such as X-ray and oral pressure techniques. Evaluating the efficiency of velopharyngeal closure through articulation testing also appears to be a clinically valuable tool. In fact, Shelton and others (1965: 42) concluded that "articulation testing appears to provide a better test of palatopharyngeal adequacy for speech than do simple measures of nasal air escape or oral breath pressure."

Some cleft-palate children may be able to achieve adequate velopharyngeal closure during single-word productions but find the exact and rapid velar adjustments required for contextual speech impossible. Therefore, the comparison of articulation proficiency between single words and connected speech may provide an estimate of velopharyngeal competence. Van Demark (1964) devised a stimulated sentence articulation test which contains at least twenty examples of fricatives, stop-plosives, glides, nasal semivowels, and blends. The test is presented below with the test consonants italicized. Errors of the stop-plosives and fricatives as well as a predominance of distortion due to excessive nasal emission may indicate inadequate velopharyngeal closure.

1. *M*os*t* *b*oy*s* li*k*e *t*o *p*lay *f*oo*t*ball.
2. *D*o you ha*v*e a *br*o*th*er or *s*i*st*er?
3. *T*ed ha*d* a *d*og wi*th* whi*t*e *f*eet.
4. *W*e *sh*ouldn'*t* *p*lay i*n* *th*e *s*treet.
5. *Pl*aying i*n* *th*e *s*now is *f*un.
6. *N*i*ck's* *gr*an*dm*o*th*er li*v*es i*n* *th*e *c*i*t*y.
7. *W*e *g*o *s*wi*m*ming o*n* a *v*ery *h*o*t* *d*ay.
8. I *l*i*k*e i*c*e *cr*eam.
9. *T*om ha*s* *h*am an*d* e*gg*s *f*or *br*ea*kf*ast.
10. *W*e *w*en*t* *t*o *t*own *y*es*t*er*d*ay.
11. *C*an you *c*ount *t*o *n*ine?
12. *D*o you *w*ant *t*o *t*ake *m*y *n*ew *c*ap?
13. *D*o you *k*now *th*e *n*ame o*f* *m*y *d*oll?

Oral mechanism. Obviously, examination of the oral mechanism is especially important in the cleft-palate child. The alveolar ridge is the contact point for 70 to 80 percent of the consonant sounds of contextual speech. Special note should be made of the contour and evenness of the ridge and the dental structure and occlusion. Berry (1949) postulated a higher incidence of lingual anomalies among the cleft-palate population; however, this thesis has been questioned by several authorities. Van Demark and Van Demark (1967) found that judges could not differentiate the articulation patterns of cleft-palate children from children with functional articulation disorders. This finding, among others, appears to substantiate the contention that lingual function in the cleft-palate population is similar to that of the normal population. However, the clinician must still examine the functioning of the oral structures. Marks (1968) indicated that cleft-palate children have a higher incidence of tongue-thrusting than the normal population; and Hochberg and Kabcenell (1967) found inferior oral stereognosis abilities among cleft-palate individuals. These factors should be evaluated with care during the oral examination.

Auditory acuity. The high incidence of auditory acuity problems among cleft-palate children has been well documented (Loeb, 1964; Sataloff and Fraser, 1952). For this reason it is absolutely essential that every cleft-palate child have a hearing examination at least once each year. These examinations should include both air- and bone-conduction testing and should be a part of every speech diagnosis.

Psychological and social adjustment. Although it has been frequently hypothesized that cleft-palate children have more adjustment problems than normal children, this thesis has not been substantiated by research (Phipps, 1965). The difference of opinion between clinicians and researchers may reflect the former's lack of confidence in the child to overcome gross physical differences or the latter's lack of research sophistication. There is no final answer to this, and each diagnostic session with a cleft-palate individual should include an evaluation of his adjusting characteristics. We have found it equally profitable to investigate the parental and family adjustment, since environmental reaction is often directly linked with the child's self-concepts.

Language assessment. Several researchers have documented the existence of a language deficit among cleft-palate children (Nation, 1970; Smith and McWilliams, 1968; Morris, 1962). The clinician should examine the child's traditional language abilities and pay particular attention to his expressive skills.

Many children with cleft palates develop language at a normal rate and in a normal sequence. Our suggestion to carefully evaluate the language component is intended to alert the clinician to the possibility of language disorder since there is some indication in the literature to suggest a higher than normal risk. The procedures discussed in Chapters 4 and 5 should be sufficient for this evaluation.

The speech clinician will wish to see the cleft-palate child as soon as possible. During this early contact the parents can be informed regarding the need for normal speech and language stimulation, what to expect from their child regarding speech production, and something of the anatomical requirements for speech. Some speech clinicians use established language-stimulation programs as a preventative measure with these children.

The diagnostic evaluation of a cleft-palate child should be comprehensive, and cover more than just certain aspects of speech. The speech clinician, as a member of the diagnostic team, must evaluate a large number of behaviors, but his responsibility does not end there. Following a careful evaluation, he must be able to accurately and concisely communicate his findings both orally and in writing. (In Chapter 10 we will discuss the report-writing process.)

PROJECTS AND QUESTIONS

1. Devise a voice analysis checklist that employs each of the vowels of the "vowel diagram" as syllable-releasers, syllable-arresters, and in isolation.
2. Vowels are sometimes classified as front-central-back, high-med-low, tense-lax, and open-closed. How might you incorporate these categorizations into your voice analysis?
3. What relevance to voice diagnosis would the following historical data have?
    a. Polio at age five
    b. Exceedingly slow metabolic rate
    c. History of drug abuse
    d. Problems of dry skin and hair
    e. Pain when swallowing
4. How does Moore (1971a) use the term compliance in vocal-fold movement? How might vocal-fold compliance be altered in the healthy mechanism, and how would those changes affect the voice?
5. When the laryngologist finds the site of the phonatory problem, he may have to identify any of the following factors: nodules, polyps, papillomas, edema, inflammation, laryngeal web, congenitally small larynx, contact ulcer, paralysis, ankylosis. Define each of these terms.
6. Michel and Wendahl (1971) suggest that sustained exhalation can be measured by having the individual blow through a straw, placing the tip of the straw just below the surface of a glass of water. The purpose of the test is to determine duration of exhalation, but does it involve other variables? What are the advantages and disadvantages of this technique?
7. Why do most speech clinicians routinely administer a hearing test to individuals with voice disorders? Categorize your responses under the headings: general precautions, therapeutic implications, and coincident variables.
8. Determine your own "natural pitch level" using the technique described by Fairbanks (1960: 122–126).
9. Perkins (1971) uses the terms pitch, loudness, voicing, constriction, mode, and focus in his discussion of voice disorders. What does he mean by these terms?
10. The abilities to produce esophageal voice and to use the electrolarynx are important to clincial success with the laryngectomee. Be sure you have developed both skills before your first meeting with a laryngectomized client.

11. Although the identification of the etiology of a voice disorder is not generally the speech clinician's task alone, it is often necessary for the clinician to know the significant attributes which characterize each disorder. Write a profile for each of the following voice disorders. We will help out by providing the first two.

Vocal Nodules

In children the syndrome includes excessive yelling, a greater than normal amount of talking, and verbal aggressiveness. The child probably comes from a family with some unresolved adjustment problems and the child may reflect these difficulties in his own feelings of self worth. The voice is husky with breathiness and the child has a history of speaking at a rather high pitch level. No pain is noted with this disorder. In adults the pattern of vocal abuse is similar to that with children. These people appear to have a high energy level and are uncomfortable in silent settings. The abuse of the voice is often associated with personal adjustment problems. Mike W. is a good example:

> Mike was a graduating senior who had experienced three very successful years with the University Theater Group. During his last quarter Mike was cast in a role which demanded little of his acting talents but required a modest amount of shouting and vocal projection. During our early discussions regarding his rather rapidly developing "hoarseness" it became evident that Mike was very unsure about his future and rather unhappy about the minor role he received in his last play as a college student. Clinical intervention included a visit with his advisor, the director of the play, and several of Mike's close associates in the Theater Department.

Contact Ulcers

This person is probably an adult male who is known as a hard worker, somewhat aggressive, with a strong feeling of purpose and drive. The voice is low in pitch, hoarse with breathiness. This person may report a pain associated with talking which radiates out from the throat area.

Spastic Dysphonia

Mutational Falsetto Voice

Aphonia

Juvenile Pappilomas

Carcinoma

12. It is difficult if not impossible to adequately describe voice quality differences. Subjective terms provide little help for the clinician. Aronson (1973) and Wilson and Rice (1977) present a series of tapes designed to train the student in identification of the various types of voice disorders. Review these tapes.
13. What are the three major causes of hoarseness in children?
14. What are the following procedures?

    a. laminography
    b. laryngography
    c. laryngoscopy
    d. cinematography
    e. cineflurography
    f. electromyography
    g. sound spectography

BIBLIOGRAPHY

ALLEY, N. (1965). "The Use of Speech Aid Prosthesis as a Diagnostic Tool." *Cleft Palate Journal*, 2: 291–292.

ARONSON, A. (1973). *Psychogenic Voice Disorders*. Philadelphia: W. B. Saunders Company.

———; J. BROWN; E. LITIN; and J. PEARSON (1968). "Spastic Dysphonia: I. Voice, Neurologic, and Psychiatric Aspects." *Journal of Speech and Hearing Disorders*, 33: 203–218.

——— (1968). "Spastic Dysphonia: II. Comparison with Essential (Voice) Tremor and Other Neurologic and Psychogenic Dysphonias." *Journal of Speech and Hearing Disorders*, 33: 219–231.

BERLIN, C. (1963). "Clinical Management of Esophageal Speech: I. Methodology and Curves of Skill Acquistion." *Journal of Speech and Hearing Disorders*, 28: 42–51.

BERRY, M. (1949). "Lingual Anomalies Associated with Palatal Clefts," *Journal of Speech and Hearing Disorders*. 14: 359–362.

——— and J. EISENSON (1956). *Speech Disorders*. New York: Appleton-Century-Crofts.

BOONE, D. (1977). *The Voice and Voice Therapy*. Englewood Cliffs, N.J.: Prentice-Hall, Inc.

BRACKETT, I. (1971). "Parameters of Voice Quality," In *Handbook of Speech Pathology and Audiology*, ed. L. Travis. New York: Appleton-Century-Crofts. Pp. 441–463.

BRADFORD, L.; A. BROOKS; and R. SHELTON (1964). "Clinical Judgment of Hypernasality in Cleft-Palate Children." *Cleft Palate Journal*, 1: 329–335.

BZOCH, K. (1971). "Measurement of Parameters of Cleft Palate Speech," in *Cleft Lip and Palate Surgical, Dental, and Speech Aspects*, ed. W. Grabb, S. Rosenstein, and K. Bzoch. Boston: Little, Brown & Co.

CHASE, R. (1960). "An Objective Evaluation of Palatopharyngeal Competence." *Plastic and Reconstructive Surgery*, 26: 23–39.

COTES, J. (1965). *Lung Function*. Philadelphia: F. A. Davis Company.

CURRY, E. (1949). "Hoarseness and Voice Change in Male Adolescents." *Journal of Speech and Hearing Disorders*. 14: 23–24.

CURTIS, J. (1968). "Acoustics of Speech Production and Nasalization." In *Cleft Palate and Communication*, eds. D. Spriestersbach and D. Sherman. New York: Academic Press, Pp. 27–60.

DAMSTE, P., and J. LERMAN, (1975). *An Introduction to Voice Pathology Functional and Organic*. Springfield, Ill.: Charles C. Thomas.

DARLEY, F. (1964). *Diagnosis and Appraisal of Communication Disorders*. Englewood Cliffs, N.J.: Prentice-Hall, Inc.

DEAL, R.; B. McCLAIN; and J. SUDDERTH (1976). "Identification, Evaluation, Therapy, and Follow-up for Children with Vocal Nodules in a Public School Setting." *Journal of Speech and Hearing Disorders*, 41: 390–397.

DIEDRICH, W., and K. YOUNGSTROM (1966). *Alaryngeal Speech*. Springfield, Ill.: Charles C. Thomas.

DIEHL, C., and C. STINNETT (1959). "Efficiency of Teacher Referrals in a School Speech Testing Program." *Journal of Speech and Hearing Disorders*, 24: 34–36.

FAIRBANKS, G., (1960). *Voice and Articulation Drillbook*, 2nd ed. New York: Harper & Row.

FOX, D., and M. BLECHMAN (1975). *Clinical Management of Voice Disorders*. Lincoln, Nebraska: Cliffs Notes, Inc.

———, and D. JOHNS (1970). "Predicting Velopharyngeal Closure with a Modified Tongue-Anchor Technique." *Journal of Speech and Hearing Disorders*, 35: 248–251.

GRAY, G., and C. WISE (1959). *The Bases of Speech*, 3rd ed. New York: Harper & Row.

GREEN, M. (1964). *The Voice and Its Disorders*. Philadelphia: J. B. Lippincott Co.

HANLEY, T., and R. PETERS (1971). "The Speech and Hearing Laboratory." In *Handbook of Speech Pathology and Audiology*, ed. L. Travis, New York: Appleton-Century-Crofts. Pp. 75–140.

————, and W. THURMAN (1970). *Developing Vocal Skills*, 2nd ed. New York: Holt, Rinehart & Winston, Inc.

HARDY, J. (1961). "Intraoral Breath Pressure in Cerebral Palsy." *Journal of Speech and Hearing Disorders*, 26: 309–319.

HARKINS, C.; B. ASA; R. HARDING; J. LONGACRE; and R. SNODGRASS (1962). "A Classification of Cleft Lip and Cleft Palate." *Plastic and Reconstructive Surgery*. 29: 31–39.

HEAVER, L. (1960) "Spastic Dysphonia: A Psychosomatic Voice Disorder," in *Psychological and Psychiatric Aspects of Speech and Hearing*, ed. D. Barbara, Springfield, Ill.: Charles C Thomas.

HOCHBERG, I., and J. KABCENELL (1967). "Oral Stereognosis in Normal and Cleft Palate Individuals." *Cleft Palate Journal*, 4: 47–57.

HOOPS, R. (1960). *Speech Science*. Springfield, Ill.: Charles C. Thomas.

JACKSON, C. (1941). "Vocal Nodules." American Laryngological Association, 63: 185.

JACOBS, R.; B. PHILIPS; and R. HARRISON (1970). "A Stimulability Test for Cleft-Palate Children." *Journal of Speech and Hearing Disorders*, 35: 354–360.

JAMES, H., and E. COOPER (1966). "Accuracy of Teacher Referral of Speech-Handicapped Children." *Exceptional Child*, 30: 29–33.

JOHNSON, W.; F. DARLEY; and D. SPRIESTERSBACH (1963). *Diagnostic Methods in Speech Pathology*. New York: Harper & Row.

KAPLAN, H. (1971). *Anatomy and Physiology of Speech*, 2nd ed. New York: McGraw-Hill.

LASS, N., and J. NOLL (1970). "A Comparative Study of Rate Characteristics in Cleft-Palate and Noncleft-Palate Speakers." *Cleft Palate Journal*, 7: 275–283.

LAUDER, E. (1971). *Self-Help for the Laryngectomee*. San Antonio, Tex.: Edmund Lauder.

LINTZ, L., and D. SHERMAN (1961). "Phonetic Elements and Perception of Nasality." *Journal of Speech and Hearing Research*, 4: 381–396.

LOEB, W. (1964). "Speech, Hearing, and the Cleft Palate." *Archives of Otolaryngology*, 79: 4–14.

LUCHSINGER, R., and G. ARNOLD (1965). *Voice-Speech-Language*. Belmont, Calif.: Wadsworth Publishing Company, Inc.

MARKS, C. (1968). "Tongue-Thrusting and Interdentalization of Speech Sounds Among Cleft-Palate and Noncleft-Palate Subjects." *Cleft Palate Journal*, 5: 48–56.

MASSENGILL, R., (1974). "Role of the Speech Pathologist in the Management of the Cleft Lip and Palate Patient," in *Symposium on Management of Cleft Lip and Palate and Associated Deformities*, ed. N. Georgiade. Saint Louis: The C. V. Mosby Company.

McDONALD, E., and B. CHANCE, JR. (1964). *Cerebral Palsy*. Englewood Cliffs, N.J.: Prentice-Hall, Inc.

McWILLIAMS, B., and D. BRADLEY (1965). "Ratings of Velopharyngeal Closure During Blowing and Speech." *Cleft Palate Journal*, 2: 46–55.

————; R. MUSGRAVE; and P. CROZIER (1968). "The Influence of Head Position Upon Velopharyngeal Closure." *Cleft Palate Journal*, 5: 117–124.

MICHEL, J., and R. WENDAHL (1971). "Correlates of Voice Production." In *Handbook of Speech Pathology and Audiology*, ed. L. Travis. New York: Appleton-Century-Crofts. Pp. 465–479.

MILLER, A. (1969). "First Experiences with the Asai Technique for Vocal Rehabilitation

After Total Laryngectomy," in *Speech Rehabilitation of the Laryngectomized*, ed. J. Snidecor. Springfield, Ill.: Charles C. Thomas. Pp. 50–57.

MOORE, G. (1971a). *Organic Voice Disorders*. Englewood Cliffs, N.J.: Prentice-Hall, Inc.

———— (1971b). "Voice Disorders Organically Based." In *Handbook of Speech Pathology and Audiology*, ed. L. Travis, New York: Appleton-Century-Crofts. Pp. 535–569.

———— (1977). "Have the Major Issues in Voice Disorders Been Answered by Research in Speech Science? A 50-Year Retrospective." *Journal of Speech and Hearing Disorders*, 42: 152–160.

MORLEY, M. (1967). *Cleft Palate and Speech*, 6th ed. Baltimore: Williams & Wilkins.

MORRIS, H. (1962). "Communication Skills of Children with Cleft Lips and Palates." *Journal of Speech and Hearing Research*, 5: 79–90.

———— (1966). "The Oral Manometer as a Diagnostic Tool in Clinical Speech Pathology," *Journal of Speech and Hearing Disorders*, 31: 362–369.

————; D. SPRIESTERSBACH; and F. DARLEY (1961). "An Articulation Test for Assessing Competency of Velopharyngeal Closure." *Journal of Speech and Hearing Research*, 4: 48–55.

MOSES, P. (1954). *The Voice of Neurosis*. New York: Grune & Stratton.

MURPHY, A. (1964). *Functional Voice Disorders*. Englewood Cliffs, N.J.: Prentice-Hall, Inc.

MYSAK, E. (1966). "Phonatory and Resonatory Problems," in *Speech Pathology: An International Study of the Science*, ed. R. Rieber and R. Brubaker. Amsterdam: North-Holland Publishing Company, Pp. 150–181.

NATION, J. (1970). "Vocabulary Comprehension and Usage in Preschool Cleft-Palate and Normal Children." *Cleft Palate Journal*, 7: 639–644.

NOLL, J. (1970). "Articulatory Assessment." In *Speech and the Dentofacial Complex: The State of the Art*, ed. R. Wertz. ASHA Reports No. 5. Washington D.C.: American Speech and Hearing Association. Pp. 283–298.

PERKINS, W. (1971a). *Speech Pathology An Applied Behavioral Science*. St. Louis: C.V. Mosby Company.

———— (1971b). "Vocal Function: Assessment and Therapy." In *Handbook of Speech Pathology and Audiology*, ed. L. Travis, New York: Appleton-Century-Crofts. Pp. 505–534.

PHILIPS, B. and R. HARRISON (1969). "Language Skills of Preschool Cleft-Palate Children." *Cleft Palate Journal*, 6: 108–119.

PHIPPS, G. (1965). "Psychosocial Aspects of Cleft Palate." In *Proceedings of the Conference: Communicative Problems in Cleft Palate*, ed. D. Green. ASHA Reports No. 1. Washington, D.C.: The American Speech and Hearing Association, Pp. 103–110.

POWERS, M. (1957). "Functional Disorders of Articulation—Symptomatology and Etiology." In *Handbook of Speech Pathology*, ed. L. Travis. New York: Appleton-Century-Crofts.

PRONOVOST, W. (1942). "An Experimental Study of Methods for Determining Natural and Habitual Pitch." *Speech Monographs*, 9: 111–123.

———— (1951). "A Survey of Services for the Speech and Hearing Handicapped in New England." *Journal of Speech and Hearing Disorders*, 16: 148–156.

PTACEK, P., and E. SANDERS (1963). "Breathiness and Phonation Length." *Journal of Speech and Hearing Disorders*, 28: 267–72.

ROBE, E.; J. BRUNLIK; and P. MOORE (1960). "A Study of Spastic Dysphonia: Neurologic and Electroencephalographic Abnormalities." *Laryngoscope*, 70: 219–245.

ROUSEY, C., and A. MORIARTY (1965). *Diagnostic Implications of Speech Sounds*. Springfield, Ill.: Charles C. Thomas.

RUSSELL, G. (1931). *Speech and Voice*. New York: Macmillan.

SATALOFF, J., and M. FRASER (1952). "Hearing Loss in Children with Cleft Palates." *Archives of Otolaryngology*, 55: 61–64.

SENTURIA, B., and F. WILSON (1968). "Otorhinolaryngic Findings in Children with Voice Disorders." *Annals of Otology, Rhinology, and Laryngology*, 77: 1027–1045.

SHELTON, R.; A. BROOKS; and K. YOUNGSTROM (1965). "Clinical Assessment of Palatopharyngeal Closure." *Journal of Speech and Hearing Disorders*, 30: 37–43.

———; E. HAHN; and H. MORRIS (1968). "Diagnosis and Therapy." In *Cleft Palate and Communication*, ed. D. Spriestersbach and D. Sherman. New York: Academic Press, Pp. 225–268.

SHERMAN, D. (1954). "The Merits of Backward Playing of Connected Speech in the Scaling of Voice Quality Disorders." *Journal of Speech and Hearing Disorders*. 19: 312–321.

SHPRINTZEN, R; G. McCALL; and M. SKOLNICK (1975). "A New Therapeutic Technique for the Treatment of Velopharyngeal Incompetence." *Journal of Speech and Hearing Disorders*, 140: 69–83.

SMITH, P.; L. KENDALL; and C. HULIN (1969). *The Measurement of Job Satisfaction in Work and Retirement; A Strategy for the Study of Attitudes*. Chicago: Rand McNally.

SMITH, R., and B. McWILLIAMS (1968). "Psycholinguistic Abilities of Children with Clefts." *Cleft Palate Journal*, 5: 238–249.

SNIDECOR, J. (1969). *Speech Rehabilitation of the Laryngectomized*. Springfield, Ill.: Charles C. Thomas.

SPRIESTERSBACH, D. (1955). "Assessing Nasal Quality in Cleft-Palate Speech of Children." *Journal of Speech and Hearing Disorders*, 20: 266–270.

———, and G. POWERS (1959). "Articulation Skills, Velopharyngeal Closure, and Oral Breath Pressure of Children with Cleft Palates." *Journal of Speech and Hearing Research*, 2: 318–325.

SUBTELNY, J.; R. McCORMACK; J. CURTIN; and K. MUSGRAVE (1970). "Speech, Intraoral Air Pressure, Nasal Airflow—Before and After Pharyngeal Flap Surgery." *Cleft Palate Journal*, 7: 68–90.

VAN DEMARK, D. (1966). "A Factor Analysis of the Speech of Children with Cleft Palate." *Cleft Palate Journal*, 3: 159–170.

——— (1964). "Misarticulations and Listener Judgments of the Speech of Individuals with Cleft Palates." *Cleft Palate Journal*, 1: 232–245.

———, and A VAN DEMARK (1967). "Misarticulations of Cleft-Palate Children Achieving Velopharyngeal Closure and Children with Functional Speech Problems." *Cleft Palate Journal*, 4: 31–37.

VAN RIPER, C. (1963). *Speech Correction Principles and Methods*, 4th ed. Englewood Cliffs, N.J.: Prentice-Hall, Inc.

———, and J. IRWIN (1958). *Voice and Articulation*. Englewood Cliffs, N.J.: Prentice-Hall, Inc.

WALDROP, W., and M. GOULD (1956). *Your New Voice*. New York: American Cancer Society.

WELLS, C. (1971). *Cleft Palate and Its Associated Speech Disorders*. New York: McGraw-Hill Book Company.

WENDAHL, R., and L. PAGE (1967). "Glottal Wave Periods in CVC Environments." *Journal of Acoustical Society of America*, 42: 1208.

WEPMAN, J.; J. MacGAHAN; J. RICKARD; and N. SHELTON (1953). "The Objective Measurement of Progressive Esophageal Speech Development." *Journal of Speech and Hearing Disorders*, 18: 247–251.

WESTLAKE, H., and D. RUTHERFORD (1966). *Cleft Palate*. Englewood Cliffs, N.J.: Prentice-Hall, Inc.

WILSON, F., and M. RICE (1977). *A Programmed Approach to Voice Therapy*. Austin, Tx.: Learning Concepts, Inc.

WITHERS, B. (1961). "Vocal Nodules." *Eye, Ear, Nose, and Throat Monthly*, 40: 35–38.

WOOD, K. (1971). "Terminology and Nomenclature," in *Handbook of Speech Pathology and Audiology*, ed. L. Travis. New York: Appleton-Century-Crofts. Pp. 3–26.

WORTHLEY, W. (1969). "The Report of a Survey for the Speech Clinician." Mimeographed manuscript.

ZEMLIN, W. (1968). *Speech and Hearing Science: Anatomy and Physiology*. Englewood Cliffs, N.J.: Prentice-Hall, Inc.

10

The Diagnostic Report

The last step in the diagnosis and evaluation procedure is to assemble the available information in a written report. The clinical interview, testing methods, results, impressions, and recommendations must now be collated and committed to paper. The raw data are of limited value to the clinician or other workers until they are assembled in a clear, precise, and orderly fashion.

A diagnostic report, then, is a written record which summarizes the relevant information we have obtained (and *how* we have obtained it) in our professional interaction with a client. It serves the following functions: (1) it acts as a guide for further services to the client—providing a clear statement of how the client was functioning at a given point in time, so that we can document change or lack of change; (2) it communicates our findings to other professional workers; and (3) it serves as a document for research purposes.

The importance of the first function should be obvious: intelligent clinical plans evolve naturally from carefully prepared reports. The second purpose of diagnostic reports is to answer questions about clients so that other professionals can plan and provide appropriate services. In addition to transmitting necessary information, a carefully prepared examination report will tend also to establish the credibility of the clinician in the eyes of other workers. To state it another way, a written document is an extension of the diagnostician, and even minor errors in spelling or grammar may cast doubt upon her accuracy and attention to detail with respect to substantive material. Although the clinician may be highly skilled in testing and interviewing, his competence may be evaluated largely by his written communications.

FORMAT

There are several ways to organize a diagnostic report (Johnson, Darley, and Spriestersbach, 1963; Irwin, 1965; Rees, Herbert, and Coates, 1969; King and Berger, 1971; Sanders, 1972; Knepflar, 1976; Nation and Aram, 1977). Since reports will vary somewhat, depending upon the intended reader, no single schema is appropriate for all circumstances; in many instances the format will be dictated by the agency the clinician serves.

Regardless of the format employed, a diagnostic report should be organized for easy retrieval of information (Pannbacker, 1975) and prepared in a manner which reflects high professional standards. Here are additional criteria we use to judge a diagnostic report: Is it *accurate?* Is it *complete?* Is it *efficiently* written (clearly and with an economy of words)? Was it prepared *promptly?*

We have found the following generic format (see Table 10-1) quite effective and recommend it to the beginning clinician. It contains several major sections.

Table 10-1   Format for Diagnostic Report

I. *Routine Information*
   Name: File No.:
   Address: Date:
                                  Phone No.:
   Birthdate: Age at Eval.:
   Parents: Referred by:
   Evaluated By:

   II. *Statement of the Problem*
  III. *Historical Information*
   IV. *Evaluation*
    V. *Clinical Impressions*
   VI. *Summary*
  VII. *Recommendations*

—————————————————————
                   Clinician

—————————————————————
                   Supervisor

Routine Information

In this first section we present basic identifying information—the client's name, address, date of birth, telephone number, parent's name where relevant, and of course the date of the examination; an undated report is of very little use. In addition to these routine data, we generally identify the referral source (parent, teacher, physician) and the evaluator.

Statement of the Problem

In this section we include a succinct statement of the presenting problem. What is the complaint and who is making it? Be sure to distinguish between the client's complaint and the problem stated by the referral source. In most instances the reason for referral is stated in the client's (or his parent's) own words—always indicated by quotation marks.

Historical Information

Information obtained from referral letters, the case history, and the intake interview are included in this section. Material regarding the client's development (general, and speech and language), his medical, educational, and familial history, and estimates of his personality and behavioral adjustments are summarized. Only the most pertinent items are included in the diagnostic report.

Evaluation

The results of the various tests and examinations are delineated in this section. Before describing the assessment procedures and results, however, we include an opening statement which describes how the client approached the clinical setting and the tasks used to evaluate his communicative abilities. Was he apprehensive, bored, fatigued, cooperative? The name of each test, an explanation of what it does and how it was administered, and the results obtained should be included. Should the clinician include statments about communicative skills that are within normal limits at the time of the evaluation? Knepflar (1976) believes that a complete diagnostic report should mention, even if briefly, all aspects of a client's speech, hearing, and language performance so that subsequent assessments can utilize the information as baseline observations. The information is simply presented, not interpreted, in this section of the report.

Clinical Impressions

In this section we summarize our impressions of the individual and his communication impairment. What type of speech or language problem does he have? How severe is it? What caused it? What factors seem to be perpetuating it? What impact has it had upon the client and his family? How much does it interfere with his everyday functioning? What are the prospects for treatment? Although we can offer interpretations here, we must still be able to support our impressions with information obtained during the interview or testing. Speculations based upon clinical experience, such as similarity between the client and other cases the diagnostician has examined, should be clearly labeled as such.

Summary

The summary should be a concise (not more than a short paragraph) statement abstracting the salient features of the whole report. What is the communicative disorder? What are the primary features of the disorder? What is the probable cause of the disorder? What is the prognosis (and general estimate of the predicted time frame) for recovery?

Recommendations

This is perhaps the most crucial portion of the report. We must now translate our findings into appropriate suggestions or directions that will help the client solve his communication and related problems. Do we recommend further speech and language evaluations? Is a medical referral necessary? Is treatment indicated? What direction should be taken? By whom, and when? The task, then, is to crystallize all the disparate interaction we have had with the individual, collate all the data, and then provide a flexible blueprint for further action. We must attempt to answer the question, "What happens now; where do we go from here?" Try to make the recommendations specific and brief. Suggestions for treatment, or a more lengthy plan of therapy, can be outlined in a letter or follow-up report. One final warning: do not recommend specific evaluations or remediation procedures to workers in other professions. It is improper, for example, to recommend a client for electroencephalography to a neurologist, or for dental braces to an orthodontist; the speech clinician would be chagrined if a physician referred a child and recommended the administration of the *ITPA*. Be sure that your referrals for additional assessment are based upon sound evidence; it is expensive, time consuming, and stressful to the client to make recommendations for comprehensive, medical or psychiatric evaluation without serious and compelling reasons:

> Early in the diagnostic session with five-year-old Mark we suspected the possibility of brain injury. Mindful of the family's limited finances, we wanted to document carefully all signs of apparent cerebral dysfunction before making a referral for a complete pediatric neurological evaluation. Observation revealed a number of serious symptoms: difficulty with motor coordination; labile emotions; rapid and slurred speech; perseveration; and blanking out spells. The necessity for referral was then obvious.

Let us now illustrate diagnostic reporting with three documents. First, a letter from a local physician referring a child for evaluation; then a report delineating our findings prepared according to the format just described; finally, we include a letter to the speech clinician selected to work with the child.

L. Emerick, Ph.D.
Speech and Hearing Clinic
Northern Michigan University

Dear Dr. Emerick:

I would appreciate it if you could evaluate a three year old girl with speech retardation. I first saw her at age 2½, with the major complaint that she would not talk. At that time she had only a single word, "ow", but seemed to comprehend commands quite well.

Physical examination at that time was completely normal; reviewing her history, it seemed that neurologically she was doing well in every respect but speech. At that time I recommended that the mother wait six months and return if the child did not develop further vocabulary. She did return and at this time Lisa has only two words. My evaluation again revealed no neurologic abnormalities. She is quite cooperative, quite responsive to verbal commands. She rides a tricycle, plays ball with her siblings and enjoys musical toys.

I would like to have this child seen for a speech and hearing evaluation at your Clinic, and, once that is completed, I plan on referring her to the local intermediate school district for treatment.

Yours truly,
Pryce Farthingwell, M.D.

Diagnostic Report

Name	*Lisa Marie Jacques*	File No.	*77-2961*
Address	*Box 32*	Date	*9-16-77*
	Tapiola, MI	Phone No.	*482-9174*
Birthdate	*11-24-73*	Age	*3.10*
Parents	*Mr. and Mrs. Robert Jacques*	Referred by	*Farthingwell*
Evaluated by	*S. Matthiasson*		
	G. Guy		

Statement of the Problem

Lisa was referred to the Speech and Hearing Clinic by Dr. Pryce Farthingwell, personal physician to the Jacques family. The concern expressed in the referral letter was that Lisa's speech and language development were not appropriate for her age. Mrs. Jacques expressed the same concern, stating that "Lisa doesn't say anything."

Historical Information

Mrs. Jacques was the sole informant. Rapport was established easily and remained good throughout the interview. Mrs. Jacques reported that she had a normal pregnancy and birth with Lisa. Lisa reached developmental milestones (sitting up, crawling, walking, babbling) within expected limits and was toilet trained at 18 months. She has had no serious illnesses or operations. Mrs. Jacques became concerned when Lisa was two years old and was not talking. She has only recently spoken her first words.

Lisa's present vocabulary consists of "no", "mama," "no way," and an attempt to say "Rodney," the name of a sibling. She allows her siblings to talk for her and makes her desires known through pointing and gesture. Mrs. Jacques stated that Lisa can relay fairly explicit messages to other siblings, but is unsure how she accomplishes this. When Lisa is unable to make herself understood, she becomes angry and walks away. Lisa follows simple directions around the home and appears to remember what she has been told.

Lisa's most frequent playmates are her brothers and sisters. However, she spends a great deal of time playing alone. Her favorite play activity is dressing and undressing her dolls.

Evaluation

On the evaluation day, Lisa initially appeared very shy and withdrawn. She sat very close to her mother and reacted to the clinician's attempts to "make friends" by hiding her face in her mother's lap. She made no sounds and remained expressionless. Although she accompanied the clinician to the audiology suite, she did not offer to cooperate. Throughout the hearing test Lisa remained tired and listless; she covered her face or put her head on the table when spoken to.

A puretone audiological evaluation was attempted but yielded inconsistent responses. The tympanogram showed normal compliance in the right ear and no compliance in the left ear at normal pressure. The bilateral stapedius reflex was not obtained in either ear.

Evaluation of speech and language abilities was accomplished in a structured play setting. Lisa willingly entered the examining room with the clinician but showed no interest or curiosity in various items around the room. Initial attempts to obtain responses using blocks and modeling clay resulted in passive acceptance of the activity but no speech behavior or change in facial expression. The first display of interest occurred when Lisa became intrigued with a doll the clinician was fashioning out of modeling clay. Following this episode, the child became a more active and willing participant in the evaluation activities.

Motor abilities. Lisa displayed good gross motor coordination in running, jumping and throwing activities. She had difficulty fitting pieces into a form board. Attempts at copying and drawing resulted in wavy lines and "jabs" with the point of the pencil.

Personal-social. Lisa appeared shy, although she was willing to be separated from her mother. Observation of her play activity revealed extensive solo play whereby she gathered blocks and toys in front of herself and structured her own play.

Language. Lisa followed one step directions but did so slowly and frequently after some delay. She ignored some commands or responded "No!" Lisa appeared to be aware of sound and responded even when she was unable to see the examiner's face. She pointed to body parts (eye, nose, mouth) on herself as well as to those of the clinician; she recognized when the clinician pointed to an incorrect body part. Lisa followed some (three of ten) directions involving a preposition or color ("Put the block on the chair," "Find the yellow puppet"), but her responses were slow.

The following words and vocalizations were noted: "me," "no," "you," "huh?," "yeah," "my" and the vowels /o/ and /i/. Spontaneous vocalization during play activity was very limited.

In response to direct stimulation, the child imitated "ma," and "mama." She responded to all other requests for imitation with "ma" or the vowel /i/. During this task Lisa's gaze was directed to the examiner's whole face rather than being focused on her mouth.

Clinicial Impressions

This child is delayed in several respects: Fine motor coordination, persnnal-social behavior, and development of oral language. The most serious delay is in terms of language. Vocalization and vocabulary development are severely limited and are at least two years below the expected level. Although Lisa seems able to comprehend simple material, her responses are erratic and immature.

The clinician has little basis for postulating probable cause but it is suspected that multiple factors, perhaps including environmental, are involved. Hearing loss cannot be ruled out. The prognosis is guarded.

Summary

This 46-month-old female shows a developmental delay in several areas, but most apparent in acquisition of oral language. Receptive abilities are more advanced than expressive abilities. Speech behavior consists of a few intelligible words and production of vowel sounds. Communicative attempts consist of pointing and gestures. The etiology is unknown and the prognosis is guarded.

Recommendations

1. Lisa should be enrolled in an intensive program of diagnostic therapy under direction of the speech clinician at the local intermediate school district. More specifically, the following goals are recommended: (a) obtain an ongoing description of Lisa's communicative performance; (b) make expressive speech a meaningful activity by employing parallel play or child centered therapy, as described in a recent article by Holland; and (c) teach her to attend to and imitate the clinician's model by providing vivid feedback.

2. Condition the child for a subsequent puretone audiological evaluation.

3. Counsel with the parents with regard to language stimulation activities they can use in the home situation.

(signed) Sandra Matthiasson
         Gina Guy

Graduate Speech Clinicians

Sharon Hextall
Ahmeek, Michigan

Dear Ms Hextall:

Enclosed is a copy of our findings regarding Lisa Jacques. Another copy was sent to Dr. Farthingwell. If you have any questions about the report, please call us on the WATTS line, 182-227-2125.

We are preparing and will send to you soon a more comprehensive treatment plan. After you have seen Lisa for a month or so, we would be happy to share your observations.

Sincerely,

(signed) Gina Guy
Graduate Speech Clinician

STYLE

An extended discussion of prose style for report writing is not possible within the scope of this text. The reader will want to consult several of the following sources for more definitive statements about common modes of report writing (Hammond and Allen, 1953; Huber, 1961; Jerger, 1962; Moore, 1969; Good, 1970; Fishbein, 1972; Pannbacker, 1975; Knepflar, 1976). In the interest of brevity, then, we shall simply enumerate several principles of style which we have found useful:

1. Make your presentation straightforward and objective, using a topical outline. Use simple, brief but complete sentences. It is often helpful to write for a specific reader; picture the reader in your mind—a classroom teacher, physician, speech clinician—and then simply tell him the story of what you observed and recommend regarding a particular client. When in doubt about a reader's level of understanding, it is better to err on the side of simplicity.

2. Use an impersonal style. Some clinicians use the first person when writing diagnostic reports; but in our view it is preferable to keep the "I" out of it; a reference to "the clinician" or "the examiner" is more in keeping with professional reports. This style also tends to encourage objectivity.

3. Edit the report carefully to make certain that spelling, use of tenses, grammar and punctuation are all accurate. Errors, even trivial ones, undermine the confidence of the reader in the diagnostician. Remember, competence is judged to a great extent by the precision of your reporting.

4. Watch your semantics. Be wary of overused or nebulous words such as "good," "beautiful," "cute," etc. Avoid pet expressions or stereotyped ways of phrasing information. One clinician used the phrase "in terms of" thirteen times in a two-page diagnostic report. Another laced his reports with currently popular words like "input," "interface," and "counterproductive." Use abbreviations sparingly. Avoid superlatives unless they are clearly indicated (Newman, 1974).

5. Avoid preparing an "Aunt Fanny" report (Sunberg and Tyler, 1962)—a bland written statement that could represent anyone, or is so filled with qualifications ("perhaps," "apparently," "tends to") that it reveals nothing; nothing, that is, except a timid diagnostician.

6. Make the report "tight". Don't leave gaps or ambiguity where it is possible to read between the lines. If findings in certain areas are unremarkable, always state this explicitly. Don't leave the reader to guess whether you have investigated all possible aspects.

7. A diagnostic report is no place to display your learning or to parade a large vocabulary. Pedantic reports are misunderstood or unread.

8. Stay close to the data until you wish to draw the observations together and make some

interpretations. For example, tell the reader which sounds were in error instead of simply stating that the child sounds infantile.

9. The very essence of good style is the willingness to take the time and energy to write and rewrite the report until it communicates what we did and what we found in the diagnostic session (Lucas, 1962).

THE WRITING PROCESS

Many students have difficulty writing reports. Most of them have found the task onerous, and a few are threatened and overwhelmed by the prospect of a blank sheet of paper in the typewriter. It has been our experience, however, that rather than a writing *deficiency* most of these students have a writing *bias*—they do not think they can do it.

> Many university educators believe there has been a decline in students' writing skills and are quick to point the finger of blame on inferior instruction in elementary and highschools. A committee at Harvard concluded that "students in high schools received nothing which can with propriety be called an education". The report was written in 1892! The current concern may be a fad rather than a crisis.

There are , of course, no quick and simple solutions; but we offer the following suggestions that have proven helpful to more than one beginning report writer.

Write on a daily basis. Each night—before retiring, for example—sit down and write a descriptive paragraph concerning something that happened to you that day. It may be easier for you to tap into your own creative power by starting with material that arouses strong feelings (see Macrorie, 1968; 1970). At first it may be halting and difficult; as in any new task, your writing "muscles" will be sore. Don't wait for an inspiration, for that magic moment when, suddenly, it will *come* to you. *Go* to it. At the end of the week, review the writing you have done; edit, revise, ask yourself what you meant by each word or phrase. The best way to learn to write, in our opinion, is to write.

Get the message out and revise it later. It is especially important in writing reports to commence work as soon as possible while the material is still fresh in your mind. A common error that some beginning writers make is to attempt to produce perfect writing in the initial draft. It doesn't matter how it looks at this point; you can always edit or have someone help you edit. When you meet barriers or mental blocks, don't linger; jump over them and go on with the rest of the report. When you come back later, you will find that your mind has filled in the blank spots.

It is helpful to have someone read and comment on the initial draft of your report. Although it is difficult to submit one's prose for dissection, ask the reader to be frank and honest in his editing. So many times, a phrase that seems clear to the writer who conceived it is vague or obscure to an objective reader. If writing continues to be a problem consult the work of Strunk and White (1959) and others

(Ferguson, 1959; Kelly, Roth and Altshuler, 1969; Jones and Faulkner, 1971; Wubben, 1971; Berke, 1972; Mayes, 1972; Leggett, Mead and Charvat, 1974).

FOLLOW-UP

The clinician's responsibilities do not end when the diagnostic report is finished and filed. A complete evaluation includes one final important task: a careful follow-up. It is the examiner's professional obligation to determine that the diagnostic activities and recommendations are translated into action; it is useless, perhaps even harmful, to identify and describe problems unless the individual is seen for further testing or treatment as soon as possible. When, as often is the case, the diagnostician is also the clinician, the follow-up can be handled directly and with a minimum of paper work. In an agency such as ours, however (a university speech and hearing clinic), we regularly refer clients to other workers for further assessment or therapy. We use the following questions as guidelines in implementing a follow-up program:

1. Did the intended readers receive the report? The best of secretaries occasionally misfile a document, so we generally call the referral source within a week after the diagnostic to determine if the report has arrived.
2. Does the reader understand the contents of the report? What questions did it raise, if any, about the client? We always log these phone calls in the client's folder.
3. What is the disposition of the client? Is he being seen for further testing? Is he on a waiting list or being seen for treatment?
4. How is the client responding to treatment? We call the local worker, usually on a monthly basis, to assess how the client is doing in therapy relative to our recommendations. Not only does this convey our interest and assistance, it also helps the diagnostic team evaluate the efficacy of their work.

We use a simple form (Table 10-2) to collate data for our follow-up program.

PROJECTS AND QUESTIONS

1. Explore the "problem-oriented" approach to report writing and record keeping by reviewing Chapter 5 in Enelow and Swisher (1972). See also the article by Bouchard and Shane (1977).
2. Several authors have described the agony and ecstasy involved in learning the craft of writing. The account in the following references are especially lucid:

S. OLSON, *Open Horizons.* (New York: Alfred A. Knopf, 1969), pp. 173–191.
J. STEINBECK, *Journal of a Novel: The East of Eden Letters.* (New York: Viking Press, 1969), pp. 3–4.

3. Review Chapter 2 in the pamphlet by Knepflar (1976). What does he refer to as the "pitfall of omnipotence."? In what sense might it be therapeutic for a client to read reports the clinician has written about him? Under what circumstances would you, or would you not, let a parent read or have a copy of a diagnostic report concerning their child?

Table 10-2 Data Sheet for Diagnostic Follow-Up

Client Information (Name, address, phone, age, etc.)	Referral Information (Date, source, reason)	Appointment (Date, time and evaluators)	Disposition & Recommendations	Follow-up
Lisa Jacques Box 32 Tapiola, MI 3.10 yrs	8-22-77 Farthingwell delayed speech	9-16-77 1 pm Matthiasson Guy	diagnostic therapy condition to audio.	10-17-77 in therapy with Sharon Hextall
Ken Lasich 621 Bluff St. Granite Harbor, MI 11 years	9-5-77 parents slow expressing self; listening problems	10-6-77 9 am Marshall	pediatric neurological training in aud. skills-awareness, focus, etc.	10-24-77 scheduled for neuro. eval.

BIBLIOGRAPPHY

BERKE, J. (1972). *Twenty Questions for the Writer*. New York: Harcourt, Brace, Jovanovich.

BOURCHARD, M., and H. SHANE (1977). "Use of the Problem-oriented Medical Record in the Speech and Hearing Profession." *Journal of the American Speech and Hearing Association,* 19: 157–159.

ENELOW, A., and S. SWISHER (1972). *Interviewing and Patient Care*. New York: Oxford University Press.

FERGUSON, C. (1959). *Say It With Words*. New York: Alfred A. Knopf.

FISHBEIN, M. (1972). *Medical Writing*. Springfield, Ill.: Charles C Thomas.

GOOD, R. (1970). "The Written Language of Rehabilitation Medicine: Meaning and Usages." *Archives of Physical Medicine and Rehabilitation,* 51: 29–36.

HAMMOND, K. and J. ALLEN (1953). *Writing Clinical Reports*. Englewood Cliffs, N.J.: Prentice-Hall, Inc.

HUBER, J. (1961). *Report Writing in Psychology and Psychiatry*. New York: Harper & Row.

IRWIN, R. (1965). *Speech and Hearing Therapy*. Pittsburgh: Stanwix House.

JERGER, J. (1962). "Scientific Writing can be Readable." *Journal of the American Speech and Hearing Association,* 4: 101–104.

JOHNSON, W.; F. DARLEY; and D. SPRIESTERSBACH (1963). *Diagnostic Methods in Speech Pathology*. New York: Harper & Row.

JONES, A., and C. FAULKNER (1971). *Writing Good Prose*. New York: Charles Scribner's Sons.

KELLY, M.; A. ROTH and T. ALTSHULER (1969). *Writing Step by Step*. Boston: Houghton Mifflin Co.

KING, R., and K. BERGER (1971). *Diagnostic Assessment and Counseling Techniques for Speech Pathologists and Audiologists*. Pittsburgh: Stanwix House.

KNEPFLAR, K. (1976). *Report Writing*. Danville, Ill.: Interstate Printers and Publishers.

LEGGETT, G.; C. MEAD; and W. CHARVAT (1974). *Handbook for Writers*. 6th ed. Englewood Cliffs, N.J.: Prentice-Hall, Inc.

LUCAS, F. (1962). *Style*. New York: Macmillan Company.

MACRORIE, K. (1968). *Writing to be Read*. Rochelle Park, N.J.: Hayden Book Company.

MACRORIE, K. (1970). *Uptaught*. Rochelle Park, N.J.: Hayden Book Company.

MAYES, J. (1972). *Writing and Rewriting*. New York: Macmillan.

MOORE, M. (1969). "Pathological Writing." *Journal of the American Speech and Hearing Association,* 11: 535–538.

NATION, J., and D. ARAM (1977). *Diagnosis of Speech and Language Disorders*. St. Louis, Mo.: C.V. Mosby Co.

NEWMAN, E. (1974). *Strictly Speaking*. New York: Bobbs-Merrill.

PANNBACKER, M. (1975). "Diagnostic Report Writing." *Journal of Speech and Hearing Disorders,* 40: 367–379.

PERLMATTER, J. (1965). *A Practical Guide to Effective Writing*. New York: Random House.

REES, M.; E. HERBERT; and N. COATES (1969). "Development of a Standard Case Record Form." *Journal of Speech and Hearing Disorders,* 34: 68–81.

SANDERS, L. (1972). *Evaluation of Speech and Language Disorders in Children*. Danville, Ill.: Interstate Printers and Publishers.

STRUNK, W. and F. WHITE (1959). *The Elements of Style*. New York: Macmillan.

SUNBERG, N., and L. TYLER (1962). *Clinical Psychology*. New York: Appleton-Century-Crofts.

WUBBEN, J. (1971). *Guided Writing*. New York: Random House.

Index